Transgender Health and Medicine

Transgender Health and Medicine

HISTORY, PRACTICE, RESEARCH, AND THE FUTURE

Dana Jennett Bevan, PhD

Essentials of Psychology and Health

PRAEGER®

An Imprint of ABC-CLIO, LLC
Santa Barbara, California • Denver, Colorado

Library of Congress Cataloging-in-Publication Data
Names: Bevan, Dana Jennett, author.
Title: Transgender health and medicine : history, practice, research, and the future / Dana Jennett Bevan, PhD.
Description: Santa Barbara, California : Praeger, [2019] | Series: Essentials of psychology and health | Includes bibliographical references and index.
Identifiers: LCCN 2019014434 (print) | LCCN 2019020616 (ebook) | ISBN 9781440866913 (print : alk. paper) | ISBN 9781440866920 (ebook)
Subjects: LCSH: Transgender people—Medical care. | Transgender people—Health and hygiene.
Classification: LCC RA564.9.T73 (ebook) | LCC RA564.9.T73 B48 2019 (print) | DDC 362.1086/7—dc23
LC record available at https://lccn.loc.gov/2019014434

ISBN: 978-1-4408-6691-3 (print)
978-1-4408-6692-0 (ebook)

23 22 21 20 19 1 2 3 4 5

This book is also available as an eBook.

Praeger
An Imprint of ABC-CLIO, LLC

ABC-CLIO, LLC
147 Castilian Drive
Santa Barbara, California 93117
www.abc-clio.com

This book is printed on acid-free paper ♾

Manufactured in the United States of America

This book discusses treatments (including types of medication and mental health therapies), diagnostic tests for various symptoms and mental health disorders, and organizations. The author has made every effort to present accurate and up-to-date information. However, the information in this book is not intended to recommend or endorse particular treatments or organizations, or substitute for the care or medical advice of a qualified health professional, or be used to alter any medical therapy without a medical doctor's advice. Specific situations may require specific therapeutic approaches not included in this book. For those reasons, we recommend that readers follow the advice of qualified health care professionals directly involved in their care. Readers who suspect they may have specific medical problems should consult a physician about any suggestions made in this book.

Contents

Series Foreword

Dozens of subfields exist in the academic disciplines of psychology and health, which help train many different types of specialists in the helping professions, from an array of counselors, social workers, and psychologists to public health scientists, medical researchers, and physicians. Yet, short of finding and completing a course concentrated on the subfield, or shadowing a particular professional at length, students and interested lay readers may have no substantial information on any particular subfield or specialty. Books in this series serve that need.

The *Essentials of Psychology and Health* series includes books that provide an introduction to, and deeper understanding of, academic subfields and resulting specialties in professions intended to understand disorders and improve physical and mental health, whether on individual or societal levels. These books are designed to be inclusive, research and case study strong, compact, and easy to use to locate particular information.

The text in these volumes includes the history of the subfield or profession, perspectives from various schools of thought, theoretical basis, demographics, roles, relationship to other fields, case studies, classic and emerging research, current events, and a look to the future of the subfield or profession. Core obstacles and, where appropriate, controversies are also addressed. Features include a glossary of terms, references, index, and a resource list for further information.

Preface

As I was researching the history of being transgender for this book, I was struck by the courage of transgender people, their care providers, and their allies in performing acts, small and large, aimed at reduced the suffering of transgender people and improving their lives.

At the time that the concept of being transgender was developed, in the early 20th century, providers Magnus Hirschfeld and Harry Benjamin walked the streets of Berlin to intercede with the police on behalf of those who would later be called transgender. At the dawn of modern anesthesia, transgender people dared to change their bodies in untried surgical procedures. Harry Benjamin risked his medical license in the United States and his reputation to find surgeons who would do transgender genital plastic surgeries to change the sex of some transgender people. In California where Benjamin practiced, based on legal opinions, the operations were considered "mayhem" and therefore illegal.

The street transgender people, who were mostly poor people, rebelled at police humiliations and harassment in the 1960s riots, which included not only New York City's Stonewall riots in 1969, but also the several other rebellions that preceded Stonewall in the prior decade. It took courage for Virginia Prince to start clandestine support groups for transgender people and to face criminal charges for letters and newsletters of which the U.S. Postal Service did not approve. It took guts for Louis Sullivan and Lin Fraser to get provider organizations to drop sexual orientation as a requirement for transgender transition and genital plastic surgeries.

In more recent times, Gavin Grimm faced off against his high school officials to gain access to the restrooms appropriate to his congruent gender. His fight continues for those transgender children behind him in school, even after he has graduated. There were transgender people and allies arrested in Charlotte to protest North Carolina's HB-2 law, which intended to make transgender people less visible by restricting public restroom access. There were also the Texas "Momma Bears," who testified across much of 11 hours of public comments in the state legislature, that lobbied against legislation that would prevent their transgender children from using restrooms and locker rooms that were not compatible with their congruent gender.

Such acts as these were made all the more courageous because there was, and is, no organized transgender movement, despite what antitransgender people say to play on conspiracy fears.

Transgender people, their providers, and their allies have committed courageous acts without any orthodox movement. It is truly a grassroots venture. We now have some organizations that advocate for transgender medical, civil, and political rights, but both our strength and our weakness is in our diversity—it is not in our lack of courage.

While transgender people are currently experiencing a dark period in the United States and elsewhere due to authoritarian populism, they have experienced such nights before and with their courage the day always comes.

Acknowledgments

I want to acknowledge all those courageous health care providers who chose to reduce the suffering of their transgender patients rather than yield to the overwhelming cultural pressure to reject them as being unworthy. I hope that the providers of today and of the future will continue this tradition.

I want to acknowledge a provider that I consulted with early in the writing of this book. He told me to be sure to tell other providers how to deal with transgender patients who had chief complaints of *nontransgender* ailments, for example, broken arms and grieving from the loss of a loved one. Such chief complaints undoubtedly represent the most frequent encounters that providers have with transgender people. They are chances for providers to show their professionalism and for patients to appreciate those providers who do.

I want to thank my daughters, both in the health professions, for their patience and understanding.

I also want to thank those in Atlanta who were friends with me when I really needed friends. Some of them are Z, Heather, Ally, Katrina, Claire, Jamie Sue, Shelly Ray, Julie, Missy, Callie, Paige, Dacey, Peggy, and all the folks at TransDecatur and Pride School. I especially want to thank Cara who brought me back.

Finally, I want to thank my providers: Virginia Erhardt, Terry Hackworth, Kathe Perez, Vincent Zubowicz, Katie Leikam, Sherman Leis, and those in my future. I know I am a difficult patient.

PART 1

Overview

1

History and Impetus

This chapter explains why providers need to understand transgender patients and discusses important definitions and history that providers need to know. Providers include mental health and medical professionals and other helping professionals that come into contact with transgender people. It is important for providers to understand transgender history because each transgender person carries with them the traditions of one of four independent demographic groups that advocated for transgender rights in the latter half of the 20th century.

THE BASICS

It is imperative for providers to understand the phenomenon of being transgender, in particular to understand the scientific background for evidence-based practice. **Transgender** people are those who do not behave according to their culturally assigned gender behavior category. This assignment is determined in Western culture entirely by natal sex, their sex assigned at birth. These gender behavior categories contain behaviors, rules, norms, and expectations defined by culture. Because people have a biological genetic predisposition about gender behaviors, they often do not "fit" within their assigned gender category. Some "fit" with another category, some cannot find a "fit," and some are fluid about the gender behavior they exhibit. Transgender people feel and behave differently from cultural expectations, and they can and do express this through verbal behavior. As children, they might say that they are a girl in a boy's body or a boy in a girl's body. Older transgender people might say that they have a **masculine** or **feminine** gender, be **genderqueer**, be **gender fluid**, or be a **crossdresser**.

Nearly all providers will come in contact with transgender people, and some providers specialize in procedures relating to being transgender. Many have already come in contact with transgender people without knowing it, because being transgender is not rare. But in the past, transgender people were reticent to talk about their status even though it might be relevant to their treatment. They did this because of potential family and cultural rejection and loss of livelihood, so their transgender status was kept a secret; their treatment and health might have suffered.

Recent survey estimates indicate that at least .7–1 percent of the population is transgender and the estimates of this population frequency have been steadily increasing. A recent study found that 2.7 percent of middle-school children were transgender (Eisenberg et al., 2017). In the past, transgender people have been reticent to tell their providers that they were transgender, but the recent trend has been for transgender people to want providers to know. Surveys indicate over 65 percent said that they wanted providers to know about their transgender status (Grant et al., 2011; Mollie, Blosnich, Dichter, Luscri, & Shipherd, 2017; Turban, Ferraiolo, Martin, & Olezeski, 2017). The physiology and anatomy of transgender people is often different from the norm because some take sex hormones and drugs to block opposing sex hormone effects. In addition to having the power to change transgender bodies, these drugs, which block the action of specific sex hormones, have other effects and medical uses. For example, the commonly used testosterone-blocking drug **spironolactone** is a potassium-sparing diuretic that is also prescribed for its effects on blood pressure and fluid balance.

In order to gain rapport with transgender people, providers need to understand trans expectations, etiquette, and language. The fact that patients are now more open about their transgender status represents an improvement in the provider-client relationship that is critical to diagnosis and treatment. *But that means that providers must understand what patients are telling them.*

Being transgender is no longer considered pathological. It is a part of natural diversity, which can be observed across a wide range of historical and geographical cultures. In recognition of this, the *Diagnostic and Statistical Manual of Mental Disorders,* 5th edition (DSM-5) recently removed being transgender as a pathological category. A nonpathological code, **gender dysphoria**, was set up in a separate section to allow for billing of situations in which a person was in severe distress or debilitation or for those going through transsexual transition. About 10 percent of transgender people are **transitioning transgender people** (previously termed **transsexuals**). Transitioning transgender people seek to modify their bodies to make them better resemble cultural expectations of the appropriate anatomy for their congruent gender behavior category. Transitioning transgender people used to be called transsexuals, but many transgender people and providers now reject this term, which will be explained further in a Chapter 6 section on etiquette. There are many different transition procedures and their selection is unique to the individual. The International Classification of Diseases (ICD) will undergo an even more radical change in the forthcoming ICD-11. It has been announced that treating transitioning transgender people will be classified under normal sexual health codes as the ICD is introduced, starting in 2019.

Standards of Care (SOC) for treating transgender people are provided by the **World Professional Association for Transgender Health (WPATH)**. This is an international organization of providers and researchers. The guidelines for transsexual transition are included in their Standards of Care document, which is currently version SOC-7 (WPATH, 2011). This document includes guidelines for treating both transgender people and the subset of transgender people who are transitioning. It is expected that SOC-8 will be completed in 2019. Complementary and coordinated guidelines have been published by the Endocrine Society (Hembree et al., 2009), American Psychological Association (APA, 2015), the American Academy of Pediatrics (Rafferty, 2018), and other professional organizations.

In order to understand being transgender, it is important to appreciate the scientific difference between sex and gender. These words are often used interchangeably in public discourse, but they have specific scientific meanings. The scientific use of the word gender was necessitated by the existence of infants with indeterminant birth sex, conditions sometimes called **intersex** or **differences in sexual development**. Providers had to distinguish between **sex** and **gender behavior categories** in order to provide proper guidance to parents for child rearing. There was and is no way of knowing the future behavior or asking an infant, so they repurposed the word gender to refer to the gender behavior category that they judged was appropriate. Today there is much confusion and confounding of sex and gender in public discourse where gender is sometimes considered to be a polite word for sex. Put simply, **sex** refers to the categorization of the biological organs of reproduction into male and female, whereas **gender** refers to cultural behavior categories. Most people never get chromosome karyotypes or genome surveys, so genital inspection at birth is the only determinant of sex that is typically used. Analysis of chromosomes and genes currently cannot predict how sex organs will be formed for a given individual because of limitations on current scientific knowledge and high variability. In Western culture, biological natal sex determination, as **male** and **female**, is automatically used to assign people to one of two **gender behavior categories** (respectively, **masculine** and **feminine**). This works for most people but not for transgender people.

The dissociation of sex and gender is demonstrated by two direct lines of scientific evidence. The first line is the existence of transgender people, whose congruent gender is different from that assigned at birth according to the Western gender system. The second line of dissociation comes from heritability studies. About 50 percent of the time if a transgender person has an identical twin, then this twin will also be transgender. However, if one member of an identical twin pair is transgender and the other is not, *they still both have the same sex.*

The **genetic gender behavior predisposition** of transgender people does not match their assigned gender behavior category at birth. Transgender people have a genetic predisposition that usually allows them to recognize their **congruent gender behavior category**, the one that "fits" them best.

Transgender people are particularly sensitive to etiquette and forms of dialogue. It is important for providers to understand this in order to have an effective provider-patient encounter. No matter what providers may think personally about transgender people, they have a professional obligation to have an effective dialogue with all their patients. In spite of cultural roadblocks, many transgender people have engaged in legal, family, and cultural struggles to change their name and pronouns. They are particularly proud of their achievements. Because transgender people experience rejection from people who deliberately address them with incorrect names and pronouns, a provider must avoid being classed with those who are deliberately trying to insult transgender people.

In the past, because so few providers were knowledgeable about transgender treatments, about 55 percent of transgender people took it on themselves to educate their providers who were willing to cooperate (Grant et al., 2011). Some providers mistakenly attempted to use their training and techniques designed around "curing" patients, which does not fit with the transgender phenomenon. A wide variety of approaches have been tried to "cure" transgender people. They all have failed—including classical psychoanalysis, prefrontal lobotomy, drugs, operant conditioning, electric shock, reparative therapy, jawboning, bullying, toy deprivation, brain stimulation, and various and sundry clinical approaches intended to be therapeutic. We now know that being transgender cannot be "cured." Being transgender is not pathological, and the medical "infectious disease" model of identifying a cause in order to select a therapeutic approach is inappropriate.

As we will see, four of the causal factors in being transgender are well established—genetics, epigenetics, Western culture, and early gender learning. These factors are embodied in an integrated Four Factors theory of transgender causation covered in Chapter 3.

Because transgender people experience cultural rejection, they *do* sometimes need help to deal with problems with family, friends, workplace, and associations, just as all other people do. Mental health professionals can help with counseling and by suggesting new approaches. But their efforts do not constitute "cures" because transgender people do not have a disorder or disease. Likewise, medical treatments including transgender transition do not represent a "cure," but some transgender people find it exceedingly difficult to present and perform in a congruent gender behavior category when their anatomy does not match cultural expectations.

The final basic to note is that **being transgender** and **sexual orientation** are quite different. Sexual orientation refers to the sex of a person to whom one is attracted and with whom one has sexual relations. Transgender people have all types of sexual orientations and these may change with transgender transition. Transgender transition is the only known process that sometimes changes sexual orientation.

IMPORTANT DEFINITIONS

Transgender people do not follow the gender behavior category to which they were assigned at birth based on their natal sex categorization as male or female. This assignment is almost universally performed on the basis of the anatomy of **external genitalia**. **Gender categories** develop in cultures, and in the Western culture there are two gender behavior categories, **masculine** and **feminine.** These categories include behaviors, roles, values, and norms. Words associated with the masculine category are **boys/men/him/his/sir** and those associated with the feminine category are **girls/women/her/hers/ma'am**. Those who are judged to be male at birth are automatically assigned to the masculine gender behavior category and those judged to be female are assigned to the feminine category. Because of this automatic assignment to gender category based on sex, the Western gender system is referred to as **cisgender**. Cisgender is the opposite of transgender. Those transgender people who are born male but whose congruent gender is feminine may be called **transwomen** or **transgirls**. Likewise, those that are born female are called **transmen** or **transboys.**

Transgender people may follow one of the two Western culture gender categories or, increasingly, they may find that neither of the two categories are congruent with their genetic gender predisposition. These transgender people may self-define as **gender fluid**, **genderqueer,** or **gender nonconforming**. Some among the genderqueer may define themselves as **transmasculine** or **transfeminine**. Females may present in a more masculine manner and males in a more feminine manner, and both may undergo some procedures usually associated with transgender transition.

Definitions of many terms pertaining to being transgender have undergone repurposing by transgender people, providers, and researchers. Although being transgender is no longer recognized as a disease or disorder, many terms we use to indicate being transgender were derived from psychiatric pathology. Indeed, the word "transgender" itself did not start out with the same definition that we now employ. Its original meaning (Oliven, 1965) was used to establish that the motivation of transitioning transgender people (previously called transsexuals) involved their congruent gender, rather than other motivations such as **sexual arousal**. Other examples are the terms "**gender identity**" and "**gender dysphoria,**" which also originated in psychiatric pathology for unobservable processes. These terms are currently being repurposed by transgender people as behavioral and sociological labels. Unfortunately, repurposing of pathological terms can be misunderstood as implying that there is still something pathological about being transgender. The term gender identity is not only pathological but can be confused with its use in sociology or intersectionalist politics. As used by many trans people, *telling someone what one's "gender identity" is is equivalent to telling them what one's "gender" is.*

The other prominent case of repurposing of words involves the words **sex** and **gender**. Sex is usually determined at birth by anatomical classification of external genitalia, some of the sex organs. Even though we might want to consider other biological definitions of sex with the advent of genetics and epigenetics, this is the most common and consistent method of sex determination. Most people never get chromosome karyotyping, genetic analysis, or hormonal analysis, and there are currently too many exceptions resulting from these methods for them to be used in application, even for such uses as sex determination for international athletics.

John Money treated patients born with indeterminate sex, and he realized in the late 1950s that he needed a new term that could be used to tell parents how to raise such children and to communicate with scientists. He repurposed the word **gender** from the language declensions of nouns to describe the masculine and feminine behavior categories or roles of Western culture. *Thus, the term sex was derived from biology and gender role or category was derived from culture.* However, in public discourse the two terms have become confounded. People who misunderstood these terms thought that gender was just a polite word for sex and the usage caught on, even among social scientists. In this book, the terms will be used in their original scientific meanings, which is actually the way most transgender people use them.

More recently, the term **genetic gender behavior predisposition** was introduced (Bevan, 2015) to indicate the formation of biological mechanisms that react to gender behaviors to establish a "fit." For transgender people, their genetic gender behavior predispositions tell them that their biology is incongruent with their culturally assigned gender behavior category because of their innate emotional experiences with the behaviors specified in these categories.

To summarize, *both sex and genetic gender behavior predisposition are biological and gender behavior categories are cultural.*

Transitioning transgender people may go through several procedures to change their bodies. **Hormone therapy (HT)** involves taking sex hormones and other drugs. **Transgender genital plastic surgery (TGPS)** involves making surgical changes to the genitalia. Other surgical procedures may be used to change the face, the breasts, and other areas of the body.

IMPETUS

The impetus for this handbook is that culture has changed enough that we are seeing a rapid increase in the visibility of transgender people. Whether or not you specialize in transgender treatment, identifiable transgender people will present for your help. From a public health perspective, this is a positive phenomenon because transgender people no longer have to suffer physical and emotional damage from living in secrecy. Most providers have already encountered or will encounter transgender people because the population frequency of transgender people is at least .7–1 percent and probably higher. (Since being transgender is no longer considered a pathological condition, **population frequency** is used here instead of **prevalence** but it is intended to be mathematically equivalent.) Although historically, transgender people were presenting to providers all along, most transgender people kept their status a secret to avoid cultural rejection, sometimes when their silence may have compromised their mental and physical health. Transgender people are found in all demographic categories. Most are law-abiding but some young people end up in dangerous street economies because they are unable to remain at home due to parental rejection of their transgender behavior. Transgender people have contributed to society in various ways including inventing the modern computer's electronic architecture, serving in the military, serving as mental health and medical professionals, practicing in the arts, and performing scientific research.

Practitioners need to adapt to this increased visibility of transgender people in order to provide effective and ethical treatment for their patients, even though being transgender may be foreign to the providers' cultural inheritance. It is not a matter of tolerance or acceptance, it is a matter of practicality and efficacy. Effective provider-transgender communication requires different rules of etiquette. Transgender people want to be called by their chosen name, even if that may not be their birth name, and studies have demonstrated that this is efficacious in reducing depression and even reducing suicide attempts (Mustanski & Liu, 2010). After changing names, transgender people sometimes refer to their birth name as their "**dead name,**" which indicates how they feel about its use.

Practitioners need to be aware of the mental and physical effects of being transgender. Secrecy can result in depression, isolation, immune suppression, and attempted suicide. These are not organic pathological conditions but rather the reactive effects of rejection and secrecy to avoid rejection. Transgender people may be reticent to reveal things that affect their physiology. For example, some transgender people may conceal the fact that they take sex hormones and other drugs, which may be obtained legally from other practitioners, from illegal sources, or from sources in countries in which such drugs do not require a prescription. Reports indicate that such drug taking is common when patients encounter delays or barriers associated with obtaining medical treatment: 22 percent of patients in the United Kingdom and 43 percent in Canada (Rotondi et al., 2013; Webberly & Webberly, 2018). Even higher estimates obtain for transgender street people, 49.1 percent in one survey (de Haan, Santos, Arayasirikul, & Raymond, 2015). Transgender people may be reticent to reveal or may not realize what drugs they are taking. Providers need to be aware of potential side effects, which include the danger of thrombosis from some estrogenic drugs and high red blood cell counts from taking testosterone. The danger of thrombosis from estrogen has declined because most providers have switched to safer estrogen compounds such as **estradiol valerate**.

As to treatment for being transgender, in the past, many practitioners have had to rely on their patients to tell them about transgender treatments, dosages, and laboratory tests. It has only been in the past few years that providers have begun to take Continuing Education Units (CEU) or learn about transgender treatment in school or internships. Some transgender people may still hide their status from providers, but the majority want their providers to know and will tell them.

Transgender people are subjected to cultural rejection and minority stress, which may need to be addressed by counseling and ultimately by more cultural change. Those who choose to stay in the closet are subject to the toxic effects of secrecy. Because of these stressors the rate of attempted suicide for transgender people is estimated as 31 to 43 percent (Bauer, Pyne, Francino, & Hammond, 2013; Clements-Nolle, Marx, & Katz, 2006; Grant et al., 2010; Liu & Mustanski, 2001; Mustanski & Liu, 2010). This does not count many of the successful attempts that we will never know about. The high suicide rate is not a result of organic pathology but a result of rejection and secrecy. As in the general population, most transgender suicide attempts occur in teenage and early adulthood years.

DEVELOPMENT OF DIVERSE GENDER SYSTEMS

The development of what we now call being transgender parallels the development of the gender system of Western culture. *You cannot be transgender unless you are in violation of the gender system of your culture.* Unlike other cultures, Western culture developed a **binary** gender system with two categories, masculine and feminine, that are automatically assigned at birth by sex classification (making the gender system **cisgender**). The Western gender system is also **inflexible** in prohibiting behaviors from the other category.

The Western gender system is somewhat unique among the ranges of historical and geographical cultures. The gender systems of other cultures have up to five gender categories, use additional criteria to assign children to gender categories other than their sex, and allow movement between categories. Many of these categories no longer exist in their original form due to conquest, Western missionary activities, and displacements resulting from, among other things, atom bomb tests in the Pacific.

Table 1.1 shows the Western gender system contrasted with some examples of non-Western gender systems. The Bugis of Indonesia are a subculture with five gender categories. In addition to third and fourth categories, the fifth category has a special spiritual significance. The fifth-category people provide spiritual guidance to their culture in spite of the fact that they are embedded in a larger Muslim culture. Muslim clerics have worked out agreements with this fifth gender so that both can coexist and serve their people.

Similarly, although the Catholic church does not accept being transgender generally, it has tacitly accepted the Muxe of Mexico, a third-category gender. The Muxe live in the extreme southern province of Mexico, which has been isolated for most of its history. And the Muxe are firmly embedded in their Zapotec Native American culture.

Over 150 Native American Plains tribes had at least three gender categories and half of these had four gender categories. Although sex at birth was used as one criterion in assignment, these tribes also used information resulting from dreams and visualizations, behavioral tendencies, and ritual

Table 1.1 Cultural Diversity

Culture Name	Subculture	Location	Time	Gender Behavior Category	Number of Category
Western	Transgender	Worldwide	Current	Transwoman	N/A
Western	Transgender	Worldwide	Current	Transman	N/A
Native American	Lakota	North America	Historical	Winkte	3
Native American	Ojibwa	North America	Historical	Agokwa	3
Native American	Mojave	North America	Historical	Hwame	4
Native American	Sauk	North America	Historical	Ickoue	4
Native American	Navajo	North America	Historical	Nadleeh	3 and 4
Native American	North Paiute	North America	Historical	Tubas	3 and 4
Native American	Zuni	North America	Historical	Llhamana	3
Native American	Zapotec	North America	Current	Muxe	3
Asian	Hijra	South Asia	Current	Hijra	3
Asian	Kathoey	Thailand	Current	Kathoey	3
Asian	Waria	Indonesia	Current	Waria	3
Asian	Bugis	Indonesia	Current	Calabai	3
Asian	Bugis	Indonesia	Current	Calalai	4
Asian	Bugis	Indonesia	Current	Bissu	5
Asian	Chuckchi	Siberia	Current	Chuckchi	3
Pacific	Hawaiian	Hawaii/Tahiti	Current	Mahu	3
Pacific	Samoa	Samoa	Current	Fa'fafane	3
Pacific	Oceania	Tonga	Current	Fakaleiti	3
Pacific	Maori	New Zealand	Current	Whakawahine	3 and 4
Pacific	Western Pacific	Phillipines	Current	Bakla	3
Middle East	Oman	Oman	Current	Xanith	3
Europe	Italian	Naples	Current	Femminiello	3

tests to assign children to gender categories. When it came to involvement in defense, third-gender males would perform leadership and strategy tasks usually assigned to first-gender category males, making the categories flexible. This flexibility was part of their culture and therefore the third- and fourth-gender categories did not constitute being transgender.

(More detail on these and other cultures is provided in Chapter 3.)

Western culture is an amalgam of Christianity and European culture resulting in a strict binary, cisgender, and inflexible gender system. Although Western culture tacitly accepted eunuchs and castrati singers, they were not assigned to separate gender behavior categories. Catholic and other religions still assert that sex and gender are the same thing. Current "defenders of their faiths" attempt to confound sex organs with gender behavior categories, substituting the term sex-type behavior for gender.

The underlying theory for the Western gender system is that sex differences caused behavior differences to evolve and become differentiated by sex in traditional hunter-gatherer clans or tribes. Males were assumed to be in charge of hunting game and defense of the group due to superior strength. Accordingly, they evolved innate aggressive behaviors. Females were assumed to be less mobile and needed to stay at home base because of pregnancy and raising the young. They also made baskets, pottery, and blankets. This division of labor helped hunter-gatherers gain individual evolutionary fitness by surviving and passing on their genes, with accompanying behavioral traits, to their offspring. This underlying theory can be termed the **traditional sex-based behavior theory**. Major proponents of this theory were European anthropologists in the 19th century who studied hunter-gatherer societies. The initial favoring of the traditional sex-based theory was likely due to these European anthropologists seeking to find examples to underpin the cultural assumptions they brought with them.

More recently, an alternative theory has developed, which can be termed the **kinship theory of gender behavior**. This theory postulates that it was not the evolutionary fitness of the individual that mattered but the evolutionary fitness of the clan or group. Members of the group contributed to the survival of the hunter-gatherer clan/tribe and shared the same genes. This resulted in a flexible, shared division of labor among males and females and greater behavioral diversity.

More recent anthropological evidence tends to support the kinship theory. It turns out that females contributed the majority of the calories to the clan/group even though they had to stay closer to home. They did this through local small game hunting and gathering tasks. When the biota around the home base no longer supported these tasks, the clan/tribe simply moved elsewhere. One could easily see how the kinship theory would give rise to third- and fourth-gender behavior categories found throughout the world. When local hunting/gathering was good at home base, some of the males had no need to go on long-distance hunting operations and could perform some of the tasks usually associated with females in the traditional sex-based theory.

Cities in the United States began to pass laws outlawing crossdressing in the mid-1850s. The growth of cities had accelerated due to immigration, mainly from Europe. This trend continued into the 20th century. The pretext for many of these laws was to prevent disguise as a means of committing crimes. But the real reasons probably had to do with the ability of people to live in cities independently of their families because of industrialization and without Old World gender constraints. This economic independence facilitated freer expression of dress and behavior. In Europe, the Napoleonic Code had been adopted in 1804 and it and Victorian society gave people more freedom in personal behavior.

Cultural backlash in response to these new economic and personal freedoms in the 19th century was in part responsible for crossdressing laws. An indication of the cultural backlash was the growth of Evangelical religions in the United States and the Evangelical Revival in England.

The effect of anticrossdressing laws decreased. Court challenges in the United States were mainly successful on the grounds of the vagueness of gender categories in terms of dress. The decisions pointed to the large overlap between masculine and feminine dressing plus continuous change due to fashion. Successful challenges were also supported by the women's movements that began in the 1840s with Amelia Bloomer. These movements advocated for allowing women to shed cumbersome garments and to wear clothing that previously only men had worn, such as pants. Eventually, the laws would become ineffective because of protections afforded by medical advocacy for transgender people. Although these challenges to anticrossdressing laws were successful, on the street and at the local level people who could not afford costly judicial appeals were still being harassed, arrested, and convicted under crossdressing laws and other laws such as loitering, being a public nuisance, and disturbing the peace.

BEING TRANSGENDER IN THE 20TH CENTURY

The concept of being transgender did not arise until the early 20th century. There are numerous examples of **crossdressing** before that time, but people crossdress for various economic, political, and theatrical reasons as well as for being transgender. For example, many females crossdressed to become soldiers in various wars including the U.S. Civil War. In Shakespeare's day when females were forbidden to act on the stage, their parts were taken by young males who crossdressed. Some believe that the term "**drag**" comes from the stage direction [Enter "Dressed as a Girl"]. Drag, which was also popular in English pantomime shows at the turn of the last century, in turn derives from European stage traditions dating back to the Middle Ages. Transgender people crossdress to feel authentic and relaxed, and to be able to behave in a gender category that fits them. Some people who engage in drag are actually transgender, but most today are homosexual males. Whether they are transgender or not depends on their off-stage behavior.

The modern idea of being transgender was developed in the early 20th century, although the word transgender was not invented until 1965 (Oliven, 1965), and it did not originally mean what it does today. Oliven used it to mean that **transitioning transgender** people (transsexuals) were not motivated by sexual arousal but by gender concerns. Undoubtedly there were people before that time whose gender behavior conflicted with the Western cultural gender system. But they were not recognized as a group with similar characteristics. Once the idea that birth sex did not explain gender behavior existed, it was probably inevitable that the idea would spread, given the fundamental biological and cultural factors involved.

Providers should note that the idea of being transgender accompanied the development of modern medicine and within it the new sciences of sexology and endocrinology. Physicians at the time felt the need to do something to help those suffering rejection, reactive depression, and shame. Shortly after the emergence of sexology, marked by the start of the *Journal of Sexology* in 1908, transgender patients began to be recognized, although the word transgender had not yet been coined. In England, Havelock Ellis and in Germany, Magnus Hirschfeld both encountered patients that we would consider transgender today. Hirschfeld called the phenomenon **transvestism** and Ellis called it **sexo-aesthetic inversion**. Both *initially* assumed the phenomenon was motivated by sexual arousal and was not gender related. Later Hirschfeld would find transgender people who showed no signs of sexual arousal while crossdressed. While it is true that crossdressing initially stimulates sexual arousal because of prior conditioning, this arousal fades with exposure because it involves Pavlovian conditioning extinction. Such conditioning extinguishes without reinforcement of unconditioned responses. Although their interpretation of the phenomenon may have been somewhat in error, sexologists began to advocate for their transgender patients, some of whom eventually went through what we would call today **transgender transition** and early **transgender genital plastic surgery**. The latter was made possible by contemporaneous improvements in anesthesia.

Realizing the cultural rejection of his patients, Hirschfeld worked with the Berlin police to reduce transgender and homosexual harassment on the street. (Hirschfeld was a homosexual himself and had been physically attacked in public.) Because transgender people were unable to find employment elsewhere, Hirschfeld hired his patients as office workers. One of them, Dora Richter, became the first recipient of "**genital transformation surgery**." Hirschfeld left Germany in 1930 and all of his records were destroyed in 1933 by a Fascist mob during one of the famous Nazi book-burning episodes. He started an extended worldwide tour, eventually arriving in France where he died in 1935.

It is important for providers to realize that transgender people may differ because of their heritages. Their characteristics, needs, and objectives may differ. The idea of being transgender spread, but it did so along four separate advocacy paths, defined by demographic groupings of transgender people. *The current increased visibility of transgender people is not a sudden phenomenon but an outcome of these four independent initiatives.* Advocacy paths for transgender people were different for the four demographics:

1. **Transitioning transwomen**: Transwomen who wanted to express their congruent gender full-time and to change their bodies by undergoing transition.
2. **Nontransitioning**: Transgender people who do not want to change their bodies but want to express their nonstereotypical gender behavior part- or full-time.
3. **Rejected by family**: Transgender people who experienced rejection by their families at an early age, experienced homelessness, and engaged in street economies.
4. **Transitioning transmen**: Transmen, assigned female at birth, who wanted to express their congruent gender full-time and to change their bodies by undergoing transition.

Transitioning Transwomen

The *first demographic* consisted of natal males who wanted to change their bodies and live full-time in their feminine congruent gender. They eventually were called transsexuals, but that term is no longer favored by transgender people or providers. This was the demographic that Hirschfeld first encountered in Germany. They were originally nearly all Caucasian natal males but later were joined by females and persons of color. Because they require medical treatment, this demographic was championed by medical and mental health providers, notably Magnus Hirschfeld and later Harry Benjamin.

Nontransitioning

The *second demographic* group consisted of those who did not want to change their bodies but wanted to express their congruent gender either full or part time but needed mutual support. They constitute about 80–90 percent of transgender people. Many had developed obligations with work, family, and community that would be compromised by public exposure. Many simply did not want to transition. This demographic started out as being primarily Caucasian natal males, but later transmen and people of color joined them with their own support groups. Their path was through semisecret, self-directed support groups starting in the 1960s. The first such group was started by Virginia Prince, whose name was a pseudonym for a PhD pharmacologist at the University of California, San Francisco who was a natal male. Some of these groups were strictly heterosexual and involved spouses, but some were open to all genders and sexual orientations. As with the first demographic, they were originally all white but later included people of color and transmen. Many such people no longer depend on support groups because of social media and more open public spaces.

Rejected by Family

The *third demographic* included those natal males who were rejected by their families for their transgender behavior and were forced to live on the street. They were predominantly poor people who engaged in risky street economies, although advocates from other demographics tried to help them. Rather than staying in hiding as the first two demographics predominately did, because they had the financial means, this demographic group was forced into the open. They reacted to cultural rejection and police harassment with direct action in the 1960s. Direct action included takeovers, picketing, and demonstrations. They started these actions with inspiration from the contemporaneous civil rights movement. After initial direct action, their path led to forming local groups to secure economic and health benefits from cities and the federal government.

Transmen

The *fourth demographic* consisted of transmen who developed their advocacy in the 1980s. These were the transmen transitioning transgender people, led by Louis Sullivan in San Francisco. They were instrumental in breaking the sexual orientation barrier, which required transitioning transgender people to be heterosexual. Until this time, transgender people were generally rejected for transitioning unless they avowed that their sexual orientation was homosexual; that is, for transmen, that they had to be attracted to the female sex. This requirement for transition was eventually abolished, championed by Lin Fraser, a psychologist in San Francisco who treated Louis Sullivan, the leader of this demographic. Fraser advocated for the independence of being transgender from sexual orientation with provider organizations.

HISTORY OF THE FOUR TRANSGENDER DEMOGRAPHICS THROUGH THE 1980s

The advocacy activities of these four demographics were and are only loosely connected. In the 1960s, if there were connections, they were in San Francisco. A linchpin in these connections was a single transgender woman, Louise Lawrence. She was a full-time transgender person and community organizer who also lectured to medical providers at the University of California, San Francisco. The providers there were and still are interested in understanding and treating transgender people. Louise was not only connected with transgender people locally but worldwide through correspondence and personal contact. This was in an age before email and social media. She was also connected with prominent sexologists, such as Alfred Kinsey and Harry Benjamin.

Historically the path of the *first demographic, transwomen who wanted to change their bodies,* began with Hirschfeld but the path eventually led to San Francisco in the United States in the 1960s. Many of Hirschfeld's strolls through the local red-light districts of Berlin to deal with police harassment were with a fellow German, Harry Benjamin. Harry Benjamin kept in contact with him because of interest in the new field of endocrinology in Germany. He later coordinated the U.S. portion of Hirschfeld's tour after Hirschfeld fled from the Nazis. Benjamin had become trapped in New York City in 1913 by the outbreak of World War I and started a consulting endocrinology practice there. Benjamin was interested in the new science of endocrinology, which had been triggered by the scientific discovery and later synthesis of sex hormones.

Benjamin became an advocate for transitioning transgender people in the United States. Although Benjamin's main practice was in New York, he spent summers in San Francisco helping transgender people and networking with local advocacy groups. It was in San Francisco that Benjamin was introduced to Louise Lawrence by none other than Alfred Kinsey, who would become probably the most famous U.S. sexologist. Benjamin treated transitioning transgender patients with hormone therapy but also arranged for several to get transgender genital plastic surgery (TGPS). Finding a surgeon to perform the operations was tricky because various European countries and U.S. states, including California, banned such surgeries from time to time. So he had to maintain worldwide connections and arrange for legal as well as illegal secret operations.

In San Francisco, Benjamin worked with Louise Lawrence. She was connected with Karl Bowman at the University of California, San Francisco and lectured to his staff. She also fostered connections between them and Alfred Kinsey on transgender issues.

Benjamin, Lawrence, Kinsey, Bowman, and Edmund Brown (then California's attorney general) became involved with a transgender case in 1949. Over the objections of Benjamin, Brown issued a legal opinion that indicated that surgical changes to genitalia constituted "mayhem" because they destroyed healthy tissue and so should be illegal. Benjamin objected to this ruling. This opinion would discourage transgender genital plastic surgery (TGPS) for some time. However, Benjamin was able to arrange for several operations under conditions of secrecy. These operations were performed mainly by Elmer Belt, a UCLA urologist.

After World War II, gender clinics were reestablished and in 1949 the American sexologist David Cauldwell coined the term **transsexual** for those undergoing transgender transition (Cauldwell, 1949). Medical advocacy for transgender people continued with the formation of university and hospital gender centers in the United States. These organizations led research on transgender issues and the development of genital plastic surgery techniques. Many of these centers in the United States eventually dissolved due to internal philosophical opposition and because a free market among providers and patients had developed outside of the clinics. The free market allowed for the development of affirmative adult treatment for transgender people and better availability of transition services and TGPS. This treatment encouraged transgender people to express themselves while keeping safe. Today, many of these clinics in universities and research hospitals have been reestablished in the United States, and new ones have been formed in order to meet the accelerating demand for services and to conduct research.

Benjamin's most famous transsexual patient was Christine Jorgensen, who had been a U.S. soldier in World War II. In 1953, after transition, Jorgensen became a performer and celebrity. She was denied transition in California, so she went to Denmark for hormone therapy and surgery. Benjamin met and treated her after her surgery. Jorgensen was the Caitlyn Jenner of her day, publicly coming out and becoming a celebrity.

Benjamin wrote a definitive book entitled *The Transsexual Phenomenon* (Benjamin, 1966), which established him as a leader in the field. He was responsible for promoting the term transsexual rather than transvestite or sexo-aesthetic inversion. In honor of Benjamin the first professional association for treating transgender people was formed—the Harry Benjamin International Gender Dysphoria Association. The organization is now called the World Professional Association for Transgender Health (WPATH). It continues to revise and publish Standards of Care documents for providers.

Progress for the *second demographic,* that of *nontransitioning transgender people,* also had its beginnings in San Francisco. The focus here was on education and the formation of self-help support groups, led not by mental health professionals but by elected peer members. After the breakup of his marriage, a person named Arnold Lowman who held a PhD in pharmacy moved to San Francisco. In California, she presented full-time in the feminine gender category. She became a lecturer at the University of California, San Francisco and changed her name to Virginia Prince because she lived locally on Prince Street. In the 1960s the self-help support group movement was all the rage. Modeled after the Alcoholics Anonymous format, groups formed on a wide variety of topics. Rather than discourage behavior as Alcoholics Anonymous tried to do, the purpose of these new support groups was to encourage and make safe the relevant behavior. Being transgender was no exception. There had been previous informal transgender groups but none went nationwide until Prince started her initiative.

Enter Louise Lawrence again. Lawrence helped Prince with her newsletters and publications both through her contacts, and with editing and production. Lawrence worked with Prince to publish the first transgender newsletter, *Transvestia.* For the newsletter, Prince wrote a lesbian fantasy story that piqued the interest of postal inspectors. She was charged and pleaded guilty to distributing pornography. The penalty was probation, which was later lifted by prosecutors. Prince organized a chain of support groups around the United States called the Society for the Second Self or Tri-Ess, which continues today. Tri-Ess was formed with the strict tenets that the participants be male, heterosexual, and nontransitioning; that they would keep discussions a secret; and that it was mandatory for their wives to participate. Although Prince argued against transgender transition, it is believed that she took hormones for breast development.

Although Tri-Ess had been the first support group for transgender people, it was just the start. Many other support groups developed that accepted pansexuals, transsexuals, and transmen as well as crossdressing heterosexuals. Many of these groups started out as "crossdressing" groups. They became formal "transgender" support groups as the term became repurposed from the original definition that John Oliven had given it in 1965. Although the term transgender was in existence, Virginia Prince actually preferred the terms "femmophile" or "transvestite." However, many people still attribute the repurposing and popularization of the word "transgender" to her.

The *third demographic* primarily involved *transwomen who had been rejected by their families and who became street people.* These people did not have the resources to be able to practice their transgender behavior in secret as could the first and second demographics. Many were forced out of their homes due to parental rejection of their transgender behavior and became homeless. To survive, they were forced into prostitution, drug pushing, and street crime. These people engaged in advocacy activities to try to improve their lives—spurred on by the concurrent civil rights and anti–Vietnam War movements in the 1960s.

Police in many areas felt that they had to crack down on these people during the 1960s in order to discourage Vietnam War soldiers from becoming patrons of the street economies in cities. There was also general civil unrest precipitated by the war and various demonstrations. This demographic of transgender people engaged in direct action in the 1960s against police harassment and brutality. They did not have the resources for legal action or to support political candidates at first. These people participated in these actions because they were often subjected to public strip search and other degrading police practices.

Although most people remember the Stonewall riots as the beginning of the gay and lesbian political movement, transgender people were at the forefront of those and other prior actions that started a decade earlier. In some cases, establishments that these people frequented were run by organized crime. Police raided them in order to obtain payoffs, harassing transgender and gay patrons, and allowing the establishments to reopen upon payment. As a token of this, the first night of the Stonewall riots in 1969 featured throwing coins at the police. This advocacy demographic engaged in direct action in the 1960s that included violent and nonviolent protests against police harassment and brutality. Although most people think of the Stonewall riots as the beginning of the GLBT political movements, the actions started a decade earlier. Actions occurred in Los Angeles at Cooper's Donuts in 1959, in Philadelphia at Dewey's Cafeteria in 1965, at Compton Cafeteria in San Francisco in 1966, and finally at Stonewall in New York City in 1969.

It was after the actions in San Francisco and New York City that local transgender rights organizations first took hold for this demographic. In San Francisco, the Tenderloin Social Justice Campaign was formed, which resulted in improvements in civil rights and restoration of financial support for local War on Poverty activities, which had been cut off by the federal government. The first transgender support group in San Francisco, called Conversion Our Goal, was formed in 1968 and led by Wendy Kohler, who had been a patient of Harry Benjamin. In New York City advocacy groups were formed in the wake of Stonewall. Silvia Rivera and Marsha P. Johnson formed the Street Transvestite Action Revolutionaries (STAR) as an educational group for people of color, especially for Hispanics.

The organization efforts in San Francisco received private donations including those from Reed Erikson, a wealthy transgender person, who had also supported Harry Benjamin in writing *The Transsexual Phenomenon*. He had been one of Benjamin's patients.

The *fourth demographic,* which involved *transitioning transmen,* started in the 1980s, much later than that of transitioning transwomen. Led by Lou Sullivan, organizations called Gateway Gender Alliance and "FTM" were formed in San Francisco. Along with his mental health provider, Sullivan and his provider, Lin Fraser, lobbied the American Psychiatric Association and the Harry Benjamin International Gender Dysphoria Association (now WPATH) for these organizations to recognize the existence of gay transmen and to remove sexual orientation requirements for transgender transition. He founded FTM International in the late 1980s, one of the first organizations to support transmen. Since then, the number of transmen has grown rapidly.

HISTORIES OF THE FOUR TRANSGENDER DEMOGRAPHICS UP TO THE EARLY 21ST CENTURY

By the end of the 1980s transgender advocacy activities by people in the four demographic categories had resulted in organized medical groups, transgender support groups, and multiracial/multigender advocacy groups in major cities. There would be ups and downs, but transgender people were here to stay. In the decades following the 1980s, the four demographics developed organizations and mechanisms at the national and international levels, which resulted in improvements in transgender tolerance, acceptance, health care, and visibility.

For the *first demographic, transitioning transwomen,* WPATH significantly liberalized the Standards of Care and expanded its activities. For example, the requirement that a person had to change their names was eliminated. The requirement for a one-year **real-life "test" (RLT)** to prove that the transitioner could maintain employment in their congruent gender behavior category was dropped. In place of the RLT, it was suggested that a **real-life experience (RLE)** would be beneficial. Even this suggestion was eventually dropped. The requirement that a person had to be attracted sexually and romantically to same-sex people was eliminated due, in large part, to influence by the *fourth demographic,* that of transitioning transmen. WPATH opposed laws requiring divorce and sterilization for transitioning transgender people, which had been adopted in some localities. Some of these laws are still in place but are gradually being repealed.

With regard to the *second demographic,* that of nontransitioning transgender people, in the 1980s the number and membership of local support groups grew rapidly. It later declined because of computer networks including the Internet, local meetups, and because of increased cultural tolerance for transgender people, allowing safe public spaces to congregate. The Internet provided information on being transgender and in recent years has allowed transgender people to form friendships and less formal associations online.

Support groups spawned transgender meetings and conventions, the largest of which was Southern Comfort, originally in Atlanta, and the largest now, Gender Odyssey in Seattle. The Be-All (as in the 1983 Army recruiting jingle "be all that you can be") Conference annually rotated between Detroit, Chicago, and Pittsburgh and was hosted by the support groups in those cities. Conferences provided how-to workshops as well as workshops dealing with transgender advocacy issues, but they primarily allowed transgender people to express their congruent gender category continuously for an extended period of time. Many of the support groups and conferences are no longer in existence due to the Internet and the formation of local meetup groups. Gender Odyssey still attracts several thousand people to Seattle, and they now have other meetings in Los Angeles and San Diego. Their offerings have expanded to sessions for providers and children.

Transgender support groups and conferences have given way to other means of expression of congruent gender, although many transgender people still do so in secret. The Internet now serves as a major networking and how-to source. A new type of transgender convention without all the trappings of a traditional convention has also evolved. For example, the Diva Las Vegas convention just provides times and places of meeting for transgender gatherings. The participants are free to stay in any hotel, to go to any restaurant in the city, and to do as they please apart from the gatherings.

The *third demographic,* those *rejected by families,* triggered the development of arrest diversion programs and civil rights legal precedents and contributed to advocacy for HIV treatment. The mistreatment of people in this group was documented in a 1995 report to the city of San Francisco written largely by Jamison Green, who connected three demographic initiatives. Jamison was a transman and later became president of WPATH. This report resulted in the formation of the San Francisco Human Rights Commission and protective ordinances. These ordinances became the legislation model for cities to deal with civil rights abuses for all people, not just transgender people.

Transgender people on the street were devastated by the HIV/AIDS epidemic in the 1980s because of their exposure through sex work and illegal drug taking. LGBT people began to fight back at the national level when the U.S. government refused to deal with the public health problem. Some of the methods of direct action that the San Francisco transgender people had used became models for the AIDS Coalition to Unleash Power (ACT-UP) organization. Four members of ACT-UP formed a national LGBT organization called Queer Nation, which advocated for LGBT rights. Although Queer Nation did not last, it spawned an organization that did last—Transgender

Nation. It was formed in 1992 by Anne Ogborne inside Queer Nation and when Queer Nation evaporated, Transgender Nation remained.

Transgender Nation used direct action to protest the exclusion of transgender people from the 1993 National Gay, Lesbian and Bisexual March on Washington. The GLB community had developed national advocacy organizations by then that voted to exclude transgender people from speaking and exclude the word "Transgender" in the march title. In the same year, Queer Nation also used direct action in a protest of the American Psychiatric Association's pathologization of transgender people

In reaction to the 1993 GLB march, a new national organization, the Transexual [*sic*] Menace, was formed by Riki Wilkins to take direct action on behalf of transgender people. They were most famous for their vigil of the court proceedings against those responsible for the brutal assault and murder of Brandon Teena, a transman. The story of Brandon Teena was subsequently dramatized in the movie *Boys Don't Cry,* which won an Academy Award. The Transexual Menace was also the subject of a documentary film. The biggest impact of the Transexual Menace was probably that it spawned GenderPAC, the first transgender national political action committee for funding political candidates.

TRANSGENDER HISTORY IN THE SECOND DECADE OF THE 21ST CENTURY

During this period, the rights that were won by transgender advocacy suffered some reversals. This has resulted in frustration, confusion, and depression among transgender people of which providers need to be aware.

Transgender advocacy organizations have partnered with GLB and other organizations to achieve their goals. Although transgender organizations have supported GLB legislation and advocacy, this support has sometimes been reciprocated and sometimes not. Transgender people supported many GLB issues such as same-sex marriage rights because GLB people are included among those who are transgender. An example of cooperative support was when the Gay and Lesbian Task Force helped set up the National Center for Transgender Equality (NCTE) in 2006. The NCTE is now the most effective organization advocating for transgender rights, although there are several others.

An example of when alliances with GLB organizations turned sour was the effort to pass the Employment Non-Discrimination Act (ENDA) in 2011. GLB organizations pledged that they would pursue a transgender-inclusive bill. But without allowing transgender organizations to fully mobilize congressional support, some GLB organizations approved of the deletion of being transgender from the bill. Because it was likely that the

Bush administration would veto this bill in any case, the deletion was unnecessary. However, there were some positive aspects of the fight. Over 200 organizations as well as some members of Congress protested the action of dropping transgender protections from this bill.

During the current decade (2010–2020) in the United States, transgender people enjoyed greater tolerance and acceptance. Advances were made in safeguarding transgender rights at the state and federal levels in many areas, including employment, education, public accommodations, prison housing, nondiscrimination in federal contracting, and health care. These advances were primarily accomplished through court case precedents and rulings by the Equal Employment Opportunity Commission. The DOJ is currently actively trying to reverse these precedents and the Supreme Court will consider such precedents in 2019. The depathologization of being transgender included the issuance of the DSM-5, which removed the pathology diagnostic category of "gender identity disorder" and added an intended nonpathological category, "gender dysphoria." During this period, many high-profile transgender celebrities emerged; among them was Caitlyn Jenner who, as a male, had won the Olympic decathlon in 1976. The affirming model for transgender treatment was developed and applied to transgender children. Reparative therapy bans were passed for transgender people in many states and localities. In 2017, an international conference was held in Yogyakarta, Indonesia to apply international human rights to transgender and sexual orientation minorities. The resulting Yogyakarta Principles Plus establishes a framework for civil and economic rights for gender and sexual orientation minorities and their intersection.

WPATH expanded their organization by forming subsidiary organizations that could function in Europe and the United States: the European Association for Transgender Health (EPATH) and the United States Professional Association for Transgender Health (USPATH). These organizations conduct their own science conferences. WPATH also began to develop courses and certification criteria, which included education and on-the-job training requirements for providers. WPATH contributed to the depathologization of being transgender. WPATH members were involved in deleting gender identity disorder from the list of mental disorders in the ***Diagnostic and Statistical Manual of Mental Disorders*** **(DSM-5)** of the American Psychiatric Association in 2017. Gender identity disorder was a pathological category that had been inserted in the DSM-III in 1980. It was based on Freudian and Eriksonian psychodynamic notions of identity and applied to transgender people in the DSM-III. WPATH also supported depathologization in the WHO International Classification of Diseases (ICD) list and the insertion of a nonpathological code for medical treatment of transitioning transgender people in a sexual health category in ICD-11, which takes effect in most countries in 2019.

In the latter part of the "teens" decade, under a new administration, pullbacks in transgender rights were pursued by U.S. department policies led by the Department of Justice. New policies were announced for allowing discrimination against transgender people on the basis of "religious freedom." Many of these policies have been blocked by litigation, at least temporarily. During this period there has been progress in depathologization of being transgender with the announced changes in the new ICD, which eliminate the "gender identity disorder" category and set up a diagnostic category in the nonpathological sexual health section that would allow medical treatment for transgender (transsexual) transition. Enactment of bans on gender change efforts, sometimes called "reparative therapy," continued at the state level in the United States. In the case of being transgender, the term **heterogenderism** was coined for discrimination based on a binary, cisgender, and inflexible gender system. Heterogenderism, along with racism, sexism, heterosexism, and their intersections, define societal minorities.

Transgender people in the United States now enjoy greater tolerance and acceptance than ever before. They now have local and national advocacy, and educational and research organizations to repel antitransgender cultural actions. More transgender people are running for office; a transgender person became a state representative in Virginia in 2018. As the civil rights movement has demonstrated, transgender people need to continue to be active to maintain their rights.

TRANSGENDER ADVOCACY OUTSIDE THE UNITED STATES

Transgender people have made gains in obtaining their rights in many countries, notably Australia and the countries of Europe and South America. The development of transgender advocacy follows a similar pattern to that of the United States with similar demographic groups.

In Australia, medical advocacy for transitioning transwomen started with the Gender Dysphoria Clinic in 1975 at Queen Victoria Hospital in Melbourne. As early as 1979 in Melbourne, the Victorian Transsexual Coalition was lobbying the government for the right to change identification documents. Australian Medicare currently provides transgender transition services.

Akin to the *second U.S. demographic* activities, the Seahorse Society was formed in 1970 in Sydney as a support group for crossdressers to provide a safe place to express their congruent gender behavior. Laws against crossdressing were still enforced at that time. The first leaders included a member of the Tri-Ess support group from the United States and a member of the Beaumont Society support group in the United Kingdom. The

Beaumont Society was, itself, a spinoff from Tri-Ess. The group was open to heterosexual transgender males who wanted to emulate women, although it stated that it did not condemn homosexuality or BDSM. The rules included good taste in dressing and secrecy. In 1975 sections of the society broke off to form their own societies in other parts of Australia and it became the Seahorse Society of New South Wales.

With regard to the *third U.S. demographic,* that of street transgender people, with government support, the Australian Transsexual Association started Tiresias House to provide semisupported housing for transsexuals and services to the wider transgender community. Tiresias House was formed in 1983 and became the Gender Centre in 1993. The New South Wales Anti-discrimination Act in 1996 gave legal recognition to transgender people. As in the United States, gender recognition, identification, and other laws are under the control of states and territories, some of which require verification of transgender genital plastic surgery. At the Australian federal level, passports and Medicare verification require only a letter from the person's doctor and do not require surgery. Once same-sex marriage was approved in 2017, the requirement for transsexuals to divorce was dropped as of 2018.

In Europe, transgender rights are guaranteed by precedents of the European Court of Justice of the European Economic Community and by legislation in the United Kingdom and Ireland. European countries are in the process of revising their transsexual policies, which until recently required sterilization and spousal divorce. Some countries still do not provide legal recognition for transitioning transgender people.

In 2005, Transgender Europe (TGEU) was formed from several transgender advocacy organizations in Europe to coordinate transgender advocacy efforts. In the United Kingdom, the first support group was a chapter of Tri-Ess in 1966, which became the Beaumont Society. Starting with Tri-Ess tenets, it has become an open group with both transwomen and transmen of all types. Mermaids, a group formed by parents of transgender children in 1995, provides support and information. The Gender Identity Research and Education Society (GIRES) provides information to policymakers and the public to improve medical, educational, legal, and other services for transgender people.

Transgender people have also made gains in recognition in South American countries, beginning in Argentina, which now has some of the most liberal transgender policies in the world. Global Action for Transgender Equality (GATE) was formed by an Argentinian transman with representation from the United Kingdom, Australia, the United States, and other countries to advocate on an international scale. Advocacy in Argentina has influenced other countries in South America, notably Uruguay and Brazil.

The struggle for transgender rights has largely been successful in many countries, although it is far from unified. This reflects diversity within the international transgender community in which multiple organizations usually team up to get things done and then go their separate ways. It confirms the idea that being transgender has a biological basis that manifests across a wide range of demographics.

TIMELINE

1908
Havelock Ellis and Magnus Hirschfeld describe being transgender.

1911
The Transvestites, a book by Hirschfeld, is published.

1922, 1931
Dora Richter has the first transgender orchiotomy and genital plastic surgery.

1933
Destruction of Hirschfeld's offices in Berlin by Nazis.

1949
"Transsexual" term coined by Cauldwell for those wanting to change their bodies.

1953
Christine Jorgensen returns from Denmark after TGPS, becomes celebrity. Patient of Harry Benjamin.

1959–1969
Transgender direct action in Los Angeles at Cooper's Donuts in 1959, in Philadelphia at Dewey's Cafeteria in 1965, Compton Cafeteria in San Francisco in 1966, and Stonewall in New York City in 1969.

1966
Publication of *The Transsexual Phenomenon* by Harry Benjamin.

1966
Term "transgender" coined by John Oliven, indicating that transitioning transgender people are not motivated by sexual arousal.

1976
First national transgender support group formed through merger of Mamselle and Foundation for Personal Expression into the Tri-Ess. Led by Virginia Prince.

1979
HBIGDA/WPATH provides Standards of Care for transgender people.

1970
Seahorse Society support group in Australia based on support groups in United States and United Kingdom.

1975
Formation of Gender Dysphoria Clinic at Queen Victoria Hospital in Melbourne.

1979
Louis Sullivan, a transman, forms FTM International and lobbies to eliminate sexual orientation as a qualifier for transgender transition.

1983
DSM-III's pathological category of gender identity disorder and depathologization of homosexuality.

1992
Transgender Nation formed by Anne Ogborne.

1993
National LGB March on Washington without transgender recognition.

2000
Lynn Conway makes first population frequency estimates of transgender transwomen (Conway, 2000–2002; Olyslager, & Conway, 2007).

2003
Employment Non-Discrimination Act bill defeated in United States.

2005
Formation of Transgender Europe (TGEU).

2006
National Center for Transgender Equality formed.

2009
First U.S. law protecting transgender people, the Matthew Shepard Act.

2017
WPATH SOC Version 7 with nonpathological category of "gender dysphoria."

2019
ICD Version 11 with nonpathological category for transition medical care.

REFERENCES

American Psychological Association. (2015, December). Guidelines for psychological practice with transgender and gender nonconforming people. *American Psychologist, 70*(9), 832–864.

Bauer, G. R., Pyne, J., Francino, M., & Hammond, R. (2013). Suicidality among trans people in Ontario: Implications for social work and social justice. *Service Signal, 59*, 35–62. http://transpulseproject.ca/wp-content/uploads/2013/09/Trans-PULSE-Suicidality-Trans-ServiceSocial-2013.pdf

Benjamin, H. (1966). *The transsexual phenomenon*. Human Outreach & Achievement Institute. http://www.mut23.de/texte/Harry%20Benjamin%20-%20The%20Transsexual%20Phenomenon.pdf

Bevan, T. (2015). *The psychobiology of transsexualism and transgenderism*. Santa Barbara, CA: Praeger.

Cauldwell, D. (1949). Psychopathia transsexualis. *Sexology, 16*, 274–280.

Clements-Nolle, K., Marx, R., & Katz, M. (2006). Attempted suicide among transgender persons. *Journal of Homosexuality, 51*(3), 53–69.

Conway, L. (2001–2002). How frequently does transsexualism occur? http://www.lynnconway.com

De Haan, G., Santos, G. M., Arayasirikul, S., & Raymond, H. F. (2015). Nonprescribed hormone use and barriers to care for transgender women in San Francisco. *LGBT Health, 2*(4), 313–323.

Eisenberg, M. E., Gower, A. L., McMorris, B. J., Rider, G. N., Shea, G., & Coleman, E. (2017). Risk and protective factors in the lives of transgender/gender nonconforming adolescents. *Journal of Adolescent Health, 64*(4), 521–526.

Grant, J. M., Mottet, L. A., Tanis, J., Harrison, J., Herman, J. L, & Keisling, M. (2011). *Injustice at every turn: A report of the national transgender discrimination survey.* Washington, DC: National Center for Transgender Equality and National Gay and Lesbian Task Force.

Hembree, W. C., Cohen-Kettenis, P., Delemarre-van de Waal, H. A., Gooren, L. J., Meyer, W. J. III, Spack, N. P., Tangpricha, V., & Montori, V. M. (2009, December). Guidelines for psychological practice with transgender and gender nonconforming people. *Journal of Endocrinology Metabolism, 94*(9), 3132–3154.

Hirschfeld, M. (1991). *Transvestites: The erotic drive to cross-dress* (M. A. Lombardi, Trans.). Amherst: Prometheus Books. (Original work published 1911)

Liu, R., & Mustanski, B. (2001). Suicidal ideation and self-harm in lesbian, gay, bisexual, and transgender people. *American Journal of Preventative Medicine, 42*, 221–228.

Mollie, R., Blosnich, J. R., Dichter, M. E., Luscri, L., & Shipherd, J. (2017). Will veterans answer sexual orientation and gender identity questions? *Medical Care, 55*, S85–S89.

Mustanski, B., & Liu, R. (2010). A longitudinal study of predictors of suicide attempt among lesbian, gay, bisexual and transgender youth. *Archives of Sexual Behavior, 42*, 437–448.

Oliven, J. (1965, June). Transgenderism = transsexualism. *Sexual Hygiene and Pathology*, 514.

Olyslager, F., & Conway, L. (2007). *On the calculation of the prevalence of transsexualism.* Presentation at 2007 WPATH Symposium, Chicago, IL.

Rafferty, J. (2018). Guidelines for ensuring comprehensive care and support for transgender and gender-diverse children and adolescents. *American Psychologist, 70*(9), 832–864.

Rotondi, N. K., Bauer, G. R., Scanlon, K., Kaay, M., Travers, R., & Travers, A. (2013). Nonprescribed hormone use and self-performing surgeries: "Do-it-yourself" transitions in transgender communities in Ontario, Canada. *American Journal of Public Health, 103*(10), 1830–1836.

Turban, J., Ferraiolo, T., Martin, A., & Olezeski, C. (2017). Ten things transgender adults and gender nonconforming youth want their doctors to know. *Journal of the American Academy of Child & Adolescent Psychiatry, 56*(4), 275–277.

Webberly, H., & Webberly, M. J. (2018). Self-medication is common in patients who face long delays in accessing NHS services in the UK. WPATH 2018 poster session.

WPATH. (2011). WPATH standards of care for the health of transsexual, transgender, and gender nonconforming people. WPATH. https://wpath.org/publications/soc

2

Perspectives on Causation and Treatment

Although being transgender is no longer considered a disorder or disease, its causal factors are important to understand and worthy of scientific definition and exploration. Providers need to know how to deal with and interact with transgender people even if a patient presents with some problem that is totally unrelated to being transgender. Those who are involved in providing transgender transition procedures especially need to know. Transgender patients and the public expect providers to know the current scientific status regarding the causal factors of being transgender, despite the fact there is more to learn about them through scientific research.

Many notions about being transgender do not rise to the level of scientific theory. In order to do so, a theory minimally must be well defined, express a causal relation, and be able to be tested empirically. Many ideas of the past did not meet these requirements because we did not have enough experience with the phenomenon or with its biology to generate theories. We now have greater ability to explore transgender science with the development of supporting sciences including genetics, epigenetics, psychology, and anthropology, and tools such as functional magnetic imaging and other technologies.

This chapter provides an overview of perspectives and schools of thought regarding transgender causation and treatment. If a perspective rises to the level of a scientific theory, it will be defined and reviewed in more detail in the next chapter.

PERSPECTIVES ON CAUSAL FACTORS

Nature versus Nurture

Nature versus nurture debates about many behavioral phenomena raged for over four centuries, but in the mid-20th century scientists started to realize that multiple factors were involved in most complex behaviors—not just two. The reason for this was that we finally developed the scientific technologies to isolate and study these factors and increasingly understand their mechanisms. Today we know that genetics, epigenetics, human learning, and culture are factors in many behavioral phenomena.

Nature versus Nurture: A False Dichotomy

The nature versus nurture debate about many behavioral phenomena raged for over four centuries, but in the mid-20th century scientists started to realize that multiple factors were involved in most complex behavioral phenomena. These factors have multiple subordinate mechanisms that influence outcomes. Knowledge of this cascade of mechanisms is beginning to create understanding of being transgender and other behavioral traits.

- We know that for complex anatomical and physiological processes as well as behavior, multiple DNA genes are typically involved.
- Among the genes in the DNA are areas we used to call "junk" DNA. We know now that these parts of the DNA molecule are involved in promoting or suppressing gene expression.
- Given that we have two sets of DNA from our parents, individual genes at each place on the DNA molecule may be activated or inactivated. For those with XX chromosomes, X-inactivation leaves cells with different configurations.
- DNA as it arrives in the fetus comes with non-DNA chemical modifiers that promote or suppress expression (e.g., methylation and histones).

- The fetus shares cells with the mother and with previous siblings as well as any fraternal twin. These cells will have different DNA. Some of these cells find a safe haven in the brain away from the immune system.
- There are genetically formed mechanisms that control hormone secretions that influence the body and indirectly the brain through neural plasticity.
- During pregnancy, the body may be exposed to teratogens, which mutate DNA or modify its expression. Diethylstilbestrol has been implicated in transgender causation but not confirmed.
- After birth, learning begins in several mechanisms (sensory, emotional, experiential, declarative, and procedural), which change brain chemistry.
- The cascade results in brain mechanisms that are associated with transgender behavior, which we are beginning to observe using brain scanners and other tools.

Genetics

It was always suspected that there was a genetic factor in being transgender during discussions in transgender support groups and informally among transgender people. Although limited by secrecy in support groups, it became known that close relatives were sometimes reported to be transgender. The genetic factor hypothesis has now been supported by heritability studies using identical and nonidentical twins. These studies are described in more detail in the next chapter. Based on data from these studies, a world-class behavioral genetics consortium (Polderman et al., 2018) has hypothesized that a polygenetic threshold model applies to being transgender, which would support the notion that close relatives of transgender people are more likely to be transgender. It should be noted that if one identical twin is transgender and the other is not transgender, they will both have the same sex, indicating dissociation of sex and gender. Partial and full genome studies indicate that there are DNA markers for being transgender, although additional studies are needed. There are also several biomarkers, believed to have genetic bases, that differ between transgender people and controls. For example, transgender people tend to be less right-handed (Watson & Coren, 1992; Wisniewski, Prendeville, & Dobs, 2005).

Epigenetics

Epigenetics has to do with non-DNA mechanisms that change (mutate) DNA and/or alter its expression. Most of these mechanisms are active after conception, but a few are initialized when parents impart non-DNA chemicals at conception to the fetus. Details of potential epigenetic mechanisms and theories are also described in the next chapter.

The idea that epigenetics can block being transgender comes from genetic twin studies. *It is commonly noticed that the traits of identical twins at birth are not identical.* Epigenetic unblocking is necessary for transgender genes to be expressed as nervous system mechanisms. If one identical twin is transgender, then the other is not always transgender, indicating a possible role of epigenetics in changing the DNA common to the twins, or changing how it is expressed.

Two epigenetic theories have been developed, which postulate that specific epigenetic mechanisms by themselves cause being transgender. These have to do with prenatal testosterone levels and exposure to teratogenic drugs.

The **Prenatal Testosterone Theory of being Transgender** (PTTT) was advanced (Dörner, 1976) based on studies of the effects of prenatal sex hormones on animal sexual behavior. This theory predicts that males (transwomen) who become transgender are exposed to lower fetal testosterone levels, while females (transmen) are exposed to higher levels than normal. The existing scientific evidence refutes this theory, although it is incorrectly assumed by some scientists and by the public. (See Chapter 3 for more detail.)

Diethylstilbestrol (DES) was a drug used ostensibly to prevent miscarriages when taken by pregnant mothers. It was prescribed in the United States and Europe from 1947 to the mid-1970s and used in animal food. Although the drug was believed to be estrogenic, it was later shown to not behave as most estrogens do and to be a teratogen that mutates DNA and probably changes how it is expressed. The results of administration of this drug have been birth defects and rare cancers in offspring into the third generation. The theory was advanced that prenatal exposure to DES was a causal factor in being a transwoman (Kerlin, 2005), but the evidence only weakly supports this notion. However, the evidence is good enough to suggest a hypothesis. The Kerlin DES study may have been biased because only those with problems may have volunteered to provide information and because the vetting of actual DES administration was weak. The possibility of using existing controlled U.S. government and private cohorts has not been pursued. (See Chapter 3 for more detail.)

Early Gender Learning and Transgender Emergence

In order for children to recognize their congruent gender, they must first learn about the gender system of the culture to which they are born.

Most children complete early gender learning by the ages of two to three (Fausto-Sterling, 2012); they will learn more about gender as they develop but will have mastered the basics by those ages. This is in contrast to learning about sex, which typically occurs later in development. Children learn to dress and comport themselves in their congruent gender by age two or three through several types of learning experiences including parental instruction and behavior modeling.

Most transgender people realize that they are transgender by the ages of four to seven, although some only know that there is something different about them until transgender behaviors emerge at later ages. From the point of emergence, they will attempt to follow the rules of behavior of their nonassigned gender behavior category through presentation and behavior including verbal behavior. These attempts are frequently conducted in secret. At young ages children may not know the word "transgender"; they may use the words "boy" and "girl" for gender categories. They may verbally express that they are supposed to be a boy but are really a girl and vice versa.

Being transgender is not a conscious choice—it is a recognition of the gender category that best fits the genetic gender predisposition of a person, and most mental processes do not require consciousness (Jaynes, 1976).

Sexual Arousal

As is discussed in Chapter 1, the early sexologists Magnus Hirschfeld and Havelock Ellis initially assumed that sexual arousal was the primary motivation for being transgender. This was from initial reports of sexual arousal in transgender people while crossdressed. It also fit theories about sex that Magnus Hirschfeld developed for homosexual people.

Since then, science has learned that although sexual arousal may be initially involved, other motivations are involved in maintaining transgender behavior. Sexual arousal declines with exposure to clothing and other features of gender behavior categories. Sexual arousal is learned and triggered by stimulus novelty. It is a learned classical conditioning or Pavlovian response. What can be learned in this paradigm can also be unlearned or extinguished. It is true that crossdressing and crosspresenting initially result in sexual arousal; this response declines over exposure and time. Reports from interviews with transgender people (Buhrich, 1978; Hirschfeld, 1991; Levitt & Ippolito, 2014) indicate that relaxation and authenticity are the primary motivations for continued crossdressing rather than sexual arousal. This was also the observation of John Oliven (1965) when he coined the term transgender in contradistinction to transsexual because he found that sexual arousal did not explain the motivation for crosspresentation and body modification.

However, the notion that sexual arousal is a causal factor in being transgender or in fetishism has not been abandoned in psychiatry, probably because of the featured role of sex in Freudian interpretations of behavior. The modern manifestation of this idea is **autogynephilia** (Blanchard, 2005), meaning love of oneself as a woman. The idea is that some transwomen are motivated to fantasize and express transgender behavior because of sexual arousal. However, the proponents of this idea have not formulated a testable theory. Instead, there are several formulations that vary between sexual arousal, idolization, and romantic love. Also, the evidence cited as proof is suspect. Autogynephilia is discussed as a controversy in Chapter 10. It is mentioned because the idea is used to sully the reputation of transgender people by transgender critics who seek to relate it exclusively to sex. Its proponents have openly attacked transgender people and others who criticized their ideas, creating ill will.

Parental Relations

There have been numerous theories regarding the potential role of parental relations in causation, but in every case where these theories were reduced to practice, the evidence did not support them (Bailey & Zucker, 1995; Cohen-Kettenis & Gooren, 1999).

These theories have triggered research studies that have refuted, not detected, a role for parental relations causation in:

- Emotional relationships with parents (Buhrich & McConaghy, 1978).
- Prenatal preferred sex preference of the mother (Zucker et al., 1994).
- Parental separation (Cohen-Kettenis & Arrindel, 1990; Freund, Langevin, Zajac, Steiner, & Zajac, 1974; Stevens, Golombok, Beveridge, & The ALSPAC Study Team, 2002; Stevenson & Black, 1998).
- Raising a child in the wrong gender category (Bradley, Oliver, Chernick, & Zucker, 1998; Colopinto, 2006; Reiner & Gearhart, 2004).
- Parental abuse and violence (Bandini et al., 2011; Ghering & Knudson, 2005; Koken, Bimbi, & Parsons, 2009; Roberts, Rosario, Corliss, Konen, & Austin, 2012).

Some clinical studies have reported that adoption among transgender children is disproportionate to the population. But no formal theory for this has been put forward as to whether it is a result of such things as maternal stress, parental relations, or presentation bias (adoptive parents may be more likely to bring transgender children to clinics) (Shumer, Abrha, Feldman, & Carswell, 2017; Zucker & Bradley, 1998).

On the other hand, studies have shown that parental acceptance and affirmation is a factor in reducing the stress of being transgender and reducing the likelihood of suicide (Ryan, Russell, Huebner, Diaz, & Sanchez, 2010; Simons, Schrager, Clark, Belzer, & Olson, 2013).

Sexual Orientation

Sexual orientation and being transgender appear to be decoupled. Sexual orientation does not appear to be a causative factor, although being transgender is often publicly sexualized to suggest an intersection. Transgender people are attracted to males, females, both, or neither, just as cisgender people are. During or after transgender (transsexual) transition, the sexual orientation of transgender people may change.

Studies, starting with Zuger (1988), have shown that there exist male children who are likely to be homosexual as adults. Some of these people crossdress as children to generate sexual interest in other people, rather than to express their congruent gender. "**Prehomosexual" children** are sexually aggressive to same-sex children and focus on "sex-type" behavior. These children do not present as transgender children do. Transgender children are generally subdued, introverted, withdrawn, and are focused on gender. In 1972, homosexuality was removed from the DSM, which made it more complicated to treat these prehomosexual children. In many cases they were treated under DSM codes intended for transgender children. Data from studies of prehomosexual children has been inappropriately used to assess the continuance or "persistence" of being transgender during maturation. This controversy is explored in Chapter 10.

Psychodynamic and Psychoanalytic Ideas

Much speculation about transgender causation has been included in psychodynamic discussions, but so far, none of these ideas constitute scientific theories. One idea is that being transgender is a result of childhood trauma. Some believe that being transgender is a form of personality dissociation, but this is contradicted by the fact that transgender people seem to remember all their experiences both while they are expressing transgender behavior and while they are not expressing it. In the classic split personality disorder, this is not usually the case. Another idea is that transwomen dress in women's clothing because of separation anxiety about leaving their mothers. And yet another is that transwomen are afraid to take on the responsibilities required of males. There are about 20 or so similar ideas, but none constitute a formal scientific theory and none are supported by objective evidence. (See Bevan, 2015, Chapter 12.)

The most common psychodynamic idea about being transgender is that it results from a malformation of gender identity. This idea was a development out of psychosexual development notions from Freud, and through the psychosocial development ideas of Erik Erikson (1968) in which it was postulated that all people develop a sense of their own identity. These ideas were synthesized by Money (Money, Epstein, & Ehrhardt, 1968) into **gender identity.** Finally, Richard Green developed the pathological term **gender identity disorder** in time for inclusion into the DSM-III (1980). The pathological idea of gender identity disorder was dismissed in the DSM-5 and will be dropped in ICD-11. The term gender identity is now in the process of being repurposed as a nonpathological term by transgender people to express recognition of their own behavior and to express membership in their congruent gender behavior category.

Psychotherapy has been used to try to change transgender behavior, but as early as 1972 the American Medical Association Committee published the medical opinion that psychotherapy was generally ineffective for changing transgender behavior (American Medical Association, 1972). Psychological counseling is clearly of value in helping transgender people with problems arising from rejection and social conflicts. Mental health professionals are also integral to guiding transgender people prior to transition and to certify that transgender individuals do not have major psychological problems prior to breast/chest surgery and transgender genital plastic surgery. The WPATH Standards of Care require letters to this effect. Surgery of the breast/chest requires one letter; TGPS requires two letters from mental health professionals. Obtaining such letters is referred to as "**gatekeeping**" by transitioning transgender people who object to the formality and expense. There is also concern that this gatekeeping function may interfere with counseling by discouraging transgender people from revealing information important to counseling success. For adults, WPATH does not require a gatekeeping letter to start hormone therapy but does for minor children.

PERSPECTIVES ON TREATMENT

There are three main schools of thought about transgender treatment:

- Transgender behavior is due to defective cultural conditioning and can be "cured" by classical counterconditioning or operant reward and punishment change efforts.
- Transgender behavior spontaneously decreases due to maturity and experience with cultural rejection, so there is no need for treatment except in persistent cases at puberty ("watchful waiting").

- Transgender behavior requires affirmative treatment and sometimes transgender (transsexual) transition to align anatomy with cultural expectations of gender.

The first school of thought was pursued because it was assumed that the human being was a *tabula rasa* and that transgender behavior is due to incomplete or incorrect learning (Zucker, Wood, & VanderLaan, 1988). This is the extreme "nurture" position in the "nature versus nurture" scientific debate, which we now know to be a false dichotomy for many behavioral phenomena. The notion was that being transgender was pathological based on the assumption that the natural state was being cisgender. Being transgender was attributed to faulty acculturation, which could be reversed. Reeducation was incorporated into gender change efforts (GCE) that have been called reparative or conversion therapy.

Consistent with this school of thought, a wide variety of "reeducation" change efforts were attempted, starting in the early 20th century. By the middle of this century it was obvious to Harry Benjamin that such efforts at change for the transgender people he treated were not effective and could be dangerous. Jan Morris, a renowned travel writer who later transitioned as a transwoman, consulted Harry Benjamin as a transgender patient. Morris summed up Harry Benjamin's findings about the transgender, mainly transsexual, people he treated:

> He had explored every aspect of the condition (transexuality) and he frankly did not know its cause; what he did know was that no true transsexual had yet been persuaded, bullied, drugged, analyzed or electrically shocked into an acceptance of his physique. It was an immutable state. (Morris, 1972, p. 52)

The first school of thought seems to have been curtailed with the closing of the Toronto gender clinic at the Canadian Centre for Addiction and Mental Health (CAMH) in 2016. Those who had been using treatments from the first school largely moved on to adopt the second school of thought. However, gender change efforts are still performed, but in many countries and U.S. states they have been made illegal.

The second school of thought developed out of the clinical misdiagnosis of prehomosexual children with transgender children. The notion was that, as they aged, transkids stopped being transgender due to increased maturity and due to increasing pressure from cultural rejection. However, most of the studies that were used until recently as evidence for this effect involved not transgender children but prehomosexual children. Prehomosexual children are known to crossdress but present quite differently from transgender children (see above). The children in most of the cited studies were prehomosexual and as adults were confirmed as being homosexual.

Only a handful were actually transgender. So, we do not actually have much outcome data for transgender children. Undoubtedly some transgender children continue to practice their transgender behavior in secret, since only about 10 percent actually transition, which requires consultation with providers. Some may discontinue transgender behavior, but we know that many come out in later life. These studies labeled children as "desisters" and "persisters," terms that have pejorative connotations in psychiatry (mental health) and social science (juvenile delinquency). The labels were deliberately repurposed from pathological psychiatric disorders (Zucker, 2018).

According to this second school of thought, the correct treatment for transgender children is "watchful waiting" until puberty (Cohen-Kettenis & Pfäfflin, 2003). No social transition is permitted until puberty. If the child continues their transgender behavior into the start of puberty, then puberty-blocking drugs may be made available until age 16 in order to complete a social transition and provide time for the child to decide whether to start sex hormone therapy. In the past decade, use of blockers for this purpose was developed by the Gender Identity Clinic at the Vrouwen University Medical Center in Amsterdam and has spread to other countries. However, this protocol is becoming increasingly difficult to follow because parents and children do not want to wait until puberty. Many parents relent when they see improvements in the mood and self-worth of transgender children who start social transition and blockers (Durwood, McLaughlin, & Olson, 2017) and are following the next school of thought—an affirmative approach.

The third school of thought, affirmative treatment (Ehrensaft, 2017), is consistent with the current predominant adult treatment but may add puberty blocker treatments for children . During the latter half of the 20th century when gender clinics were largely abandoned in favor of free market treatment, affirmative treatment evolved for transgender adults. Counselors encouraged transgender adults to explore their transgender behavior in safe environments. The main purpose of counseling was to deal with social problems that the transgender adult may have and to determine if they want to explore transgender transition. The affirmative approach includes **gatekeeping** for some transgender transition surgeries by mental health professionals, which involves confirmation that the person does not have a serious mental health disorder or one that will interfere with transition. This gatekeeping role pertains mainly to TGPS and chest/breast surgeries. Such letters may also be used to support obtaining patient insurance coverage, so some surgeons require letters for additional procedures, such as cosmetic surgeries.

This affirming approach may lead to continuation of the behavior as part-time or full-time, to transgender (transsexual) transition, or to discontinuation of the behavior.

In the past decade, the affirming approach for adults has been extended to transchildren. The affirmative treatment school for children advocates treatment as soon as it is recognized and confirmed that a child is consistent, insistent, and persistent in their congruent gender. At this point, social transition is started and puberty-blocking drugs may be administered starting at the early signs of puberty. The blockers continue until age 16 when the child and their team of parents and providers must decide whether the child should transition using sex hormone therapy. This school of thought emerged in the United States as an adaptation of the VU University Medical Center's "watchful waiting" approach. As currently implemented, along with blockers, the child may take low doses of sex hormones in order to regulate bone growth and encourage growth of external genitalia tissue. The concern is that there should be sufficient external genitalia tissue to facilitate transgender genital plastic surgery, although new surgical techniques to "borrow" tissue from other locations are now established.

For the most part, the affirmative approach is supported in the current WPATH Standards of Care. Affirmative treatment involves encouraging the transgender person to safely explore their transgender behavior while providing supportive counseling

Both the "watchful waiting" school and the affirmative school for children employ hormone blocker drugs in off-label fashion. The use of these drugs is therefore controversial and is discussed in Chapter 10.

Classical Counterconditioning and Operant Conditioning Change Efforts

As the quote from Jan Morris about Harry Benjamin (see page 41) indicates, by the 1960s the *tabula rasa* school of thought had already tried a wide range of counterconditioning techniques including aversion therapy, shock therapy, and drug therapy, which were ineffective and sometimes dangerous.

Aversion therapy has been tried on transgender people but the behavior continued. Aversion therapy uses nausea-producing drugs or electric shock to attempt to create a second learned response, nausea, that will conflict with the conditioned response to be suppressed (sexual arousal) and change classical conditioned learning. As Garcia and Kolling (1967) have shown, not all unconditioned stimuli can be successfully paired with unconditioned stimuli to produce learning. And in the case of being transgender, it is not clear which stimuli to use. The effects also deteriorate rapidly once the patient leaves the conditioning environment.

Operant conditioning and **jawboning** are two of the standard techniques used in reparative or conversion "therapies," but these therapies have not been shown to permanently change behavior. A change effort approach for transchildren has involved operant conditioning. In such efforts, poker chip tokens were used to reinforce behaviors associated with assigned gender and discourage behaviors in congruent gender categories. A white token indicated "appropriate" behavior, a blue token "inappropriate" behavior and loss of a white token. The white tokens were redeemable for treats. As with other counterconditioning approaches, the behavior was not sustainable outside of the conditioning space, even when that space was the home and the parents administered the conditioning. "Jawboning" involves the counselor and parents trying to convince the child that they will have a hard time in later life if their transgender behavior continues.

It has been demonstrated that reparative or conversion therapy is ineffective and may cause physical or psychological injury because it uses techniques such as physiological stress, sleep deprivation, and physical bullying for change efforts for homosexuality. Such change efforts have been rejected by professional societies (American Psychological Association, 2009) and are banned in many U.S. states and several countries. Yet they still continue in some practices and religious organizations. Shock therapy to erase memory has been tried without success. Even internal stimulation of the brain through electrodes has been tried to stop transgender behavior (O'Neal, Baker, Glenn, Conner, & Sughrue, 2017), but was ineffective. Lobotomy has also been tried to disrupt memory, but its side effects are now rightfully considered to be unacceptable.

WATCHFUL WAITING APPROACH FOR CHILDREN

The "watchful waiting" school of thought was developed in the VU University Medical Center in Amsterdam. It features intense observation of transkids until puberty without intervention. It was hoped that the child would spontaneously change their behavior due to social rejection and maturation as predicted by "desistence" studies on prehomosexual children conducted at CAMH and in the Netherlands.

At signs of puberty, if the child was still behaving in their congruent gender behavior category, interventions can begin under this approach. These included a social transition, puberty blockers, and potentially later transgender transition. Social transition means living full-time in their congruent gender behavior category with support by parents and the provider team. Affirmative procedures are described in Chapter 7.

The "watchful waiting" approach is fading in its use because parents and children are anxious to get on with transition and children circumvent providers' health care suggestions to go immediately into social transition.

Parents see their children and other children flourishing in social transition and are unwilling to halt it.

Change Effort/"Watchful Waiting" Variant: "Live in Your Own Skin"

A variant of the "watchful waiting" approach combined operant conditioning with jawboning and environmental control before signs of puberty. This was to reinforce the supposed natural tendency for being transgender to fade with maturity and social rejection. Operant conditioning was practiced. Also, in this approach, forceful language was used to try to convince transgender children during counseling that continuing to behave in other than their assigned gender category would negatively influence their future lives. They were told that they would be rejected at school and in their adult lives. Parents were urged to continue operant conditioning and jawboning as well as to control the home environment with the removal of "inappropriate" toys and activities associated with the child's congruent gender category. This included the choice of only "appropriate" playmates and toys. Psychotherapy for child and parent was also encouraged, although previously it had been shown to be ineffective. Clinics using this approach claimed a high level of transgender discontinuation, but it has subsequently been revealed that most of the children in this clinic were prehomosexual, not transgender at all. Many were shown to be nontransgender homosexuals in adulthood.

After all this discouragement, if the child continued to insist on their congruent behavior by the time of puberty, then they were offered puberty blockers and transgender transition as in the "watchful waiting" approach described in the previous section.

AFFIRMATIVE APPROACHES

Affirmative approaches for both adults and children allow exploration of the "fit" of their congruent gender behavior category. They are encouraged to gradually increase the time spent in their congruent gender to determine if there are problems with living in this gender. Problems of work and family are identified and addressed. The provider should provide patient management help in terms of finding safe sources for things like clothing and social activity. In the case of transgender children, when it becomes clear from behavior and verbal expression that the child is likely to be transgender, then the child will be allowed to pursue a social transition. This determination is made by children, parents, and a team of providers. The children must be insistent, consistent, and persistent in their presentation and verbal behavior, although presentation may lag behind somewhat. Social transition typically requires some interventions with family, school, and the community to reduce rejection and deal with problems

If social transitions are successful, then adults may start transgender transition, usually with hormone therapy. In the case of children, they may take blocking drugs to delay puberty until age 16. At this age, the children may start transgender transition, usually with hormone therapy. This approach is described in Chapter 7 in more detail.

Medical Therapies

At least 10 percent of transgender people desire to change their bodies to reshape them into anatomies that are closer to what people would expect for their gender. Procedures for these changes are outlined in the WPATH Standards of Care and they appear to be efficacious and relatively safe. Transition is highly individualized with respect to choice and order of procedures. The general philosophy is to perform desired procedures in order of easiest to hardest reversibility. Studies indicate that counseling should be available both during and after transition, because transition is not a panacea. Problems may continue to occur that involve rejection and social relations. Critics of transgender transition assert that many who undergo transgender genital plastic surgery regret their decision, although the actual rate of regret is less than 1 percent. These procedures are described in more detail in Chapter 7.

Flight to Marriage or the Military

Many transgender people have believed that flight into marriage or the military will "cure" them. With regard to marriage, many transgender people have believed that receiving/giving love/sex would reduce their transgender behavior. Transwomen join the military at a rate twice their peers (Blosnich et al., 2013), and transmen at a rate over three times that of their peers (Gates & Herman, 2014). Hypothesized reasons for military flight include hypermasculinity (Brown, 1988), distraction from the urge for transgender behavior due to the demands of military life, and potential concealment (Kennedy & Mark, 2010).

REFERENCES

American Medical Association. Committee on Human Sexuality. (1972). *Human sexuality.* Chicago: American Medical Association.

American Psychiatric Association. (1980). *Diagnostic and statistical manual of mental disorders* (3rd ed.). Washington, DC: Author.

American Psychological Association. (2009). American Psychological Association task force on appropriate therapeutic responses to sexual orientation. https://www.apa.org/pi/lgbt/resources/therapeutic-response.pdf

Bailey, M., & Zucker, K. (1995). Childhood sex-typed behavior and sexual judgements: A conceptual analysis and quantitative review. *Developmental Psychology, 31*, 43–55.

Bandini, E., et al. (2011). Childhood maltreatment in subjects with male to female gender identity disorder. *International Journal of Impotence Research, 23*, 276–285.

Bevan, T. (2015). *The psychobiology of transsexualism and transgenderism.* Santa Barbara, CA: Praeger.

Blanchard, R. (2005). Early history of the concept of autogynephilia. *Archives of Sexual Behavior, 34*(4), 439–446.

Blosnich, J., Brown, G., Shipherd, J., Kauth, M., Plegari, M., & Bossarte, R. (2013). Prevalence of gender identity disorder and suicide risk among transgender veterans utilizing veterans' health administration care. *American Journal of Public Health, 103*, E27–E32.

Bradley, S., Oliver, G., Chernick, A., & Zucker, K. J. (1998). Experiment of nurture: Ablato penis at 2 months, sex reassignment at 7 months, a psychosexual follow-up in young adulthood. *Pediatrics, 102*, 1–5.

Brown, G. (1988). Transsexuals in the military: Flight into hypermasculinity. *Archives of Sexual Behavior, 17*, 527–537.

Buhrich, N. (1978). Motivation for cross-dressing in heterosexual transvestism. *Acta Psychiatrica Scandinavica, 57*, 145–152.

Buhrich, N., & McConaghy, N. (1978). Parental relationships during childhood in homosexuality, transvestism and transsexualism. *Australian and New Zealand Journal of Psychiatry, 12*, 103–108.

Cohen-Kettenis, P. T., & Arrindel, W. (1990). Perceived parental rearing style, parental divorce and transsexualism: A controlled study. *Psychological Medicine, 20*, 613–620.

Cohen-Kettenis, P. T., & Gooren, L. J. G. (1999). Transsexualism: A review of etiology, diagnosis and treatment. *Journal of Psychosomatic Research, 40*, 315–333.

Cohen-Kettenis, P. T., & Pfäfflin, F. (2003). *Transgenderism and intersexuality in childhood and adolescence.* Thousand Oaks, CA: Sage Publications.

Colopinto, J. (2006). *As nature made him: The boy that was raised as a girl.* New York: Harper Perennial.

Dörner, G. (1976). *Hormones and brain differentiation.* New York: Elsevier.

Durwood L., McLaughlin, K. A., & Olson, K. R. (2017). Mental health and self-worth in socially transitioned transgender youth. *Journal of the American Academy of Child & Adolescent Psychiatry, 56*(2), 116–123.

Ehrensaft, D. (2017). Gender nonconforming youth: Current perspectives. *Adolescent Health, Medicine and Therapeutics, 8*, 57–67.

Erikson, E. H. (1968; 1994). *Identity: Youth and crisis.* New York: W. W. Norton.

Fausto-Sterling, A. (2012). The dynamic development of gender variability. *Journal of Homosexuality, 59*, 393–421.

Freund, K., Langevin, R., Zajac, Y., Steiner, B., & Zajac, A. (1974). Parental-child relations in transsexual and non-transsexual homosexual males. *British Journal of Psychiatry, 124*, 22–23.

Garcia, J., & Kolling, R. A. (1967). A comparison of aversions induced by x-rays, toxins, and drugs in the rat. *Radiation Research Supplement, 7*, 439–450.

Gates, G. J., & Herman, J. L. (2014). *Transgender military service in the United States*. Williams Institute, UCLA School of Law.

Ghering, D., & Knudson, G. (2005). Prevalence of childhood trauma in a clinical population of transsexual people. *International Journal of Transgenderism, 8*, 23–30.

Hirschfeld, M. (1991). *Transvestites: The erotic drive to cross-dress* (M. A. Lombardi, Trans.). Amherst: Prometheus Books. (Original work published 1911.)

Jaynes, J. (1976). *The origin of consciousness in the breakdown of the bicameral mind*. New York: Houghton Mifflin.

Kennedy, N., & Mark, H. (2010). Transgender children: More than a theoretical challenge. *Graduate Journal of Social Science, 7*, 25–42.

Kerlin, S. (2005). *Prenatal exposure to diethylstilbestrol (DES) in males and gender-related disorders: Results from a 5-year study*. Paper prepared for the International Behavioral Development Symposium. Retrieved from http://e.hormone.tulane.edu.

Koken, J., Bimbi, D., & Parsons, J. (2009). Experiences of familial acceptance-rejection among transwomen of color. *Journal of Family Psychology, 23*, 853–860.

Levitt, H. M., & Ippolito, M. R. (2014). Being transgender: The experience of transgender identity development. *Journal of Homosexuality, 61*(12), 1727–1758.

Money, J., Epstein, R., & Ehrhardt, A. A. (1968). Fetal androgens and female gender identity in the early-treated adrenogenital syndrome. *Johns Hopkins Medical Journal, 122*(3), 160–167.

Morris, J. (1972). *Conundrum*. New York: Harcourt Brace.

Oliven, J. (1965, June). Transgenderism = transsexualism. *Sexual Hygiene and Pathology*, 514.

O'Neal, C. M., Baker, C. M., Glenn, C. A., Conner, A. K., & Sughrue, M. E. (2017). Dr. Robert G. Heath: A controversial figure in the history of deep brain stimulation. *Neurosurgical Focus, 43*(3), E12.

Polderman, T. J. C., et al. (2018). The biological contributions to gender identity and gender diversity: Bringing data to the table. *Behavioral Genetics, 48*, 95–108.

Reiner, W., & Gearhart, J. (2004). Discordant sexual identity in some genetic males with cloacal exstrophy assigned to female sex at birth. *New England Journal of Medicine, 350*, 333–343.

Roberts, A., Rosario, M., Corliss, H., Konen, K., & Austin, B. (2012). Childhood gender non-conformity: A risk indicator for childhood abuse and post-traumatic stress in youth. *Pediatrics, 129*, 410–418.

Ryan, C., Russell, S. T., Huebner, D., Diaz, R., & Sanchez, J. (2010). Family acceptance in adolescence and the health of LGBT young adults. *Journal of Child and Adolescent Psychiatric Nursing, 23*(4), 205–213.

Shumer, D. E., Abrha, A., Feldman, H. A., & Carswell, J. (2017). Overrepresentation of adopted adolescents at a hospital-based gender dysphoria clinic. *Transgender Health, 12*(1), 76–79.

Simons, L., Schrager, S. M., Clark, L. F., Belzer, M., & Olson, J. (2013). Parental support and mental health among transgender adolescents. *Journal of Adolescent Health, 53*(6), 791–793.

Stevens, M., Golombok, S., Beveridge, M., & The ALSPAC Study Team. (2002). Does father absence influence children's gender development? Findings from a general population study of preschool children. *Parenting Science and Practice, 2*, 47–60.

Stevenson, M., & Black, K. (1998). Paternal absence and sex-role development: A meta-analysis. *Child Development, 59*, 793–814.

Watson, D. B., & Coren, S. (1992). Left-handedness in male-to-female transsexuals. *Journal of the American Medical Association, 267*, 10, 1342.

Wisniewski, A. B., Prendeville, M. T., & Dobs, A. S. (2005). Handedness, functional cerebral hemispheric lateralization, and cognition in male-to-female transsexuals receiving cross-sex hormone treatment. *Archives of Sexual Behavior, 34*(2), 167–172.

Zucker, K. J., et al. (1994). Prenatal gender preference of mothers of feminine and masculine boys. *Journal of Abnormal Child Psychology, 22*, 1–13.

Zucker, K. J. (2018). The myth of persistence: Response to "A critical commentary on follow-up studies and 'desistance' theories about transgender and gender nonconforming children" by Temple Newhook et al. *International Journal of Transgenderism*, https://doi.org/10.1080/15532739.2018.1468293

Zucker, K. J., & Bradley, S. J. (1998). Adoptee overrepresentation among clinic-referred boys with gender identity disorder. *Canadian Journal of Psychiatry, 43*(10), 1040–1043.

Zucker, K. J., Wood, H., & VanderLaan, D. P. (1988). Models of psychopathology in children and adolescents with gender dysphoria. In B. P. C. Kreukels, T. D. Steensma, & A. L. C. de Vries (Eds.), *Gender dysphoria and disorders of sex development* (pp. 171–192). New York: Springer.

Zuger, B. (1988). Is early effeminate behavior in boys early homosexuality? *Comparative Psychiatry, 29*(5), 509–519.

3

Theories

This chapter provides more detailed discussion of scientific theories pertaining to transgender causation that emerge from the schools of thought described in Chapter 2. These are the theories that conform to the requirements defined in that chapter. A theory, at a minimum, must be well defined, express a causal relation, and be able to be tested empirically according to the scientific method.

Most transgender causation theories have been conceptualized and studied as individual theories, although most researchers believe that multiple factors are involved and typically begin their research articles with that explanation. The four that seem to be supported by the most evidence are formalized and combined into the integrated Four Factors theory (Bevan, 2015, 2017a, 2017b, 2018). These are woven together by adding the concept of gender behavior predisposition and the concept of recognition of congruent gender behavior category. The Four Factors theory is claimed only as a working theory, as all theories are, because research in this area is far from complete. But the theory and its components are testable at the next level of detail.

INTEGRATED FOUR FACTORS CAUSATION THEORY

It is important to note that the dichotomy of nature versus nurture of the 19th century has largely been replaced with our understanding that causation of human physical and behavioral phenomena is multifactorial. For example, we know that genes that might result in particular traits may be mutated or may not be expressed because of epigenetic and environmental factors. It is well established that genes can result in a predisposition for traits that may not be expressed. We also know that a human is not a *tabula rasa* for learning because people are born with genetic predispositions for particular phenomena, including behavior. We also know that our biology does not completely determine our behavior. We commonly sense these predispositions in the personalities of people, which are biologically innate and differ between individuals, but, of course, are somewhat modifiable by learning during maturation. Behavior emerges as the interaction of genetics, epigenetics, and learning. Gender behaviors also involve culture because culture categorizes and assigns value to them. Humans are bound to culture because they developed a gregarious trait that facilitated survival by living in groups.

The Four Factors theory postulates that there is a **genetic gender predisposition** formed by inherited genes instantiated in nervous system mechanisms. The predisposition is not fully instantiated until **epigenetic mechanisms** have a chance during fetal development to modify the genes or to modify how they are expressed. This predisposition is particular to the behaviors that are contained in culturally defined **gender behavior categories**, which vary from culture to culture and over time. **Western culture** gender categories (masculine, feminine) are **binary, cisgender, and rigid** compared with gender categories of some other cultures. Those determined to be male at birth are automatically assigned to the masculine category and those determined to be females to the feminine category. These categories contain the behaviors, rules, and norms for behavior with regard to those behaviors classed as gender behaviors by culture. Almost all children easily learn these gender behavior categories through **early gender learning**. By age two or three, they have learned these categories from modeling of parents and people with which they come in contact, as well as through declarative learning explanations wherein they learn to dress and present themselves. With the advent of modern media, they also receive this training by watching video representations. Most children accept their assigned gender behavior category, but may at ages four or five start reacting differently to these behaviors and categories and sense that their assigned gender behavior category does not fit them. The reactions are subconscious based on the mechanisms resulting from gender behavior predisposition and not a conscious choice. They may say that they are a girl, not a boy, or vice versa. They may only sense that something is wrong and only later emerge as transgender. Some will find that their congruent gender category, the one that "fits," is the one to which they were not assigned. Some will be unable to establish a fit with either a masculine or feminine gender category. They may start behaving in their congruent category immediately or maybe later in life. As they express transgender behavior or verbalize their congruent gender, they find that our rigid Western culture will punish and reject them for violating the gender system. To be transgender is to be a **cultural outlaw**, a violator of cultural norms.

The evidence for this integrated theory currently resides in four factors, each of which will be discussed in turn: genetics, epigenetics, culture, and early learning.

Support for the Four Factors theory of transgender causation includes the following:

- Timing of the emergence of being transgender at ages three to four is compatible with the activity of prenatal early genetic, epigenetic, and early learning factors.
- Biological evidence of genetics and epigenetics factors in DNA markers, biomarkers, and co-occurrences.
- Heritability evidence from twin studies, genetic markers, and biomarkers.
- Heritability estimates from twin studies indicate that if one identical twin is transgender, then the other will be about 50 percent of the time. This is in the range of strong heritability for things like adult height.
- Twin heritability studies support an epigenetics factor in that twin pairs with one transgender twin only contain two transgender individuals about 50 percent of the time, indicating that epigenetics mechanisms sometimes interfere with genetic gender predisposition formation. Unblocking by these mechanisms is required to form a predisposition leading to being transgender.
- Evidence that refutes other theories or offers weak support. The Prenatal Testosterone Theory of being Transgender (PTTT) is refuted by the evidence. Family dynamics have been thoroughly studied and evidence refutes it. Diethylstilbestrol theory evidence is weak because of potential self-selection bias.

- The failure of many ideas and schools of thought to reach the level of scientific theory that is precise and can be tested. These ideas include many psychodynamics notions. In the future, some of these ideas may be testable as we learn more about the brain and instrumentation improves.
- Transgender people do not exist in cultures or subcultures that offer more than two gender behavior categories. Most other cultures base gender behavior category assignment on early behavior as well as sex. They may be deemed transgender cultural outlaws from the perspective of their subculture being in a larger (usually Western) culture that conflicts and has the power to impose economic and social discrimination.

Genetic Causal Factor

Prior to the development of modern genomic analysis, many genetic phenomena were first conceived as being caused by a single gene, but today we know that multiple genes are involved in many or most traits. The DNA mechanism supporting many behaviors including gender behavior predisposition is generally believed to involve multiple genes (polygenetic). After reviewing all the available genetic heritability evidence on being transgender, a polygenetic threshold model for being transgender was proposed in which if enough of the associated genes are set to contribute, a threshold will be crossed and the trait will be expressed (Polderman et al., 2018).

Genetic predisposition determines how people react unconsciously to various behaviors that have been identified in a culture as being gender behaviors. For most people, their genetic predisposition is in alignment with their assigned gender behavior category according to cisgender cultural rules, but for transgender people it is not.

The Four Factors theory predicts that DNA can be expressed to form a genetic predisposition for gender behaviors, instantiated in mechanisms of the nervous system, so-called **aptic structures** (Jaynes, 1976) because a person is more apt to react in a certain way or perform certain behaviors. This can be tested empirically through heritability (twin) studies, by genome analysis that identifies genetic markers on the DNA molecule, indirectly by correlating biomarkers known to be genetic in origin, and by looking for neuroanatomical and neurophysiological mechanisms using brain scanning devices. It is consistent with findings on personality traits that influence behavior, are strongly linked to genetics, and endure throughout a lifetime (Briley & Tucker-Drob, 2014). For transgender people, it has been found that the gender-related personality traits of transgender people are more similar to those of the opposite birth sex than of the same birth sex (Lippa, 2001).

Heritability

Heritability of a trait is typically assessed by twin studies in which the behavior of identical twins who possess identical DNA at conception are compared with one another. These comparisons can also be contrasted with nonidentical twins and with nontwin siblings, and with the very rare identical-twins-reared-apart subjects. Such studies are a staple of the genetic contribution to traits, and many organizations and governments have developed twin registries to identify large samples of twins for study. Factor analysis models have been developed to analyze this data that takes heritability and family environment into account by partitioning the variance. Heritability assesses the amount of variance accounted for by DNA information in a Western cultural environment.

At least 23 transgender twin studies have been conducted with 14 using transitioning transgender (transsexual) people and the remainder with nontransitioned transgender people. They have been summarized (Bevan, 2015; Polderman, 2018). Nine of these studies involved small numbers of twin pairs. They are remarkable incidental reports in which identical twins were encountered who were transgender (in one case, identical triplets who were all transgender).

Seven moderate-size studies were conducted for transitioning transgender twin pairs. Four retrospective studies (27–39 twin monozygotic pairs) found that if one twin was transitioning transgender, then the other was also transitioning transgender in about 37 percent of the cases (range 23–52%). These studies may underestimate heritability because they involved providers consulting their records retrospectively when there was no requirement to capture such information at the time.

Eight twin studies of monozygotic transgender identical twins were conducted with large numbers of twin pairs (96–14,000). Heritability correlations loadings ranged from .26 to .70, indicating a genetic factor. The .70 correlation came from the study with 14,000 twin pairs (van Beijseveldt et al., 2006). A study using the Australian National Health and Medical Research Twin Registry in which 312 MTF twin pairs had at least one transgender (gender nonconforming) member found a loading of .54 with a 95 percent confidence interval of .45–.65 (Bailey, Dunne, & Martin, 2000). In a parallel study involving 668 FTM transgender twins, the loading was .42 with a 95 percent confidence interval of .31–.49.

There were two studies of fraternal twins (dizygotic). Dizygotic twins, in general, do not share the same DNA at conception. These studies with over

300 twin pairs indicated that a fraternal twin pair with one transitioned transgender person were both transitioned twin pairs only .63 percent of the time, which is what one would expect if the effect was genetic and did not involve family environments.

In summary, the empirical data indicates that heritability for being transgender is approximately 31–70 percent, that is, if one identical twin is transgender, then the other will be transgender about 50 percent of the time. This rate is well above the estimated population frequency of 1 percent for unrelated people. The population frequency for nonidentical twins is less than 1 percent. It needs to be said that these estimates may be lower than the actual heritability because transgender people and their parents may have been reticent about reporting being transgender. Factor analysis shows that environment plays little or no role in contributing to being transgender. By way of benchmarking, the highest loading for heritability is body height, which is loaded at 65–70 percent, which indicates that heritability for being transgender is reasonably strong.

The data from these studies was recently reviewed by a group of experts in genetics (Polderman, 2018), and they theorized that a polygenetic threshold model might obtain for being transgender. In such a model, there are multiple genes that contribute to being transgender. As they are switched on, a threshold is reached and the person will be transgender if unblocked by epigenetics. This model is consistent with ideas about a gender spectrum with incremental steps across the spectrum. It also may explain why being transgender seems to run in families because families tend to share some of the same genes.

DNA Genetic Markers

The genetic factor theory predicts that there should be genetic markers for being transgender. There have been seven such studies comparing transgender people with controls, all of which were conducted on samples from transitioning transgender people. Until recently, it was prohibitive in cost and time to perform genome-wide studies. For this reason, all but the most recent study looked at only a few places on the DNA molecule. Some of the results were not replicated, in particular for those from Asian samples. Early studies that looked at specific sites found markers on the androgen receptor site Xq11-12. Hengschlager et al. (2003) found microdeletions on the Y chromosome for 30 transwomen but could not get more specific. Studies by Hennigsson et al. (2005) found markers in the androgen receptor (Xq11-12), **estrogen receptor AR** repeat lengths (14q21-22), and aromatase gene repeat lengths (15q21.1). **Aromatase** is the enzyme that converts testosterone into dihydrotestosterone, which has much greater male effects on the body.

Studies by Hare et al. (2009) replicated the finding of longer AR repeat lengths in the X androreceptor gene (Xq11-12) but failed to replicate markers at 14q21-22 and 15q21.1. Bentz et al. (2008) replicated the finding of a T>C SNP allele frequency marker in MTF at 15q21 for aromatase but found no marker for transmen at the same location. Certain types of repeat length anomalies (CAG) are believed to be due to "slippage" during DNA pauses in replication.

For Asian samples, Ujike et al. (2009) found for either transwomen or transmen no markers at Xq11-12, 11q13, an estrogen receptor site, 15q21.1 and PGR 11q22. The authors attributed this to their common findings of differences in Asian DNA results, compared with DNA from other regions of the world.

Most recently Foreman et al. (2018) looked at 12 sex hormone signaling genes in 380 transwomen and 344 control males. A significant association was identified in the ER-alpha, SRD5A2, and STS allelles as well as ER-*alpha* and SULT2A1 genotypes. For transwomen, several allele patterns were also overrepresented in the androgen receptor (AR-ER *beta*, ARPGR, AR-COMT), cytochrome CYP17-SRD5A2. They suggested that multiple genes are involved in transgender inheritance.

The most recent study conducted a full genome scan (Theisen et al., 2018) and found 20 genetic markers in 14 transmen and 16 transwomen transitioning transgender people, but their identification remains for future analysis and reporting.

In summary, DNA markers for being transgender have been found but future genome-wide surveys and other genetic studies will still be needed to replicate and explore the results. The international expert team responsible for the Polderman et al. (2018) report and other teams continue to propose such surveys. This team has already collected the genetic samples needed, but sponsorship is required to process and analyze these samples.

Biomarkers

There are several biomarkers that transgender people possess that are believed to have a genetic origin. It is not established that these biomarkers are due to shared genetic or epigenetic mechanisms with being transgender.

Biomarkers of interest include:

- Less right-handedness in both transwomen and transmen
- Transmen biomarkers (tooth shape, hip-girdle structure)
- Finger length ratio
- Personality
- Activity level

Transitioning transgender (transsexual) people have been shown to be less right-handed than controls (Green & Young, 2001; Orlebeke, Boomsma, Gooren, Verschoor, & Van Den Bree, 1992; Watson & Coren, 1992; Wisniewski et al., 2009; Zucker, Beaulieu, Bradley, Grimshaw, & Wilcox, 2001). This is true for both transwomen and transmen. It has been suggested that being transgender and handedness may have similar origins (Ellis & Ebertz, 1997). Handedness in 24–26 percent of cases has been shown to have a genetic basis, although the genetic markers are still in dispute. For example, if both parents tend to use their left hand, they are more likely to produce left-handed offspring.

No one is purely left- or right-handed. Handedness is measured on a continuum based on whether people use their right or left hands for common tasks (e.g., writing, cutting food with a knife, swinging a bat, drawing, brushing teeth, etc.). The Edinburgh scale consists of 20 such common tasks and should be more sensitive than simply categorizing someone as left- or right-handed. It is sometimes used in handedness trait assessments. But many studies only use an abbreviated handedness scale or simply ask which hand people use to write. This latter assessment may be misleading because there are still people in the population who were forced in school to write with their right hand instead of naturally with their left. Non-right-handedness is linked to the same DNA marker on the androgen receptor gene (Xq11-12) as being transgender (Medland et al., 2005) in transwomen.

Studies suggest that transmen have biomarkers that are generally believed to be influenced by genetics. There are biomarkers for tooth diameter and pelvic bone structure. Researchers who measured tooth diameter in 12 different tooth shape types in adults found that diameters were intermediate between people determined to be male at birth versus those determined to be female (Antoszewski, Kruk-Jeromin, & Malinowski, 1998; Antoszewski, Zadzinska, & Foczpanski, 2009). Measurements of pelvic bone structure was more similar to persons born male than female (Sitek, Fijałkowska, Zadzinska, & Antoszewski, 2012).

The 2D:4D finger length ratio (index to ring finger) has been found to correlate with being transgender. (Kraemer et al., 2009; Schneider, Pickel, & Stalla, 2006; Wallien, Zucker, Steensma, & Cohen-Kettenis, 2008). In these studies, the ratio was higher in transwomen. Other results did not find a statistically significant difference (Wallien et al., 2008). But still other reports (Hisasue, Sasaki, Tsukamoto, & Horie, 2012) found that the ratio was lower. The 2D:4D has been found to have a high degree of heritability, approaching 66 percent (Gobrogge, Breedlove, & Klump, 2008; Hiraishi, Sasaki, Shikishima, & Ando, 2012; Paul, Kato, Cherkas, Andrew, & Spector, 2006). It is believed that finger length is controlled by 39 genes (HOX) on chromosomes 2, 7, 12, and 17. Differences in ratios between regions of the world support heritability (Loehlin, McFadden, Medland, & Martin, 2006; Maia, Thomis, & Beunen, 2002).

Lippa (2001) found through measurement of personality variables on psychometric tests that transwomen scored more like females and transmen more like males. These personality variables included occupational and hobby preferences, instrumentality, expressiveness, and self-ascribed masculinity and femininity. These "gender diagnosticity" variables are supposed to assess gender interests and were derived from the Big Five personality dimensions across "people versus things" interests, which show strong heritability differences between males and females (Lippa, 1998). On average females are more interested in occupations that feature contact with people (e.g., teachers, nurses) while males are more interested in occupations that involve manipulation of things (e.g., engineers, mechanics).

Building on the findings that males tend to have higher activity levels than females (Campbell & Eaton, 1999; Eaton & Enns, 1986), Zucker and Bradley (1995) found that transwomen tended to have activity levels that were closer to female levels and that transmen had activity levels that were closer to that of males. In fact, transmen on average had higher levels of activity than control males. Activity level has been shown to have a strong heritability level and DNA markers have been identified (Rankinen & Bouchard, 2012).

Epigenetics

Epigenetics involves the study of mechanisms that modify DNA or change DNA expression external to the DNA molecule itself. Expression refers to the transfer of information contained in the cell nucleus and mitochondria, in the form of DNA, to other parts of the cell. Such mechanisms may be active prior to conception or during fetal development, or even later in life. During conception, transcription factors and chromatin-blocking factors (methyl groups, histones) are transferred in the female gamete along with DNA. In utero, teratogens may alter DNA and/or its expression. Because being transgender emerges as soon as four or five years old, we will concentrate on those mechanisms that are active prenatally or in early life.

Epigenetic mechanisms can interfere or promote the genes involved with forming a genetic gender predisposition. We know this from the twin studies described earlier. Although some identical twin pairs are both transgender, most only have one transgender member. It is common for a given trait to be blocked in one member of a twin pair. Indeed, at birth, identical twins usually have many traits that differ.

Genetic **imprinting** is an epigenetic mechanism in which a fetus receives a non-DNA chemical from one of its forebears that might be responsible for silencing or enhancing particular gene expression. Green and Keverne (2000), studying a sample of 417 transitioning transwomen, found that a significant number had more maternal aunts than uncles. They attributed this to a non-DNA inheritance from the mother of a chemical on one of her X-chromosomes that selectively reduced the survival of prenatal males but not females. No such a phenomenon was found in 96 transitioning transmen. These findings have not been replicated or extended. It was initially thought that this might be associated with **sibling sex ratio** or **sibling order** (Green & Keverne, 2000), but these were shown to be predictive of homosexuality in males, rather than transwomen, once experiments were conducted with appropriate control groups.

The DNA molecule is far from static. Every time it is copied in making a new cell, spontaneous mutations occur; enough **spontaneous mutations** that it is possible to determine a "copy number" for each neuron (McConnell et al., 2013). And there are mechanisms that are constantly changing DNA, which are viewed as "repair" mechanisms. Some gene sequences, termed **transposons**, are constantly jumping to locations around the DNA molecule, which affects development (McClintock, 1950) and complicates the search for genetic markers.

Toxic substances can change DNA or its expression. One has been studied with respect to being transgender—**diethylstilbestrol (DES)**. There is some evidence that DES might be associated with the development of transwomen (Kerlin, 2005; Kerlin & Beyer, 2002), but the research was conducted through an online website. The participants were not qualified as to confirmatory evidence that their mothers took DES nor confirmed their mothers' dosages, as in established DES cohorts maintained by the CDC and NIH. These latter cohorts contain several thousand people. DES was given to pregnant mothers during the period 1947 through 1972 and used in food supplies until later in the 1970s as a "synthetic estrogen." However, DES has been shown to be a teratogen that mutates DNA to cause rare genetic diseases into the third generation, including diseases affecting male genitalia. The results of the website survey were potentially affected by selection bias because those who had complaints might be more likely to register. More than 150 of the approximately 500 males who registered at the site claimed to be transgender. Although the U.S. government by law is charged with making regular follow-up studies on those exposed to DES, investigators have never asked whether the people in their CDC and NIH cohorts are transgender (Titus-Ernstoff, 2012). It has performed behavioral studies but questions on being transgender have never been included (Titus-Ernstoff et al., 2003).

Because of widespread genetic testing we are learning that not all cells in the body contain the same DNA, and there is reason to believe that the brain is a "safe haven" for foreign cells that survive attacks by the immune system in the periphery. There is not yet evidence that such cells alter behavior, but it is a hypothesis for future research. A fetus receives "foreign cells" from its mother, who also may share cells from the fetuses from her previous births. Fraternal twins sometimes share cells, depending on the placental circulation. Cells containing Y chromosomes have been found in the brains (hippocampus) of postmortem females after these females received bone marrow transplants from males and 1 percent of these were neurons, the remainder being astrocytes and microglia (Cogle et al., 2004). Very rare but existent are **humans who are their own twins**, inappropriately called "**chimeras**," which is a reference to a Greek monster composed of more than one animal. This phenomenon is due to the merger of two fertilized fetuses within a few days of conception. It is usually undetected when both fertilized eggs are the same sex, but in even rarer cases they can be of opposite sex.

Potential Epigenetic Correlations

There is evidence to show that being transgender, handedness, and autism have genetic bases but their co-occurrences indicate possible epigenetic involvement rather than DNA involvement. Transgender people are less right-handed than controls (Green & Young, 2001; Orlebeke et al., 1992; Watson & Coren, 1992; Wisniewski et al., 2009; Zucker et al., 2001), and research has indicated that being transgender and being on the autism spectrum overlap by 8–20 percent (de Vries, Noens, Cohen-Kettenis, van Berckelaer-Onnes, & Doreleijers, 2010; reviewed in Strang et al., 2018). People on the autism spectrum are less right-handed. Those exposed to DES are less right-handed (Roberts et al., 1994; Schachter, 1994; Scheirs & Vingerhoets, 1995), and there is weak evidence that DES may be involved in facilitating being transgender (Kerlin, 2005; Kerlin & Beyer, 2002). Although these are correlations and do not imply causation, they may form the basis for future research hypotheses into the commonality of epigenetic mechanisms involved with these behavioral phenomena.

Culture

It is important to know that Western culture, although currently dominant in most of the world, is different from many historical and contemporary cultures with regard to gender system characteristics. Table 1.1 shows the range of such gender systems as documented by anthropologists and journalists compared with the current Western gender system. Most of these non-Western cultures have been obliterated by Western culture and those that still exist are currently under pressure. (These categories are described in more detail in Bevan, 2015, 2017b.)

Western culture is binary, cisgender, and inflexible with regard to moving between gender categories. Other cultures have more than two gender categories, do not require automatic assignment to gender behavior category based on natal sex determination, and allow movement between categories. Some of the Native American cultures had people who were termed Two-Spirit, meaning that they could move readily between gender behavior categories.

It should be noted that all of the gender categories in Table 1.1 were not outlawed by their cultures and technically people who remain in them are not transgender. There are no records available that indicate that people would behave out of their category. The anthropologists who studied many of these cultures insisted that those in the nonbinary categories were not deviant, but instead that these categories were "a way for society to recognize and assimilate some atypical individuals without imposing a change on them or stigmatizing them as deviant" (Williams, 1986, p. 74).

By definition, being transgender requires violation of a gender behavior category set up by a cultural gender system. People in these other categories shown in Table 1.1 were not outlaws because they were just following the gender system of their cultures. Transgender people do not behave in their culturally assigned gender behavior category. This violation is, in part, the basis for rejection of transgender people.

Early Gender Learning and Transgender Emergence

In order for children to recognize their congruent gender, they must first learn about the gender system of their culture. Children learn basic gender concepts by 18 months (Fausto-Sterling, 2012). Although male children prefer human and doll images to images of trucks and cars at six months, just as female children do (Escudero, Robbins, & Johnson, 2013), learning about stereotypes proceeds quickly. They learn cultural gender stereotypes in toys and in household tasks by age two to three (Eichstedt, Serbin, Poulin-Dubois, & Sen, 2002; Serbin, Poulin-Dubois, Colburne, Sen, & Eichstedt, 2001), although this learning may be facilitated by personality traits. They continue to learn about gender-stereotyped clothing and presentation as they develop from 5 to 10 years of age.

Transgender children show no learning deficits in gender category learning (Chiu et al., 2006; Maccoby, 1990). Many learn how to behave in *two* gender categories as they are forced to behave in their noncongruent gender. Children learn about gender from their parents, the media, and their preschool teachers (Hilliard & Liben, 2010), through primary types of learning experiences including parental instruction and behavior modeling.

Children are fully knowledgeable to make important decisions about gender by age eight (Martin, 1993), which is when female puberty usually starts. For males, puberty starts around age nine.

Children realize that they are transgender starting at ages three to four (Green, 1976). Retrospective data indicates that half of children realize that they are transgender before age six, with a peak at age five. At those ages, they may not know the word "transgender" but they may verbally express that they are supposed to be a boy but are really a girl or vice versa. At about age eight, they will attempt to follow the rules of their nonassigned gender behavior category through crossdressing and crosspresentation behavior (Kennedy, 2008; Kennedy & Hellen, 2010). Many children will realize something is amiss about their gender but will not realize that they are transgender until their teenage years or adulthood. Most will learn the word transgender by age nine (Kennedy, 2008; Kennedy & Hellen, 2010). Only 31 percent of transgender children will tell their parents, which means that most keep their transgender behavior a secret. Only 2 percent of transgirls will present in public, but 33 percent of transboys will be allowed to present in public because they are believed to be "tomboys" (Kennedy, 2008; Kennedy & Hellen, 2010).

Secrecy starts in childhood and continues into adulthood with adverse consequences (Kelly, 2002). With increasing tolerance for being transgender, more and more children are coming out at earlier ages. Some will delay until their teens and some will delay until adulthood. That is why teenage emergence in the rapid onset gender dysphoria study (Littman, 2018) was not a surprise to most researchers and providers. (See Chapter 10 for a discussion of ROGD).

Transgender emergence does not require a conscious choice, only recognition of the gender behavior category that fits best and is congruent with a person's gender behavior predisposition. The feeling of conscious choice is only one of many illusions created by our nervous system (Jaynes, 1976). The real processing goes on at subconscious levels. The Wurzberg school of psychology discovered this in the 19th century but Freud sexualized it and applied it to mental health.

Starting in the 1980s, researchers began to make physiological measurements and correlate them with the sensation of conscious choice and actual choice. Libet and his colleagues found that they could predict what decision would be made using EEG recordings before the subject had the conscious sensation that they had actually made the decision. This result was replicated by Keller and Heckhausen (1990). These results were extended to functional magnetic resonance imaging (fMRI) (Soon, Brass, Heinze, & Haynes, 2008) and decisions seemed to be made in the frontal and parietal lobes, which is consistent with lesion studies (Bechara & Van Der Linden, 2005; Fellows, 2006, 2011).

Children are aware of their own behavior and they know how they feel when they observe or perform various gender behaviors. It turns out that observing behaviors causes the same brain processes to be involved as performing behaviors, supporting a learning paradigm known as modeling (Walters & Bandura, 1963). Learning that occurs through this modeling paradigm is augmented through declaratory and procedural learning. Humans have a subconscious learning system that attaches emotions to various stimuli and behavior based on their innate reactions. The emotional system is very old, evolutionarily speaking, and some of our emotions are governed by predispositions. Culture identifies and categorizes gender behaviors and children learn this categorization. They thus have a net emotional valence toward one gender category or another or neither gender category based on the emotional responses to the behaviors in those categories. These behavior-by-behavior reactions give rise to the notion that gender behavior predisposition is a continuous spectrum, although it may actually be incremental.

Learning about gender behavior does not required consciousness but it is eventually conveyed to verbal processes, which we might consider consciousness. People can tell whether a particular behavior is compatible with their personality and gender behavior predisposition.

Many transchildren seek refuge in secrecy only to come out in later life. They represent a reservoir of potential visible transgender people, some of whom go through transgender transition. They will practice their transgender behavior in private by wearing their parents' clothing. Transwomen will also apply makeup and perfume in private when their parents go out. All clothing must be meticulously replaced and remnants of such chemicals must be purged before their parents come back. As adults, transgender people will practice in secret, if living alone, or will practice on business and other trips. It is very common for transgender people to keep an "extra" suitcase filled with items needed for presenting in their congruent gender on a trip.

Transgender people who practice their congruent gender in secret are highly stressed. As Jennifer Finney Boylan, English professor, best-selling author, and *New York Times* columnist, wrote:

> I was sitting on top of a mountain of secrets so high it was almost impossible to see the earth anymore. For one thing, now that I lived alone, I was living as a woman half the time. I would come home and go female and pay the bills and write and watch television, and then I would go back to boy mode and teach my classes. I did not venture out into the world much *en femme* [dressed in a feminine manner], although I did get out now and then. It was unbelievably frightening. . . .
>
> At every waking moment now, I was plagued by the thought that I was living a lie. (Boylan, 2013, p. 70)

Keeping a secret is stressful both mentally and physically (Kelly, 2002). Secrecy results in active defense by lying, and lying creates large increases in mental workload, which interfere with relationships and performance. Such a simple thing as talking around the water cooler on Monday and reciting the weekend's activities becomes a Herculean mental feat. A transgender person must be careful about events and pronouns and must have "cover stories." For closeted transwomen, these cover stories may include hypermasculine activities to distract from episodes of transgender behavior.

Avoiding being caught and increased mental workload is reduced by isolation. A transgender person does not want to get too close to a friend, in case the friend discovers the secret of their being transgender by correlating conflicting information. Transgender people, living in secret, compartmentalize their friends and activities. They deliberately avoid making and keeping friends. Avoiding people results in loneliness. Transgender people already experience reactive depression from cultural rejection during the periods that they are out in public. Guilt over lies also contributes to depression. Loneliness, reactive depression, and guilt increase depression and contribute to suicide attempts. Secrecy also prevents transgender people from seeking help from providers with their transgender chief complaints. Most part-time transgender people never seek help for this reason. Until recently, transgender people in the military and those working for the military were prohibited from seeking counseling help on transgender issues with the threat that their security clearances might be suspended.

Part-time transgender people are prone to **purging**, which consists of getting rid of clothing, makeup, or other things involved in practicing transgender behavior. They do this because concealing such things represents yet another stressful burden from which they need relief. But there is a cycle of purging and reacquisition. In several weeks, the transgender person has acquired a new "kit" of objects that they will need to practice their transgender behavior. This purge cycle occurs so frequently that support groups and friends often hold the "kit" for a person for a time, until they are ready to practice their transgender behavior again.

NEUROANATOMY AND NEUROPHYSIOLOGY MECHANISMS

The Four Factors theory predicts that there should be differences in neural mechanisms (aptic structures) for transgender people versus nontransgender people that might be reflected in neuroanatomy and neurophysiology. These differences are set up and form genetic gender predispositions. Anatomical and neurophysiological studies confirm that such differences exist but do not permit understanding them in detail as yet. Because there are so many anatomical loci and physiological mechanisms, one has to be careful that they are correlated by chance with being transgender in particular experiments.

Neuroanatomical differences have been observed in transgender people using postmortem specimens and high-resolution MRI. In general, we can detect microscopic differences in neuroanatomy that result from differences in neural activity. The general idea is that those structures that are actively functioning grow bigger. This is called neuroplasticity. We know neuroplasticity exists from various studies including the "London cab driver" study (Woollett, Spiers, & Maguire, 2009) using MRI, in which it was found that parts of a particular structure (the hippocampus) were larger in cabbies who had to memorize all the routes and addresses in London to get their licenses. From animal studies, these structures are the ones that are believed to be involved in storage and processing of internal geographical "cognitive maps." For some phenomena, we can observe neural changes that are close to inputs or outputs from the nervous system and we can make some educated guesses as to functionality.

Neurophysiology mechanisms have been studied using functional MRI and other scanners, which confirm that the anatomy of neurophysiological mechanisms is different in those people who are transgender compared with controls; although, given our current state of learning about the nervous system, it is sometimes hard to interpret their significance. Again, for the phenomena we can observe that are close to inputs or outputs from the nervous system, we can make some educated guesses.

The first neuroanatomical structures that were found to be different in transgender people were in the anterior hypothalamus using postmortem specimens. Figure 3.1 shows, schematically, the location of these structures.

Two structures in this area, in particular, have shown differences. One is the **bed nucleus of the stria terminalis (BNST)**, which is the home nucleus for a fiber bundle that connects the amygdala with the hypothalamus in a roundabout way. See Figure 3.2.

Zhou, Hofman, Gooren, and Swaab (1995) and Kruijver et al. (2000) found that this structure and the number of its cells was smaller in transitioning transwomen who had been on HT than in either nontransgender males or females. This result was facilitated by tracing techniques for vasoactive intestinal peptide and somatostatin in seven postmortem human specimens. One of the seven postmortem specimens was not on HT and acted as a control. In this specimen, the BNST was also reduced in size. This study is described in more detail in Chapter 11, "Classic Research."

In another anterior hypothalamic structure, the **interstitial nucleus of the anterior hypothalamus number 3 (INAH3)**, Garcia-Falgueras and Swaab (2008) found that it was smaller in transitioning transwomen than

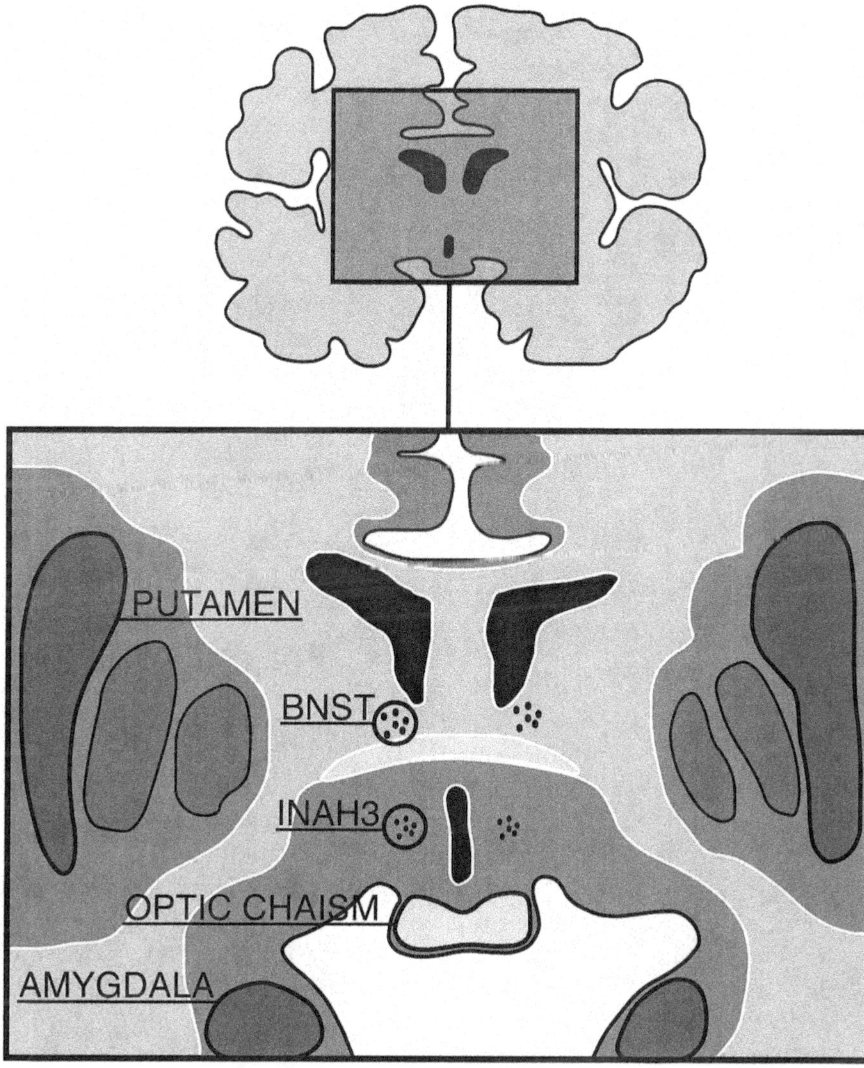

Figure 3.1 Structures at the level of the BNST.

in control postmortem male specimens; the one transman had similar size structures as control males. MRI anatomical research in humans (Pol et al., 2006) confirmed that after six months of HT, structures in this anterior hypothalamic region were reduced in size and the third ventricle was increased in size. The instrument that they used did not have enough resolution to look for changes in individual structures, but this change typically involves shrinkage or damage to nearby hypothalamic structures.

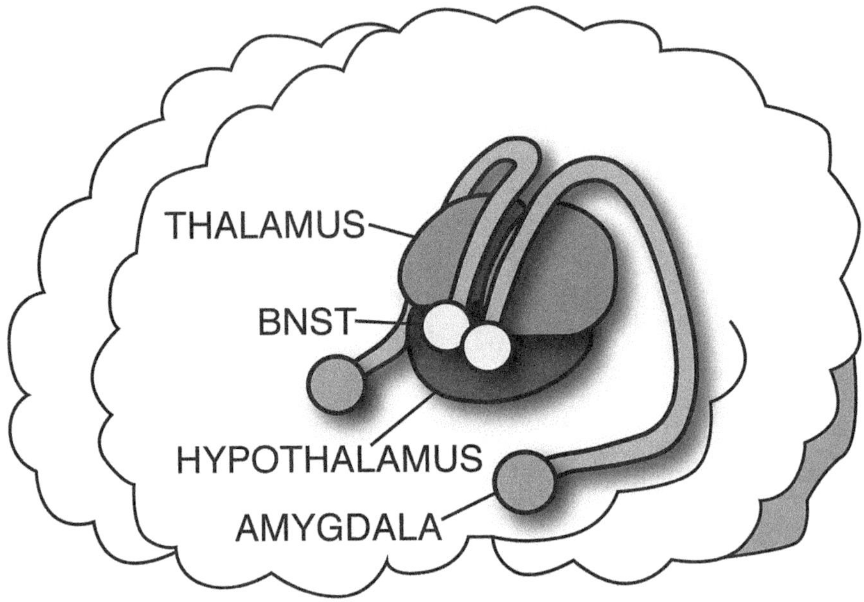

Figure 3.2 Connection from BNST to Amygdala.

The **corpus callosum (CC)** size (Emory, Williams, Cole, Amparo, & Meyer, 1991) and shape (Yokota, Kawamura, & Kameya, 2005) has been found to show differences in transitioning transwomen and transmen, but interpretation of the results was found to be difficult. (See Figure 3.3.) It was hard to describe the differences, just as it is hard to describe the shape of the CC. Interpretations due to handedness are problematic because of conflicting results indicating that the CC was either larger (Witelson, 1985) or showed no difference (Luders et al., 2009; Preuss et al., 2002) with regard to those who are less right-handed.

MRI gray matter surveys indicated that the **right putamen** structures of transwomen were larger compared with controls. This structure is involved with motor control of the left hand, so this result correlates with less right-handedness difference in transgender people (see the "Biomarkers" section of this chapter).

White matter surveys of transgender people have been conducted using MRI diffuse tensor imaging, which is believed to be selective for water molecules moving in fiber bundles. Findings for pre-HT transwomen (Rametti et al., 2011a) indicated that the cortical spinal tract of transwomen was different from that of both male and female controls. Surveys done with transwomen after initiation of HT showed differences in several structures including the cortical spinal tract (Rametti et al.,

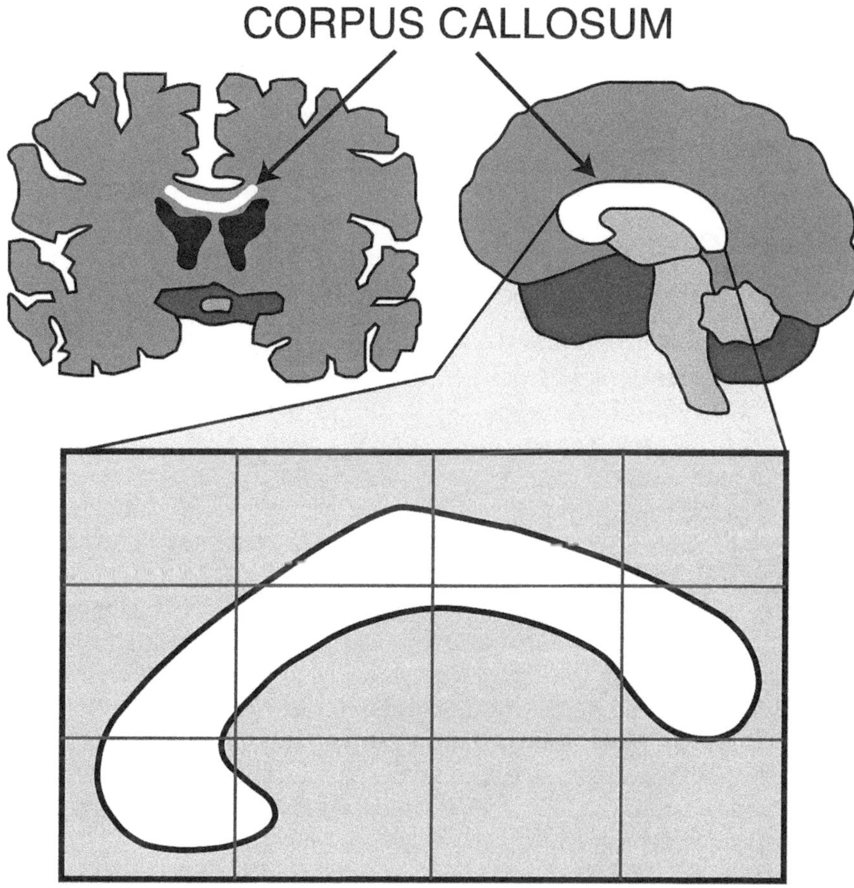

Figure 3.3 Corpus Callosum.

2011b). Nauert (2018) found differences for both transwomen and transmen in the **insula** brain structure, but this was not due to HT. Nauert had included a control group, which had not yet started formal HT.

fMRI studies also indicate anatomical differences in responses. Ku et al. (2013) found functional circuits for both transwomen and transmen with fMRI. They found functional circuits involving the ventral tegmental area, the anterior cingulate, and genital representation. The study used both erotic and nonerotic stimulus materials. Using the putative sex pheromones AND and EST, Berglund, Lindstrom, Dhejne-Helmy, and Savic (2008) found that nonhomosexual transwomen respond to both pheromones, whereas nontransgender males responded to EST and nontransgender females to AND.

Neuroanatomical and neurophysiological research for transgender people support the idea that different neural mechanisms are formed as a result of genetic gender predispositions and that these mechanisms are found all over the brain and not just in one location. There does not appear to be a "gender" center.

OTHER THEORIES

Prenatal Testosterone Theory of Being Transgender (PTTT)

The **prenatal testosterone theory of being transgender (PTTT)** was suggested and researched by Dörner and his colleagues in East Germany starting in the 1960s (Dörner, 1967, 1968, 1976; Dörner et al., 2001; Dörner, Poppe, Stahl, Kolzsch, & Uebelhack, 1991). It states that female fetuses exposed to high levels of testosterone become transitioning transmen and male fetuses exposed to low levels of testosterone become transitioning transwomen. Since direct measurement of fetal testosterone levels was beyond the state of the art, and still is, absolute levels of testosterone have never been specified. This theory was originally developed for homosexuality. Dörner believed that homosexuality was required for being transgender (Dörner, 1976). At the time, this was not at variance with clinical doctrine that required being homosexual in order to transition. That is, a person designated male at birth had to be sexually oriented to males in order to transition and likewise females designated at birth had to be sexually oriented to females. The theory is widely mentioned today even though evidence refutes the theory.

While it is certainly conceivable that hormones influence prenatal brain development, the current evidence does not support testosterone as being directly involved. Actually, there is evidence that brain mechanisms of maleness, so-called sex dichotomous structures, are facilitated by estradiol, which does not readily cross the blood brain barrier. Estradiol influences brain development only where estradiol receptors are found. Estradiol can be manufactured from testosterone but the reaction only takes place where the enzyme aromatase is present. So, during development, the brain is somewhat protected from direct testosterone influence. Furthermore, during gestation, the brain mechanisms of maleness begin to form by genetic influences before gonads start to secret testosterone.

The PTTT was based on animal studies, which provided evidence for the **Organization-Activation theory (Org-Act)** of sexual behavior. The evidence for this theory was based on studies of sexual behavior in rats and guinea pigs (Phoenix, Goy, Gerall, & Young, 1959) in which these animals were given testosterone prenatally or castrated immediately after birth, which is believed to be similar in developmental period to the last fetal stages of human beings. The animals were then tested as adults with or without hormonal administration in situations in which they could have sex with an estrous female. If testosterone had been administrated prenatally or in early life, male sexual behavior was facilitated. The results seemed to confirm that the sexual behavior of the animals was determined during early organization and activated by hormones in adulthood. Dörner and his colleagues continued experimentation on the Org-Act theory (Dörner, 1967, 1976; Dörner et al., 2001; Dörner et al., 1991; Dörner et al., 1968). Without confirming evidence, the authors first tried to extrapolate theoretically from animal sexual research to homosexuality and later to transitioning transgender people (Dörner, 1976).

Dörner advocated for administration of testosterone to mothers during gestation of a male child and administration of testosterone blockers if a mother was carrying a female child (Dörner, 1976) in order to block being transgender and homosexuality. But at that time, sexing of prenatal children was beyond the state of the art through amniocentesis or ultrasound, so as far as can be determined historically, administration of these drugs was not actually performed with humans. However, at that point in history the East Germans were experimenting with hormones to increase athletic performance and it is possible that a female athlete might have been dosed.

Evidence that refutes the PTTT includes the following:

- Human sex and gender behavior are not the same, although there are some overlaps. Some gender behaviors do result in sexual arousal, which facilitates sexual behavior but many change with "fashion" because novelty stimulates sexual arousal (Ford & Beach, 1952). Gender behaviors are identified by human culture, not by biology.
- Animal *sexual* behavior is *not* the same as human *gender* behavior. Testosterone does influence the brain directly or indirectly in humans, but it seems to influence functions related to sexual behavior and aggression (McCarthy, 2008). As far as we know, animals have not developed behaviors that we would actually consider gender behavior. Human gender behavior requires cognitive capability that infrahuman species lack (Meyer-Bahlburg et al., 2004). The PTTT cannot be proven through animal behavior experimentation.
- During early prenatal periods, genes are expressed to form specific brain reflex structures before the gonads are mature enough to secrete sex hormones (Davies & Wilkinson, 2006; Dewing, Shia, Horvath, & Vilain, 2004). The original Org-Act theory was modified to include genetics (Arnold, van Haus, & Lusis, 2009).
- **Kallmann's syndrome** is a phenomenon that is caused by a gene that controls expression of gonadotropin-releasing factor, resulting in low testosterone from conception until treatment begins. Only two people

with Kallmann's syndrome who are transgender have been reported in the past 70 years (Meyenburg & Sigusch, 2001). Transwomen do not have chronically low testosterone levels before transition.

- **Congenital adrenal hyperplasia (CAH)** is a phenomenon in which there is a failure to produce cortisol in the adrenal glands, which causes the pituitary to emit ACTH, which, in turn, influences the adrenal glands to greatly increase the release of testosterone. This results in increased testosterone levels from early fetal development until treatment, which usually begins in adolescence. *Females with CAH are not transgender* (Meyer-Bahlburg, 2004). Out of 281 cases reported in the literature, there are only four reports of CAH females, when asked, being interested in transgender behavior (1.7%), but no reports that they actually pursued it (Dessens, Slijper, & Drop, 2005). There is one report of interest in transition but there was no follow-up information (Zucker et al., 1996). Surveys of CAH females indicate that these people behave in the feminine behavior category (Berenbaum & Bailey, 2003; Dessens et al., 2005; Meyer-Bahlburg, et al., 2004).
- Although **2D:4D finger length ratio** is cited as an indicator of prenatal testosterone levels, and transgender people do have finger length ratios that are different from controls, it appears that such ratios are genetically determined by the HOX gene complex.
- Direct measurement of fetal testosterone blood levels is still beyond the state of the art.
- **Androgen insensitivity syndrome (AIS)** research is often cited in support of the PTTT because both low testosterone levels and behavior in the feminine gender category occur. AIS comes from a difference in the androgen receptor gene, which results in ineffectiveness of testosterone and dihydrotestosterone to masculinize the body. This is one of the same genes that shows DNA markers for being transgender, resulting in transwomen. Differences in the androgen receptor gene are common to both AIS and being transgender, but there is no evidence that low testosterone effectiveness is a factor in being transgender.

Parental Relations and Child Rearing

There have been schools of thought that say that parental relations and child rearing are causative factors for being transgender, but in every case where this theory was reduced to practice, the evidence does not support it (Bailey & Zucker, 1995; Cohen-Kettenis & Gooren, 1999).

Stoller hypothesized that a causative factor in being transgender pertained to the emotional relationships between children and parents (Stoller,

1968; Uddenberg, Wålinder, & Höjerback, 1979). Buhrich and McConaghy (1978) found that there was no pathological relationship between transitioning transwomen or transmen that could account for being transgender. They did find that fathers were less interested in their transgender children, presumably because of their rejection of transgender, but this was also true for fathers of homosexuals. Transmen and transwomen rate their mothers the same as control subjects on emotional relations but their fathers were more protective and less caring.

No emotional disruption of families has been found that could contribute to being transgender, although there is some evidence that adopted transgender children present at hospital-based gender dysphoria clinics at a rate higher than population rates for adoption (Shumer, Abrha, Feldman, & Carswell, 2017).

Another hypothesis put forward for being transgender was that mothers originally wanted a child of a different sex and would treat those children differently (Buhrich & McConaghy, 1978). However, researchers have found that mothers' prebirth choices were not predictive of offspring being transgender (Zucker et al., 1994).

It was suggested by Buhrich and McConaghy (1978) that parental separation might be a contributory cause of being transgender. Subsequent investigations have found no such relationship (Cohen-Kettenis & Arrindell, 1990; Stevens, Golombok, Beveridge, & The ALSPAC Study Team, 2009).

It is well established that the parents of transgender children often physically and psychologically reject these children because of their behavior, but there is no evidence that trauma from parents is a causative factor in being transgender (Bandini et al., 2011; Gehring & Knudson, 2005; Roberts, Rosario, Corliss, Koenen & Austin, 2012). As a result of this physical and psychological abuse, many transgender children are forced into homelessness and may engage in illegal street economies. Some transgender children suffer from post-traumatic stress disorder because of this abuse (Roberts et al., 2012).

REFERENCES

Antoszewski, B., Kruk-Jeromin, J., & Malinowski, A. (1998). Body structure of female-to-male transsexuals. *Acta Chirurgiae Plasticae*, *40*(2), 54–58.

Antoszewski, B., Zadzinska, E., & Foczpanski, J. (2009). The metric features of teeth in female-to-male transsexuals. *Archives of Sexual Behavior*, *38*, 351–358.

Arnold, A. P., van Nas, A., & Lusis, A. J. (2009). Systems biology asks new questions about sex differences. *Trends in Endocrinology and Metabolism*, *20*(10), 471–476.

Bailey, J., Dunne, M., & Martin, N. (2000). Genetic and environmental influences on sexual orientation and its correlates in an Australian twin sample. *Journal of Personality and Social Psychology, 78*, 524–536.

Bailey, J. M., & Zucker, K. J. (1995). Childhood sex-typed behavior and sexual orientation: A conceptual analysis and quantitative review. *Developmental Psychology, 31*(1), 43–55.

Bandini, E., Fisher, A. D., Ricca, V., Ristori, J., Meriggiola, M. C., Jannini, E. A., . . . Maggi, M. (2011). Childhood maltreatment in subjects with male-to-female gender identity disorder. *International Journal of Impotence, 23*(6), 276–285.

Bechara, A., & Van Der Linden, M. (2005). Decision-making and impulse control after frontal lobe injuries. *Current Opinion in Neurology, 18*(16), 734–739.

Bentz, E. K., Hefler, L. A., Kaufmann, U., Huber, J. C., Kolbus, A., & Tempfer, C. B. (2008). A polymorphism of the CYP17 gene related to sex steroid metabolism is associated with female-to-male but not male-to-female transsexualism. *Fertility and Sterility, 90*(1), 56–59.

Berenbaum, S. A., & Bailey, J. M. (2003). Effects on gender identity of prenatal androgens and genital appearance: Evidence from girls with congenital adrenal hyperplasia. *Journal of Clinical Endocrinology and Metabolism, 88*(3), 1102–1106.

Berglund, H., Lindstrom, P., Dhejne-Helmy, C., & Savic, I. (2008). Male-to-female transsexuals show sex-atypical hypothalamus activation when smelling odorous steroids. *Cerebral Cortex, 18*(8), 1900–1908.

Bevan, T. (2015). *The psychobiology of transsexualism and transgenderism.* Santa Barbara, CA: Praeger.

Bevan, T. (2017a). Biological theories of gender development. In *Sage encyclopedia of psychology and gender* (pp. 182–186).

Bevan, T. (2017b). *Being transgender: What you should know.* Santa Barbara, CA: Praeger.

Bevan, T. (2018, March 4). The science factors that create transgender people. The Transgender Scientist Podcast, http://www.blogtalkradio.com/thetrans genderscientist

Boylan, J. F. (2013). *She's not there: A life in two genders.* New York: Broadway.

Briley, D. A., & Tucker-Drob, E. (2014). Genetic and environmental continuity in personality development: A meta-analysis. *Psychological Bulletin, 140*(5), 1303–1331.

Buhrich, N. (1978). Motivation for cross-dressing in heterosexual transvestism. *Acta Psychiatrica Scandinavia, 57*, 53–69.

Buhrich, N., & McConaghy, N. (1978). Parental relationships during childhood in homosexuality, transvestism and transsexualism. *Australia and New Zealand Journal of Psychiatry, 57*, 53–69.

Campbell, D. W., & Eaton, W. O. (1999). Sex differences in the activity level of infants. *Infant and Child Development, 8*, 1–17.

Chiu, S. W., Geran, S., Fairbrother, C., Johnson, L., Owen-Anderson, A., & Bradley, S. (2006). Sex-dimorphic color preference in children with gender identity disorder. *Sex Roles, 55*, 385–395.

Cogle, C. R., Yachnis, A. T., Laywell, E. D., Zander, D. S., Wingard, J. R., Steindler, D. A., & Scott, E. W. (2004, May 1). Bone marrow transdifferentiation in brain after transplantation: A retrospective study. *Lancet, 363*(9419), 1432–1437.

Cohen-Kettenis, P. T., & Arrindell, W. A. (1990). Perceived parental rearing style, parental divorce and transsexualism: A controlled study. *Psychological Medicine, 20*(3), 613–620.

Cohen-Kettenis, P. T., & Gooren, L. J. (1999). Transsexualism: A review of etiology, diagnosis and treatment. *Journal of Psychosomatic Research, 46*(4), 315–333.

Davies, W., & Wilkinson, L. S. (2006). It is not all hormones: Alternative explanations for sexual differentiation of the brain. *Brain Research, 18*, 1126, 36–45.

Dessens, A. B, Slijper, F. M, & Drop, S. L. (2005). Gender dysphoria and gender change in chromosomal females with congenital adrenal hyperplasia. *Archives of Sexual Behavior, 34*(4), 389–397.

de Vries, A. L. C., Noens, I. L. J., Cohen-Kettenis, P. T., van Berckelaer-Onnes, I. A., & Doreleijers, T. A. (2010). Autism spectrum disorders in gender dysphoric children and adolescents. *Journal of Autism and Developmental Disorders, 40*(8), 930–936.

Dewing, P., Shia, T., Horvath, S., & Vilain, E. (2004). Sexually dimorphic gene expression in mouse brain precedes gonadal differentiation. *Molecular Brain Research, 118*, 82–90.

Dörner, G. (1967). Animal experimental studies on the problem of hormone pathogenesis of homosexuality. *Acta Biologica et Medica Germanica, 19*, 569–584.

Dörner, G. (1976). *Hormones and brain differentiation.* New York: Elsevier.

Dörner, G., Döcke, F., & Moustafa, S. (1968). Homosexuality in female rats following testosterone implantation in the anterior hypothalamus. *Journal of Reproduction and Fertility, 17*(1), 173–175.

Dörner, G., Gotz, F., Rhode, W., Plagemann, P., Lindner, R., & Hartmut, P. (2001). Genetic and epigenetic effects on sexual brain organization mediated by sex hormones. *Neuroendocrinology Letters, 22*, 403–409.

Dörner, G., Poppe, F., Stahl, F., Kolzsch, J., & Uebelhack, R. (1991). Gene and environmental-dependent neuroendocrine etiogenesis of homosexuality and transsexualism. *Experimental and Clinical Endocrinology, 98*, 141–150.

Eaton, W. O., & Enns, L. R. (1986). Sex differences in human motor activity level. *Psychological Bulletin, 100*(1), 19–28.

Eichstedt, J., Serbin, L., Poulin-Dubois, D., & Sen, M. (2002). Of bears and men: Infant's knowledge of conventional and metaphorical gender stereotypes. *Infant Behavior and Development, 25*, 296–310.

Ellis, L., & Ebertz, L. (1997). *Sexual orientation: Toward biological understanding.* Westport, CT: Praeger.

Emory, L. E., Williams, D. H., Cole, C. M., Amparo, E. G., & Meyer, W. J. (1991). Anatomic variation of the corpus callosum in persons with gender dysphoria. *Archives of Sexual Behavior, 20*(4), 409–417.

Escudero, P., Robbins, R. A., & Johnson, S. P. (2013). Sex-related preferences for real and doll faces versus real and toy objects in young infants and adults. *Journal of Experimental Child Psychology, 116*(2), 367–379.

Fausto-Sterling, A. (2012). The dynamic development of gender variability. *Journal of Homosexuality, 59*, 393–421.

Fellows, L. K. (2006). Deciding how to decide: Ventromedial frontal lobe damage affects information acquisition in multi-attribute decision making. *Brain, 129*(4), 944–952.

Fellows, L. K. (2011). Orbitofrontal contributions to value-base decision-making: Evidence from humans with frontal lobe damage. *Annals of the New York Academy of Science, 1239*, 51–58.

Ford, C. S., & Beach, F. A. (1952). *Patterns of sexual behavior.* Harper and Brothers.

Foreman, M., Hare, L., York, K., Balakrishnan, K., Sanchez, F. J., Harte, F., . . . Harley, V. R. (2018). A genetic link between gender dysphoria and sex hormone signaling. *Journal of Clinical Endocrinology and Metabolism, 104*(2), 390–396.

Garcia-Falgueras, A., & Swaab, D. F. (2008). A sex difference in the hypothalamic uncinate nucleus: Relationship to gender identity. *Brain, 131*, 3132–3146.

Gehring, D., & Knudson, G. (2005). Prevalence of childhood trauma in a clinical population of transsexual people. *International Journal of Transgenderism, 8*, 23–30.

Gobrogge, K. L., Breedlove, S. M., & Klump, K. L. (2008). Genetic and environmental influences on 2D:4D finger length ratios: A study of monozygotic and dizygotic male and female twins. *Archives of Sexual Behavior, 37*(1), 112–118.

Green, R. (1976). One-hundred ten feminine and masculine boys: Behavioral contrasts and demographic similarities. *Archives of Sexual Behavior, 5*(5), 425–426.

Green, R., & Keverne, E. B. (2000). The disparate maternal aunt-uncle ratio in male transsexuals: An explanation invoking genomic imprinting. *Journal of Theoretical Biology, 202*, 55–63.

Green, R., & Young, R. (2001). Hand preference, sexual preference, and transsexualism. *Archives of Sexual Behavior, 30*(6), 565–574.

Hare, L., Bernard, P., Sanchez, F. J., Baird, P. N., Vilain, E., Kennedy, T., & Harley, V. R. (2009). Androgen repeat length polymorphism associated with male-to-female transsexualism. *Biological Psychiatry, 65*, 93–96.

Hengschlager, M., von Trostburg, M., Repa, C., Marton, E., Huber, J. C., & Bernaschek, G. (2003). Sex chromosome aberrations and transsexualism. *Psychoneuroendocrinology, 30*, 657–664.

Henningsson, S., Westberg, L., Nilsson, S., Lundstrom, B., Ekeliusd, L., & Bodlunde, O. (2005). Sex steroid-related genes and male-to-female transsexualism. *Psychoneuroendocrinology, 30*, 657–664.

Hilliard, L. J., & Liben, L. S. (2010). Differing levels of gender salience in preschool classrooms: Effects on children's gender attitudes and intergroup bias. *Child Development, 81*(6), 1787. https://doi.org/10.1111/j.1467-8624.2010.01510.x

Hiraishi, K., Sasaki, S., Shikishima, C., & Ando, J. (2012, June). The second to fourth digit ratio (2D:4D) in a Japanese twin sample: Heritability, prenatal hormone transfer, and association with sexual orientation. *Archives of Sexual Behavior, 41*, 711–724.

Hisasue, S., Sasaki S., Tsukamoto, T., & Horie, S. (2012). The relationship between second-to-fourth digit ratio and female gender identity. *Journal of Sexual Medicine, 9*(11), 2903–2910.

Jaynes, J. (1976). *The origin of consciousness in the breakdown of the bicameral mind.* Boston: Houghton Mifflin.

Keller, I., & Heckhausen, H. (1990). Readiness potentials preceding spontaneous motor acts: Voluntary vs. involuntary control. *Electroencephalogram and Clinical Neurophysiology, 76*(4), 351–361.

Kelly, A. E. (2002). *The psychology of secrets.* New York: Springer Science and Business Media.

Kennedy, N. 2008. Transgender children in schools: A critical review of homophobic bullying: Safe to learn—embedding anti-bullying work in schools. *Forum, 50*, 383–396.

Kennedy, N., & Hellen, M. (2010). Transgender children: More than a theoretical challenge. *Graduate Journal of Social Science, 7*, 25–42.

Kerlin, S. (2005). Prenatal exposure to diethylstilbestrol (DES) in males and gender-related disorders: Results from a 5-year study. Paper prepared for the International Behavioral Development Symposium. http://e.hormone.tulane.edu (Confirmed January 22, 2019)

Kerlin, S., & Beyer, D. (2002). The DES Sons online discussion network. *Transgender Tapestry, 100*, 18.

Kraemer, B., Noll, T., Delsignore, A., Milos, G., Schnyder, U., & Hepp, U. (2009). Finger length ratio (2D:4D) in adults with gender identity disorder. *Archives of Sexual Behavior, 38*(3), 359–363.

Kruijver, F. P., Zhou, J. N., Pool, C. W., Hofman, M. A., Gooren, L. J., & Swaab, D. F. (2000). Male-to-female transsexuals have female neuron numbers in a limbic nucleus. *Journal of Clinical Endocrinology and Metabolism, 85*(5), 2034–2041.

Ku, H. L., Lin, C. S., Chao, H. T., Tu, P. C., Li, C. T., & Cheng, C. M. (2013). Brain signature characterizing the body-brain-mind axis of transsexuals. *Plos One.* 8e70808.

Lippa, R. A. (1998). Gender-related individual differences and the structure of vocational interests: The importance of the "People-Things" dimension. *Journal of Personality and Social Psychology, 74*, 996–1009.

Lippa, R. A. (2001). Gender-related traits in transsexuals and nontranssexuals. *Archives of Sexual Behavior, 30*(6), 603–614.

Littman, L. (2018). Rapid-onset gender dysphoria in adolescents and young adults: A study of parental reports. *PLoS ONE, 13*(8), e0202330. https://doi.org/10.1371/journal.pone.0202330

Loehlin, J. C., McFadden, D., Medland, S. E., & Martin, N. G. (2006, December). Population differences in finger-length ratios: Ethnicity or latitude? *Archives of Sexual Behavior, 35*(6), 739–742.

Luders, E., Sanchez, F. J., Gaser, C., Toga, A. W., Narr, K. L., Hamilton, L. S., & Vilain, E. (2009). Regional gray matter variation in male-to-female transsexualism. *Neuroimage, 46*(4), 904–907.

Maccoby, E. E. (1990). The role of gender identity and gender constancy in sex-differentiated development. *New Directions in Child Development, 47,* 5–20.

Maia, J. A. R., Thomis, M., & Beunen, G. (2002). Genetic factors in physical activity levels: A twin study. *American Journal of Preventative Medicine, 23*(2), Supplement.

Martin, C. (1993). New directions for investigating children's gender knowledge. *Developmental Review, 13,* 184–204.

McCarthy, M. (2008). Estradiol and the developing brain. *Physiological Review, 88,* 91–134.

McClintock, B. J. (1950). The origin and behavior of mutable loci in maize. *Proceedings of the National Academy of Science, 36*(6), 344–355.

McConnell, M. J., Lindberg, M. R., Brennand, K. J., Piper, J. C., Cowing-Zitron, C., Shumillina, S., . . . Gage, F. H. (2013). Mosaic copy number in human neurons. *Science, 342,* 6158, 6320637.

Medland, S. E., Duffy, D. L., Spurdle, A. B., Wright, M. J., Geffen, G. M., Montgomery, G. W., & Martin, N. G. (2005). Opposite effects of androgen receptor CAG repeat length on increased risk of left-handedness in males and females. *Behavioral Genetics, 35*(6), 735–744.

Meyenburg, B., & Sigusch, V. (2001). Kallmann's syndrome and transsexualism. *Archives of Sexual Behavior, 30*(1), 75–81.

Meyer-Bahlburg, H. F., Dolezal, C., Baker, S. W., Carlson, A. D., Obeid, J. S., & New, M. I. (2004). Cognitive and motor development of children with and without congenital adrenal hyperplasia after early-prenatal dexamethasone. *Journal of Clinical Endocrinology and Metabolism, 89*(2), 610–614.

Nauert, R. (2018, June 12). Structural brain differences for transgender people. *Psychology Central,* E133802. https://psychcentral.com/news/2018/03/16/structural-brain-differences-fortransgender-people/133802.html (Confirmed January 22, 2019).

Orlebeke, J., Boomsma, D. I., Gooren, L. K. G., Verschoor, A. M., & Van Den Bree, M. J. M. (1992). Elevated sinistrality in transsexuals. *Neuropsychology, 6,* 351–355.

Paul, S. N., Kato, B. S., Cherkas, L. F., Andrew, T., & Spector, T. D. (2006). Heritability of the second to fourth digit ratio (2d:4d): A twin study. *Twin Research and Human Genetics, 9*(2), 215–219.

Phoenix, C., Goy, R., Gerall, A., & Young, W. (1959). Organizing action of prenatally administered testosterone proportionate on the tissues mediating mating behavior in the female guinea pig. *Endocrinology, 65,* 369–382.

Pol, H. E. H., Cohen-Kettenis, P. T., Van Haren, N. E. M., Peper, J. S., Brans, R. G. H., Cahn, W., . . . Kahen, R. S. (2006). Changing your sex changes your brain: Influences of testosterone and estrogen on adult human brain structure. *European Journal of Endocrinology, 155,* S107–S114.

Polderman, T. J. C., et al. (2018). The biological contributions to gender identity and gender diversity: Bringing data to the table. *Behavioral Genetics, 48,* 95–108.

Preuss, U. W., Meisenzahl, E. M., Frodl, T., Zetzsche, T., Holder, J., Leinsinger, G., . . . Moller, H. J. (2002). Handedness and corpus callosum morphology. *Psychiatry Research, 30*(116), 1–2, 33–42.

Rametti, G., Carrillo, B., Gomez-Gil, E., Junque, C., Segovia, S., Gomez, A., & Guillamon, A. (2011a). White matter microstructure in female to male transsexuals before cross-sex hormonal treatment. A diffusion tensor imaging study. *Journal of Psychiatric Research, 45*(2), 199–204.

Rametti, G., Carrillo, B., Gomez-Gil, E., Junque, C., Zubiarre-Elorza, L., Segovia, S., . . . Guillamon, A. (2011b). The microstructure of white matter in male to female transsexuals before cross-sex hormonal treatment. A DTI study. *Journal of Psychiatric Research, 45*(7), 949–954.

Rankinen, T., & Bouchard, C. (2012). Chapter 24: Genetic differences in the relationships among physical activity, fitness and health. In C. Bouchard, S. N. Blair, & W. Haskell (Eds.), *Physical activity and health.* New York: Human Kinetics.

Roberts, A. L., Rosario, M., Corliss, H. L., Koenen, K. C., & Austin, S. B. (2012). Childhood gender nonconformity: A risk indicator for childhood abuse and posttraumatic stress in youth. *Pediatrics, 129*(3), 410–417.

Schachter, S. C. (1994). Handedness in women with intrauterine exposure to diethylstilbestrol. *Neuropsychologia, 32*(5), 619–623.

Scheirs, J. G., & Vingerhoets, A. J. (1995). Handedness and other laterality indices in women prenatally exposed to DES. *Journal of Clinical and Experimental Neuropsychology, 17*(5), 725–730.

Schneider, H. J., Pickel, J., & Stalla, G. K. (2006). Typical female 2nd-4th finger length (2D:4D) ratios in male-to-female transsexuals: Possible implications for prenatal androgen exposure. *Psychoneuroendocrinology, 32*(2), 265–259.

Serbin, L., Poulin-Dubois, D., Colburne, K., Sen, M., & Eichstedt, J. (2001). Gender stereotyping in infancy: Visual preference for and knowledge of gender-stereotyped toys in the second year. *International Journal of Behavioral Development, 25*, 7–15.

Shumer, D. E., Abrha, A., Feldman, H. A., & Carswell, J. (2017, May 1). Overrepresentation of adopted adolescents at a hospital-based gender dysphoria clinic. *Transgender Health, 2*(1), 76–79.

Sitek, A., Fijałkowska, M., Zadzinska, E., & Antoszewski, B. (2012). Biometric characteristics of the pelvis in female-to-male transsexuals. *Archives of Sexual Behavior, 41*(5), 1303–1313.

Soon, C. S., Brass, M., Heinze, H. J., & Haynes, J. D. (2008). Unconscious determinants of free decisions in the human brain. *Nature Neuroscience, 11*(5), 543–545.

Stevens, M., Golombok, S., Beveridge, M., & The ALSPAC Study Team. (2009). Does father absence influence children's gender development? Findings from a general population study of preschool children. *Parenting: Science and Practice, 2*, 47–60.

Stoller, R. (1968). *Differential diagnoses: Transvestism and transsexualism.* In J. Sutherland (Ed.), *Sex and Gender* (pp. 220–226). London: Hogarth.

Strang, J. F., et al. (2018). Initial clinical guidelines for co-occurring autism spectrum disorder and gender dysphoria or incongruence in adolescents. *Journal of Clinical Child and Adolescent Psychology, 47*(1), 105–115.

Theisen, J. G., Filchak, M. S., Sundaram, V., Chorich, L. P., Sullivan, M. E., Friez, M. J., . . . Lay, L. C. (2018, March 18). *Transgender identity, gender dysphoria, whole exome sequencing*. Society for Reproductive Investigation Conference.

Titus-Ernstoff, L. (2012). Personal communication. Titus-Ernstoff conducted the last follow-up study on sexual behavior in 2003 for those exposed to DES (see next reference).

Titus-Ernstoff, L., et al. (2003). Psychosexual characteristics of men and women exposed prenatally to diethylstilbestrol. *Epidemiology, 14*(2), 155–160.

Uddenberg, N., Wålinder, J., & Höjerback, T. (1979). Parental contact in male and female transsexuals. *Acta Psychiatrica Scandinavia, 60*(1), 113–120.

Ujike, H., Otani, K., Nakatsuka, M., Ishii, K., Sasaki, A., Oishi, T., . . . Kuroda, S. (2009). Association study of gender identity disorder and sex-hormone related genes. Progress in *Neuropsychopharmacology and Biological Psychiatry, 48*, 1116–1117.

van Beijsterveldt, C.E., Hudziak, J.J., & Boomsma, D.I. (2006). Genetic and environmental influences on cross-gender behavior and relation to behavior problems: a study of Dutch twins at ages 7 and 10 years. *Archives of Sexual Behavior*, 35, 6, 647–658.

Wallien, M. S., Zucker, K. J., Steensma, T. D., & Cohen-Kettenis, P. T. (2008). 2D:4D finger-length ratios in children and adults with gender identity disorder. *Hormones and Behavior, 54*(3), 450–454.

Walters, A., & Bandura, R. H. (1963). *Social learning and personality development*. New York: Holt, Rinehart and Winston.

Watson, D. B., & Coren, S. (1992). Left-handedness in male-to-female transsexuals. *Journal of the American Medical Association, 267*(10), 1342.

Williams, W. (1986). *The spirit and the flesh: Sexual diversity in American Indian culture*. Boston, MA: Beacon.

Wisniewski, A. B., Prendeville, M. T., & Dobs, A. S. (2009). Handedness, functional cerebral hemispheric lateralization, and cognition in male-to-female transsexuals receiving cross-sex hormone treatment. *Archives of Sexual Behavior, 34*(2), 167–172.

Witelson, S. F. (1985). The brain connection: The corpus callosum is larger in left-handers. *Science, 229*(4714), 665–668.

Woollett, K., Spiers, H. K., & Maguire, E. A. (2009, May). Talent in the taxi: A model for exploring expertise. *Royal Society Transactions B, 364*, 1522.

Yokota, Y., Kawamura, Y., & Kameya, Y. (2005). Callosal shapes at the midsagittal plane: MRI differences of normal males, normal females, and GID. *Conference Proceedings IEEE Medical and Biological Science, 3*, 3055–3058.

Zhou, J. N., Hofman, M. A., Gooren, L. J., & Swaab, D. F. (1995). A sex difference in the human brain and its relation to transsexuality. *Nature, 378*(6552), 68–70.

Zucker, K. J., Beaulieu, N., Bradley, S. J., Grimshaw, G. M., & Wilcox, A. (2001). Handedness in boys with gender identity disorder. *Journal of Child Psychology and Psychiatry, 42*(6), 767–776.

Zucker, K. J., & Bradley, S. J. (1995). *Gender identity disorder and psychosexual problems in children and adolescents* (pp. 189–193). New York: Guilford Press.

Zucker, K. J., Bradley, S. J., Oliver, G., Blake, J., Fleming, S., & Hood, J. (1996). Psychosexual development of women with congenital adrenal hyperplasia. *Hormones and Behavior, 30*(4), 300–318.

Zucker, K. J., Green, R., Garofano, C., Bradley, S., Williams, K., Rebach, H., & Sullivan, C. B. (1994). Prenatal preferences of mothers of feminine and masculine boys. *Journal of Abnormal Child Psychology, 22*, 1–13.

4

Relationships to Other Health Care Fields

Providers should know how being transgender compares with other similar phenomena in terms of understanding and treatment. Two medical fields that relate to behavior, have been the subject of sexology, have been depathologized by virtue of changes in the DSM, and have often been confused with being transgender are being gay (**homosexuality**) and **BDSM** (bondage, discipline, sadism, masochism), sometimes called kink. Being transgender is totally independent from these behavioral phenomena. Transgender people come in all types of sexual orientations, and there is no reason to believe that transgender people practice fetish/BDSM more than their peers. One way of imposing cultural rejection on transgender people is to try to associate being gay and practicing BDSM with being transgender in order to associate being transgender with sex. Sex and gender are two different things, sex having to do with sex organs associated with reproduction and gender having to do with culturally defined behavior categories.

Being gay involves sexual arousal and pair bonding with a person of the same sex; BDSM involves sexual arousal from unconventional, culturally disapproved stimuli. Although transgender people initially become sexually aroused by crossdressing and crosspresentation, it is not sufficient motivation to maintain the behaviors. Transgender people continue to crossdress and crosspresent in order to express their congruent gender, feel relaxed, and feel authentic (Buhrich, 1978; Hirschfeld, 1911; Levitt & Ippolito, 2014). Some cannot find a congruent gender and so express themselves in a mixture or alternation of behaviors that culture has deemed to be gender behaviors.

One thing that being transgender has in common with these two other phenomena is that all three came under study by early sexologists. In order to legitimize their study for culture, sexologists had to pathologize these phenomena, although most early sexologists deemed them to be natural phenomena. Medicine developed the medical model in the early 20th century as these phenomena came under investigation, which requires understanding the origin of a disease state before treatment. This was based on the popular "germ" theory of disease in the 19th century. But these three phenomena are naturally occurring behaviors that have no pathological basis. We have now come around to the idea that unless these phenomena cause distress or impairment by themselves, they are not pathological.

Similarities and Differences between Being Transgender, Homosexuality, and BDSM

Similarities

1. All involve identified behaviors.
2. All three independent from one another.
3. All three studied by early sexologists Havelock Ellis and Magnus Hirschfeld at beginning of 20th century, who believed them to be natural phenomena and not pathological.
4. All three included in DSM-I sexual deviation category in 1952, developed largely by military psychiatrists as a result of World War II mobilization.
5. All three eventually depathologized in DSM.
6. All three have "cures" that were tried: psychoanalysis, lobotomy, aversion therapy, jawboning, shock therapy, operant conditioning. All were ineffective and some were dangerous.
7. For all three, accepted treatment is affirmative model to practice safely.
8. All three spawned support groups.

9. For all three, no confirmed causal factor for parental interactions and child rearing.
10. For all three, no confirmed causal factor of trauma demonstrated.

Differences

1. Being transgender has to do with gender. Transitioning transgender people modify their bodies to be compatible with what people expect from their gender. Homosexuality involves same-sex attraction and pair bonding. BDSM involves culturally taboo sexual stimuli.
2. Being transgender was depathologized in 2017 (DSM-5), homosexuality in 1974 (DSM-II-6), BDSM in 1994 (DSM-IV).
3. Population frequencies: being transgender >1 percent, homosexuality 1.6–4.5 percent, BDSM >1.2 percent.
4. Suspected causal factors of being transgender and homosexuality are genetics, epigenetics; BDSM is an extension of normal sexual arousal learning.
5. Evolutionary model for being transgender and homosexuality is kinship theory; model for BDSM is sexual stimulation for reproduction.
6. No animal model for being transgender but confirmed animal models exist for homosexuality and BDSM.

All three phenomena have in common their inclusion in the same diagnostic category in the old DSM-I (1952) under the heading of "Sexual Deviation," but they later diverged into their own categories and medical fields:

> This diagnosis is reserved for deviant sexuality which is not symptomatic of more extensive syndromes, such as schizophrenic and obsessional reactions. The term includes most of the cases formerly classed as "psychopathic personality with pathological sexuality." The diagnosis will specify the type of the pathological behavior, such as homosexuality, transvestism, pedophilia, fetishism and sexual sadism (including rape, sexual assault, mutilation). (DSM-I, pp. 38–39)

The DSM-I was fashioned largely by U.S. military psychiatrists based on primitive hospital classification schemes. Such hospital schemes were found to be inadequate for induction physicals of the millions of U.S. servicemen during World War II. Subsequently, the DSM-I was heavily influenced by U.S. Army and U.S. Navy schemes ostensibly used for classification to screen people for service and security clearances. Thus, the DSM started out as a document that was very strict and designed to eliminate people who could not be expected to live in close quarters with others. But, in fact, the policy was put in place more to reassure parents and families of

Table 4.1 Comparisons of Three Medical Fields

Comparison/Independent Medical Field		Transgender	Homosexualism	Fetish and BDSM
	Phenomenon Involves	Behavior not in assigned natal gender category	Same-sex sexual behavior and pair bonding	Unconventional or unusual sexual arousal stimuli
History	Sexologist Study Beginning	1920s	1920s	1920s
	Demographics Support Group	1970s	1950s	1970s
	Demographics Street Action	Starting 1965-1969	Starting 1965-1969	1980s
	National Advocacy Groups	2000s	1970s	1990s
Pathology/Depathology	DSM I (1952)	Sexual Deviation	Sexual Deviation	Sexual Deviation
	DSM-II (1968)	Sexual Deviation	Sociopathic personality disturbance	Sexual Deviation
	DSM-II-6 (1974)	Sexual Deviation	Sexual orientation disturbance	Sexual Deviation
	DSM III (1980)	Gender Identity Disorder	Ego-dystonic homosexuality	Sexual Deviation
	DSM-III-R (1987)	Gender Identity Disorder	Sexual disorder not specified–personal distress or impairment required	Sexual Sadism and Sexual Masochism paraphilia disorders
	DSM IV (1994)	Gender Identity Disorder requiring personal distress or impairment required	Sexual disorder not specified–personal distress or impairment required	Paraphilic disorder–personal distress or impairment required

	DSM IV-TR (2000)	Gender Identity Disorder requiring personal distress or impairment required	Sexual disorder not specified–personal distress or impairment required	Paraphilic disorder–personal distress or impairment required
	DSM 5 (2013)	Gender dysphoria–personal distress or impairment required	Sexual disorder not specified–personal distress or impairment required	Paraphilias unusual sex interest–disorder requires non-consensual sex
	ICD 10 (1990)	Gender Identity Disorder	Deleted 1990	Paraphilia
	ICD 11 (2019)	Sexual Health-non-pathological	Deleted	Consensual BDSM excluded–personal distress or impairment required
Population		At least 1% of males, Conway (2003)	3.5% Williams Institute (2011)	1.2% male; 1.3% female practice Australian Study; more interested
Frequency		.6% Williams Institute (2017)	LG 1.6% CDC, Bi .7% (2013)	
Estimates			4.5% Williams Institute (2017,	
	Causal Factor Theories			
		Genetics-twin studies, DNA markers	Genetics-twin studies, DNA markers	N/A
		Epigenetics Unblocking	Epigenetics–Possible Imprinting from Mother; Epi-marks	N/A

(continued)

Table 4.1 (continued)

Comparison/Independent Medical Field	Transgender	Homosexualism	Fetish and BDSM
	Possible Prenatal Teratogens and DNA Mutation (e.g. DES)	N/A	N/A
	Childhood Gender Learning	Childhood Sex Learning	Classical Conditioning Learning
	Current Western Binary Cisgender Inflexible Culture	N/A	N/A
	Not Prenatal Sex Hormones-Evidence Refutes	N/A	N/A
	Sexual Arousal Motivation-Evidence Refutes	Sexual Arousal	Sexual Arousal
	No Animal Model	Animal models in over 500 species	Animal model of Classical conditioning of sexual arousal but not BDSM stimuli
	Parenting–refuted by evidence	Parenting–No Evidence	Parenting–No Evidence
	Trauma-no evidence	Trauma-no evidence	Trauma-no evidence
Evolution	Kinship theory over Traditional Heterogenderist Theory	Kinship theory over Traditional Heterosexist Theory; Epi-marks	Stimulates sex and reproduction
	N/A	Increased Maternal fertility associated with homosexuality	N/A

Ineffective Treatments	Psychoanalysis	Psychoanalysis	Psychoanalysis
	Aversion Therapy	Aversion Therapy	Aversion Therapy
	Operant Conditioning (Reparative Therapy)	Operant Conditioning (Reparative Therapy)	N/A
	Jawboning (Reparative Therapy)	Jawboning (Reparative Therapy)	N/A
	Shock Therapy	Shock Therapy	N/A
	Lobotomy	Lobotomy	Lobotomy
	Implanted Electrode Stimulation		
Effective Treatments	Affirmative Counseling for Social Problems	Affirmative Counseling for Social Problems	Affirmative Counseling for Social Problems
	Medical Transition (Transsexual Transition)	N/A	N/A
	Counseling for TGPS Gatekeeping (Transsexual Transition)	N/A	N/A

service men and women. It is ironic that the modern BDSM interest was patterned after homosexual BDSM practitioners in the military in World War II. This strict approach was echoed in the recent debates over whether gay or transgender people can serve in the military. The DSM-I was also published in the midst of a British spy scandal involving several gay males. Because of this experience, exclusion of homosexuals and transgender people from the U.S. and U.K. military and intelligence services persisted well into the late 20th century but has now been relaxed.

Table 4.1 shows a comparison of the three independent fields of study. The following sections compare being transgender to homosexuality and to BDSM.

BEING TRANSGENDER CONTRASTED TO HOMOSEXUALITY

Unlike being transgender, which was not recognized until the early 20th century, being gay was known to the 5th–4th-century BCE Greeks. In fact, being gay or **pederasty** as it was called was an important social factor that contributed to military cohesion in all-male Greek armies. Many Greek army units consisted of numerous same-sex couples, usually of an older and younger pair-bond. At this time females also had same-sex partners. This continued into the Roman era, through the Renaissance, and into the 19th century. Being gay was largely ignored as a social phenomenon in Europe until the 12th century when the three Abrahamic religions all condemned it. It remains outlawed in many Middle Eastern countries (punishable by death) and in many countries visited by Christian missionaries.

Before Magnus Hirschfeld gave being transgender a name (transvestism) in the early 20th century, in 1880 Karl-Maria Kertbeny, a human rights advocate, coined the terms "**homosexual**" and "**heterosexual**." Krafft-Ebing, an Austro-German sexologist, began popularizing these terms with the publication of his book *Psychopathia Sexualis* (1886). Krafft-Ebing believed that being gay was a natural phenomenon and not pathological. He pointed out the many contributions of gay people to society.

Hirschfeld was himself a gay person who did not believe that being gay or being transgender should be pathologized. In this, he agreed with the U.K. sexologist Havelock Ellis who had contributed to a European initiative against sodomy laws. But modern medicine began to pathologize being gay to offer it protection from being considered a crime and to bring it under scientific study and medical control. All of the early sexologists believed that being gay was different from being transgender.

After World War II, research on homosexuality began in earnest, although the DSM-I had categorized it as a sexual deviation. Frank Beach (1949) found that testosterone and estrogen levels in male gays were normal. In reaction to the pathologization in the DSM-I in 1952, the U.S. National Institutes of Health began to sponsor research that would ultimately lead to depathologization of being gay. By comparison, basic research sponsorship on being transgender was not pursued in the United States but was pursued abroad.

In 1948 Kinsey studied both homosexuality and being transgender and reported that both were more common than most people believed. Kinsey developed a sexual orientation scale that is still in use today (Kinsey, Pomeroy, & Martin, 1948).

Depathologization of homosexuality in the DSM and ICD began with a 1957 study by Hooker, which found that there was no difference in psychological adjustment for homosexuality using standard psychological clinical tests. Investigators found that most homosexuals were satisfied with their sexual orientation and not impaired in judgment, social capability, or in distress. These scientific findings supported the advocacy for depathologizing homosexuality, which began by a temporizing move in the DSM-II-6 (1973) when homosexuality was changed to ego-dystonic homosexuality (thoughts in conflict with a person's ideal self-image). This change occurred because of the accumulation of scientific evidence about being homosexual but also because of considerable pressure from advocacy groups. Pressure also came from behavioral psychology, sociology, and from mental health professionals.

The diagnosis of homosexuality required patient distress and no indicated arousal to heterosexual stimuli. Homosexuality was finally removed from the DSM-III-R release in 1987. But the DSM-III-R still retained a "sexual disorder not otherwise specified" requiring "persistent and marked distress about one's sexual orientation." This category continues in the DSM-5 (2017).

Until 1993 the World Health Organization's ICD listed homosexuality as a mental illness, but it was removed entirely from the ICD in 1994 with ICD-10. The DSM's depathologization of being transgender followed the same pattern as that of homosexuality but delayed by 44 years. First a temporizing category, gender dysphoria (transgender), and ego-dystonic homosexuality in the DSM, then final depathologization in the next edition of the ICD.

The depathologization of homosexuality left providers with the problem of how to bill for treatments for so-called "prehomosexual children." Adults could be counseled or treated under existing DSM billing codes. Prehomosexual children presented as sexually aggressive with same-sex children and it was established that they became homosexual in adulthood. Since homosexuality was no longer an accepted diagnosis, some providers billed using the DSM codes for treatment of transgender children. Some of these prehomosexual children do crossdress, but transgender children present quite differently. The problem comes when one tries to determine outcomes for transkids. Using data from prehomosexual kids would force a prediction that transgender kids would no longer be transgender in adulthood because the prehomosexual children are not transgender in adulthood but, instead, will become homosexual. This "desister" controversy will be explored in Chapter 10.

Although bans on homosexual sexual behavior were repealed by some states, it was not until the *Lawrence v. Texas* (2003) decision that gay sexual behavior became legal throughout the United States. And it was not until *Obergefell v. Hodges* (2015) that same-sex marriage became legal throughout the United States. Transgender people also benefited by this decision because many were married before transition, leaving them in an inconvenient legal status. By that time, WPATH guidelines requiring gay sexual orientation and/or divorce for transition had been relaxed. The decision allowed transitioned transgender people as well as gays the freedom to marry or remain married to people with any type of sexual orientation.

Estimates of population frequency indicate that there are several times more gay people than transgender people. Estimates for transgender people indicate that the lower bound population frequency for being transgender is a least .7–1 percent of males; these frequency estimates from surveys have increased in percentage over time. Estimates for the population frequency of homosexual people puts it at about 2.3–4.5 percent from the Williams Institute based on CDC data (Flores, Herman, Gates, & Brown, 2016). Neither transgender nor gay people have ever been included in the U.S. Census, although the number of same-sex households can be estimated.

With regard to causal factors, there are more studies providing evidence on being transgender than being gay, but the evidence supports a genetic factor for both. The evidence for a genetic factor and heritability for being transgender is summarized in Chapter 3. The evidence for a genetic factor for being gay is based on twin studies and DNA marker studies (Bailey & Bell, 1993; Kendler, Thornton, Gilman, & Kessler, 2000; Mustanski et al., 2005; Rahman, 2005; Sanders et al., 2014) for chromosome 8 and location Xq28. Extreme skewing of maternal X-inactivation has also been reported (Bocklandt, Horvath, Vilain, & Hamer, 2006). A polygenetic threshold model seems to fit the evidence for being transgender, but no similar model has emerged for homosexuality. Epigenetics can interfere with the genetic predisposition for being transgender because heritability, as for many traits, is not 100 percent. Birth order studies were done with "transgender homosexual" samples, but studies with nonhomosexual transgender control groups indicate that the effect was actually due to homosexuality. Some have suggested that gay genes continue because they are associated with increased family fecundity (Camperio-Ciani, Battaglia, Cesare, Camperio-Ciani, & Capiluppi, 2018; Camperio-Ciani, Coma, & Capiluppi, 2004; Ganna et al., 2018).

A fraternal birth order effect has been reported for homosexuality, which indicates that the probability of being a gay male increases with male birth order (Blanchard, 1997). This "genetic imprinting" effect is believed to be due to acquired immunity by the mother, which increases as she has more male children. Replications of this study have not been reported. It has been suggested that exposure to high levels of testosterone in females and low levels in males may lead to both being transgender and homosexual (Dörner, 1976), but current evidence refutes this theory. In fact, Dörner believed that being transgender required being homosexual, which was a requirement for transgender transition at the time. There have been inconclusive studies that being transgender might be due to exposure to teratogens, which cause prenatal genetic mutations and interfere with DNA expression, but there have been no such studies for being gay. Recent work has focused on epigenetic theories for being gay (Ngun & Vilain, 2014; Rice, Friberg, & Gavrilets, 2012) and has featured "epi-marks," which are non-DNA chemicals that bind to DNA and turn gene expression on or off for particular genes. There is no equivalent theory about being transgender.

Just as childhood gender learning appears to be required for being transgender, sex learning in late childhood and adolescence is required for being gay. Being transgender requires knowledge of the gender system of gender behavior categories. Homosexuality requires knowledge of sex and sexual behavior.

The current Western binary, cisgender, and inflexible gender system forces transgender people to violate cultural norms for expressing congruent gender behavior in public. Transgender people are therefore cultural outlaws. Since gay behavior does not necessarily require public expression, Western culture is less of a factor in rejecting public expression; it involves violation of heterosexism cultural rules.

Although sexual arousal does not appear to be the long-term motivation for transgender behavior, clearly sexual arousal is involved in gay sexual behavior. Transgender people often experience sexual arousal in initial experiences with crossdressing and crosspresentation, but this fades with exposure due to classical conditioning extinction. For gay people, same-sex stimuli evoke sexual arousal based on classical conditioning learning about sex based on a sexual orientation predisposition, and this appears to be reinforced throughout life.

There is evidence that refutes parental relations as a causal factor in being transgender, and there is no evidence that it is a factor in homosexuality. It was originally suggested for both behavioral phenomena that a controlling "smother" mother and absent father were possibly involved in causation, but that does not appear to be correct (Bailey et al., 2016).

In contrast to the 500 species of animals that have same-sex relationships (Bailey & Zuk, 2009; Roughgarden, 2004), there is no infrahuman animal model for being transgender. Human gender behavior categories were developed by human culture, and human gender is much more complicated, sophisticated, and different from infrahuman animal sexual behavior.

Evolutionary theory to identify the reasons why both being transgender and being gay have not died out during evolution has been advanced. Kinship evolutionary theory as opposed to traditional heterosexist/heterogenderist theory indicates that it is the evolutionary fitness of the family, tribe, clan, or group that allowed humans to survive. Both transgender people and gay people contributed to the overall fitness of the family and tribe who all shared the same genes, thus the behavioral predisposition would be passed on.

Many similar treatments for both transgender people and homosexuals have been tried and shown to be ineffective, as shown in Table 4.1. Some of them caused physical and psychological injury. They followed the trending ideas of the times in psychiatry, which included Freudian ideas, aversion counter conditioning, classical conditioning, and operant conditioning. Psychoanalysis is ineffective as a "cure" for both phenomena, but psychiatric and psychological counseling can help both homosexuals and transgender people with social problems. Like being transgender, being gay is not due to trauma (Perrin, 2002), which undermines several psychodynamic ideas as well as **sexual orientation change efforts (SOCE)**. Aversion therapy has been tried on both transgender and homosexual people, but the behaviors recover. Aversion therapy uses nausea-producing drugs or electric shock to attempt to change classical conditioned learning. As Garcia and Kolling (1967) have shown, not all unconditioned stimuli can be successfully paired with unconditioned stimuli to produce learning. Aversion therapy also seems to fade outside of the conditioning site. Operant conditioning and jawboning are two of the standard techniques used in reparative or conversion "therapies," but these therapies have not been shown to permanently change behavior. These therapies have been rejected by professional societies (APA, 2009) and are banned in many U.S. states and countries. Shock therapy (Tran et al., 2017) and lobotomy (Rieber & Sigusch, 1979; Schmidt & Schorsch, 1981) have been tried without success. Internal stimulation of the brain through electrodes has been tried for being transgender without long-term effect (O'Neal, Baker, Glenn, Conner, & Sughrue, 2017).

Affirmative psychological counseling has been shown to be an effective treatment for both transgender and gay people, but this treatment is concerned with how to deal with social problems resulting from stigma and rejection, particularly family problems. It is not concerned with curtailing behavior. Counseling also helps people deal with depression, loneliness, and suicidal thoughts.

Affirmative medical transgender transition has been shown to improve the lives of transgender people. Transgender people who are denied transition and TGPS are more likely to attempt suicide. Family acceptance, use of chosen name, and access to transitioning lower the risks from depression and suicide (Camperio-Ciani et al., 2018; Russell, Pollitt, Li, & Grossman, 2018). Psychological counseling has been beneficial in "gatekeeping" for those who want chest/breast or transgender genital plastic surgery, which is required by WPATH guidelines. The purpose of gatekeeping is to ensure that the person has no major mental illness, such as a psychosis, that would interfere with successful outcomes. It is believed that this requirement along with counseling has been instrumental in reducing the frequency of surgical regret.

COMPARISON OF BEING TRANSGENDER WITH BDSM

Various stimuli trigger sexual arousal in humans and culture attempts to control which ones are socially condoned and legalized. Culture does not typically discourage sexual behavior for procreation (unless families grow too large) but prohibits sexual abuse, harassment, or injury to a nonconsenting person. This is considered violent behavior, which is punishable under criminal and civil statutes. Today in some U.S. states, BDSM is protected by law if consent can be demonstrated.

There is a wide range of stimuli that trigger sexual arousal that are perfectly legal but may be discouraged by culture, and they vary from time to time and culture to culture. For example, people in Western culture kiss on the lips for sexual arousal but Indigenous people of the north polar regions rub noses. The very idea that some customs are cultural taboos may be a turn-on for some people.

A fetish is an object or practice that results in sexual arousal that is deemed by culture to be unusual or unconventional. In 1991 the initialism BDSM was created but before that it was called **fetishism**, one of the **paraphilia disorders**. The current definition in DSM-5 says that BDSM is not a disorder unless a person suffers from impairment or distress because of their fetish feelings and behavior, but during World War II and until recently it was classified as a pathological disorder. Some pathological definitions also included the requirement that it was only a fetish if it was required for consummation of sexual behavior.

Fetishism was known to the ancient Sumerians (2000 BCE) and can be traced through many cultures up to today. BDSM is a more recent idea that came into being only in the late 20th century. BDSM stands for bondage, discipline, sadism, and masochism and is strongly associated with support group subcultures whose members engage in such practices for sexual arousal under strict rules of engagement. Bondage is physical restraint. Discipline is psychological restraint and control. Together they involve dominance and submission. Sadism is inflicting pain or control for sexual arousal. Masochism is voluntary submission to pain or control. In these support group subcultures the initial rules of engagement were that such practices must be safe, sane, and consensual (SSC). Because some felt that this did not reflect risk understanding and consensus well enough, the "risk-aware consensus kink" (RACK) rules of engagement were developed. These rules ensure that both partners are aware of the risks, both are able to give initial consensus, and both are aware of the legal risks that they are about to undertake with alternative sex practices. Initial consensus involves rules that allow both parties to slow or stop by indicating verbally (safe words) or nonverbally that they are unwilling to continue. Both of these rules of engagement sets are intended to avoid legal sexual abuse, rape, or sexual harassment.

Engagement in BDSM activities still poses legal risks to jobs and family court decisions, so many people engaged in BDSM are not out. In contrast, many people now openly acknowledge being transgender, including those who transitioned and followed previously closeted "stealth" status.

In this discussion, we need to bear in mind two things about sexual arousal. The first is that novelty can trigger sexual arousal. We know this from research on the Coolidge effect (Ford & Beach, 1952) in infrahuman species. It is also the case that stimuli such as novel human clothing and other fashions may be sexually arousing. The second is that it is learned through classical, sometimes called Pavlovian conditioning (Lalumiere & Quinsey, 1998; Letourneau & O'Donohue, 1997; O'Donohue & Plaud, 1994). BDSM seems to have all the properties of classical conditioning including acquisition, chaining from one stimulus to the next, extinction, and spontaneous recovery. As in classical conditioning, arousal can be chained from stimulus to stimulus, resulting in what John Money (1986) called a "lovemap." This process involves pairing a new stimulus with one that invokes sexual arousal. Lovemaps are not specific to BDSM but occur in all people.

As with being transgender, early sexologists regarded fetishism, what we call BDSM today, as nonpathological and a normal variation of human behavior. Krafft-Ebing defined masochism and sadism in his work *Psychopathical Sexualis* (1886). In the early 20th century, Magnus Hirschfeld and Havelock Ellis both concluded that BDSM was a learned phenomenon, probably influenced by the earlier work of Ivan Pavlov. Hirschfeld concluded in his partial attractiveness theory (Hirschfeld, 1911) that fetishism is common to most people and that particular stimuli from a partner stimulate arousal. Kinsey (1953) later found that 12 percent of females and 22 percent of males reported sexual arousal from the reading of a sadomasochistic story. Although Freud developed complicated psychodynamic processes to account for fetishism, his case studies clearly indicated that learning was involved because culture influenced the particular triggering stimuli.

As with being transgender, BDSM support groups were formed in major U.S. and European cities in the 1970s. Support groups were in vogue for many activities at the time and continue today. The first support group was The Eulenspiegel Society in 1971 in New York City. The Society of Janus was formed in 1974 in San Francisco. These support groups were influenced by gay leather groups, which formed after contacts were made during World War II military service, although these new support groups were typically pansexual. The overlap continued in 1980 with the group Gay Male Sexual Activists, which became Folsom Street East and now runs the annual Folsom Street Fair. As with transgender support groups, many local BDSM groups put on convention meetings.

Support groups have proliferated even to smaller cities and universities. BDSM parties were arranged, and still are, for both nonprofit and for-profit venues. People who participate in these events typically arrange short BDSM experiences known as "scenes." Participation in BDSM is known as being in the "scene." Group meetings center around presentations on various BDSM techniques and how to perform them safely with consenting adults. They also allow BDSM people to meet each other and form relationships. BDSM "munches" are commonly arranged online. Munches are dinners or lunches in public places in which people meet each other outside of the scene. BDSM people also network through Internet websites such as the secure site, FetLife.

An outgrowth of these support groups were national groups that began to lobby for changes in the DSM and the law. The National Coalition for Sexual Freedom (NCSF), which was formed in 1997 in New York City, included many of the local groups including the groups mentioned above as well as the Black Rose in Washington, DC, and the National Leather Association. At that time, adults could easily lose their children because of their BDSM activities or be vulnerable to accusations of violence because their activities were deemed to be pathological by virtue of the DSM. The NCSF advocated for BDSM sexual freedom and privacy rights. In its advocacy, the NCSF has been supported by the Woodhull Freedom Foundation. At the international level the Federal Association for Sadomasochism was formed in 2003 in Germany, which included affiliations with over 600 local groups.

There were also providers who treated those with BDSM behaviors in the mental health and legal communities who formed a group called Kink

Aware Professionals in 1987. This group had been formed to provide listings of those providers who specialized in helping BDSM people through counseling. They also advocated for changes in the DSM and for legal changes.

As with homosexuality and being transgender, fetishism appeared in the 1952 DSM-I as a pathological state of sexual deviation. It continued in this way until 1994 when it was removed from the DSM-IV, putting it on the same footing as being transgender in 2013.

The classification of pathological sexual deviation continued until 1987 when the DSM-III-R classified BDSM as a **paraphilia** disorder. Paraphilia disorders were defined as those pathological conditions involving intense sexual urges and acting on them. Advocates for the change to paraphilia also believed that many people who conducted BDSM behavior were not mentally ill, and in the next version of the DSM, in 1994, they qualified the requirements for a paraphilia mental illness to require distress or impairment. This change essentially said that it was not mental illness unless it interfered with work, family, friendships, or other activities. This change represented a depathologization from previous classifications and was due to accumulated scientific evidence but also to the efforts of national advocacy groups.

In DSM-5 in 2013 the paraphilias were defined as "unusual sex interests," but a paraphilic disorder or mental illness required nonconsensual sex or deliberately causing harm to themselves or others. This was a result of surveys by national advocacy groups indicating the economic, legal, and social harm done by stereotyping those into BDSM. Buttressing these surveys was a report from emergency rooms that did *not* indicate a higher incidence of injury from BDSM as opposed to nonkink sex (Barker, Iantaffi, & Gupta, 2007). Expert analysis was also used as evidence (Karasic & Drescher, 2005; Moser, 2009; Moser & Kleinplatz, 2005).

The ICD followed a delayed but similar pattern as the DSM with BDSM as a paraphilia until 2017 (ICD-11) when consensual BDSM was excluded and personal distress or impairment was required.

The most representative survey indicates that those who practice BDSM represent 2.5 percent of the population (Richters et al., 2008), although some surveys report up to 15 percent of the population. This is considerably higher than the estimates for being transgender.

From the early sexologist studies, it has been assumed that classical conditioning learning is a causal factor in BDSM. A number of studies have demonstrated classical conditioning of sexual arousal (Both et al., 2008; Both, Brauer, & Laan, 2011; Hoffman, Janssen, & Turner, 2004). This has also been demonstrated in animals (Koksal et al., 2004). In the latter study, a neutral stimulus, a terrycloth object, was paired with the opportunity to copulate. However, definitive studies for the stimuli involved in BDSM have not been performed.

In contrast, being transgender does involve learning, but the learning is primarily about gender norms and behaviors learned in early childhood from parental modeling, not sexual arousal conditioning. There are some who attribute psychopathology to being transgender and the idea that sexual arousal motivations for transgender behavior depend on sexual arousal as a result of love of oneself as a woman (see Chapter 10 for autogynephilia). Love, in this context, devolves to sexual fetish. This idea is controversial. Although early traumatization and abusive parenting have been suggested as causal factors for BDSM, there is no evidence of these.

Sexual behavior clearly has a role in maintaining the species and therefore there should be selective evolutionary pressure to encourage sexual arousal. In contrast, sexual arousal plays a minor role in being transgender during the initial stages of crossdressing and crosspresentation, and it extinguishes according to the rules of classical conditioning.

As with transgender behavior, there is no evidence that BDSM behavior decreases with psychoanalysis treatment. Medical treatment for fetishism was tried using aversion therapy. Aversion therapy involves pairing an aversive state with stimuli that trigger unwanted sexual arousal. The aversive state can be induced by administration of a drug that causes nausea (apomorphine) or by electric shock. The results indicated that this procedure is not effective in permanently reducing the classical conditioned connection between the stimulus and sexual arousal. In most cases, results did not persist outside of the treatment facility. As Garcia and Kolling (1967) have shown, not every stimulus can be conditioned to every unconditioned response, and it is not clear what conditioned response to use to conflict with BDSM stimuli, since BDSM actually involves aversive stimuli (e.g., pain, bondage).

As with being transgender, the best treatment found is affirmative treatment with counseling. Most people involved in both being transgender and BDSM do not want to decrease their behavior but want help to deal with cultural rejection and social problems.

REFERENCES

American Psychological Association. (2009). Report of the American Psychological Association Task Force on Appropriate Therapeutic Responses to Sexual Orientation. http://www.apa.org/about/policy/sexual-orientation.pdf, https://www.apa.org/pi/lgbt/resources/therapeutic-response.pdf

Bailey, J. M., & Bell, A. P. (1993). Familiality of male and female homosexuality. *Behavioral Genetics, 23*, 313–322.

Bailey, J. M., et al. (2016). Sexual orientation, controversy, and science. *Psychological Science in the Public Interest, 17*(2), 45–101.

Bailey, N., & Zuk, M. (2009). Same-sex sexual behavior and evolution. *Cell: Trends in Ecological Evolution, 24*(8), 439–446.

Barker, M., Iantaffi, A., & Gupta, C. (2007). Kinky clients, kinky counselling? The challenges and potentials of BDSM. In L. Moon (Ed.), *Feeling queer or queer feelings: Radical approaches to counselling sex, sexualities and genders* (pp. 106–124). London: Routledge.

Blanchard, R. (1997). Birth order and sibling sex ratio in homosexual versus heterosexual males and females. *Annual Review of Sex Research, 8*, 27–67.

Bocklandt, S., Horvath, S., Vilain, E., & Hamer, D. H. (2006). Extreme skewing of X chromosome inactivation in mothers of homosexual men. *Human Genetics, 118*(6), 691–694.

Both, S., Brauer, M., & Laan, E. (2001, November). Classical conditioning of sexual response in women: A replication study. *Journal of Sexual Medicine, 8*, 3116–3131.

Both, S., Spiering, M., Laan, E., Belcome, S., van den Heuvel, B., & Everaerd, W. (2008). Unconscious classical conditioning of sexual arousal: Evidence for the condition of female genital arousal to subliminally presented sexual stimuli, *Journal of Sexual Medicine, 5*, 100–109.

Buhrich, N. (1978). Motivation for cross-dressing in heterosexual transvestism. *Acta Psychiatrica Scandinavia, 57*, 145–152.

Camperio-Ciani, A., Battaglia, U., Cesare, L., Camperio-Ciani, G., & Capiluppi, C. (2018). Possible balancing selection in human female homosexuality. *Human Nature, 29*(1), 14–32.

Camperio-Ciani, A., Coma, F., & Capiluppi, C. (2004). Evidence for maternally inherited factors favoring male homosexuality and promoting fecundity. *Proceedings of Biological Science, 7*(271), 1554, 2217–2221.

Chaladze, G. (2016). Heterosexual male carriers could explain persistence of homosexuality in men: Individual-based simulations of an X-linked inheritance model. *Archives of Sexual Behavior, 45*(7), 1705–1711.

Conway, L. (2002). How frequently does transsexualism occur? Retrieved from http://www.lynnconway.com.

Dörner, G. (1976). *Hormones and brain differentiation* (p. 227). New York: Elsevier.

Flores, A. R., Herman, J. L., Gates, G. J., & Brown, T. N. T. (2016). *How many adults identify as transgender in the United States?* Los Angeles, CA: Williams Institute.

Ganna, A., et al. (2018). Large genome-wide analysis of sexual orientation identifies for the first time variants associated with non-heterosexual behavior and reveals overlap with heterosexual reproductive traits. *Archive Today, 278*. https://archive.is/B6o23#selection-73.0-58.50

Garcia, J., & Kolling, R. A. (1967). A comparison of aversions induced by x-rays, toxins, and drugs in the rat. *Radiation Research Supplement, 7*, 439–450.

Gates, G. (2011). How many people are LGBT? Williams Institute. http://williamsinstitute.law.ucla/wp-contenct/uploads/Gates-How-Many-People_LGBT-apri-2011.pdf

Hirschfeld, M. (1991). *Transvestites: The erotic drive to cross-dress* (M. A. Lombardi, Trans.). Amherst: Prometheus Books. (Original work published 1911.)

Hoffman, H., Janssen, E., & Turner, S. (2004). Classical conditioning of sexual arousal in women and men: Effects of varying awareness and biological relevance of the conditioned stimulus. *Archives of Sexual Behavior, 33*, 43–53.

Karasic, D., & Drescher, J. (2005). Sexual and gender diagnoses of the *Diagnostic and Statistical Manual* (DSM). *Journal of Psychology and Human Sexuality, 17*, 91–109.

Kendler, K. S., Thornton, L. M., Gilman, S. E., & Kessler, R. C. (2000). Sexual orientation in a U.S. national sample of twin and nontwin sibling pairs. *American Journal of Psychiatry, 157*(11), 1843–1846.

Kinsey, A. C., Pomeroy, W. B., & Martin, C. E. (1948). *Sexual behavior in the human male*. Philadelphia: Saunders.

Kinsey, A. C., Pomeroy, W. B., Martin, C. E., & Gebhard, P. H. (1953). *Sexual behavior in the human female* (pp. 677–678). Indiana University Press.

Koksal, F., Domjan, M., Kurt, A., Sertel, O., Orung, S., Bowers, R., et al. (2004). An animal model of fetishism. *Behavioral Research Therapy, 42*, 1421–1434.

Krafft-Ebing, R. (1886/2010). *Psychopathia sexualis*. FQ Legacy Books.

Lalumiere, M. L., & Quinsey, V. L. (1998). Pavlovian conditioning of sexual interests in human males. *Archives of Sexual Behavior, 17*(3), 241–252.

Letourneau, E. J. & O'Donohue, W. (1997). Classical conditioning of female sexual arousal. *Archives of Sexual Behavior, 26*(1), 1997.

Levitt, H. M., & Ippolito, M. R. (2014). Being transgender: The experience of transgender identity development. *Journal of Homosexuality, 61*(12), 1727–1758.

Money, J. (1986). *Lovemaps: Clinical concepts of sexual/erotic health and pathology, paraphilia, and gender transposition in childhood, adolescence and maturity*. New York: Prometheus Books.

Moser, C. (2009). When is an unusual sex interest a mental disorder? *Archives of Sexual Behavior, 38*, 323–325.

Moser, C., & Klienplatz, P. J. (2005). DSM-IV-TR and the Paraphilias: An argument for removal. *Journal of Psychology and Human Sexuality, 17*(3/4), 91–109.

Mustanski, B. S., et al. (2005). A genome wide scan of male sexual orientation. *Human Genetics, 116*, 272–278.

Ngun, T. C., & Vilain, E. (2014.) The biological basis of human sexual orientation: Is there a role for epigenetics? *Advances in Genetics, 86*, 167–184.

O'Donohue, W., & Plaud, J. J. (1994).The conditioning of human sexual arousal. *Archives of Sexual Behavior, 23*(3), 321.

O'Neal, C. M., Baker, C. M., Glenn, C. A., Conner, A. K., & Sughrue, M. E. (2017). Dr. Robert G. Heath: A controversial figure in the history of deep brain stimulation. *Neurosurgical Focus, 43*(3), E12.

Perrin, E. C. (2002). *Sexual orientation in child and adolescent health care* (pp. 1–14). New York: Kluwer Academic/Plenum.

Rahman, Q. (2005) The neurodevelopment of human sexual orientation. *Neuroscience and Biobehavioral Reviews*, 29, 1057–1066.

Rice, R., Friberg, U., & Gavrilets, G. (2012). Homosexuality as a consequence of epigenetically canalized sexual development. *Quarterly Review of Biology, 87*, 4.

Rice, W. R., Friberg, U., & Gavrilets, S. (2013). Homosexuality via canalized sexual development: A testing protocol for a new epigenetic model. *Bioessays, 9*, 764–770.

Richters, J., et al. (2008). Demographic and psychosocial features of participants in bondage and discipline, "sadomasochism" or dominance and submission (BDSM): Data from a national survey. *Journal of Sex Medicine, 5*(7), 1660–1608.

Rieber, I., & Sigusch, V. (1979). Psychosurgery on sex offenders and sexual "deviants" in West Germany. *Archives of Sexual Behavior, 8*(6), 523–527.

Roughgarden, J. (2004). *Evolution's rainbow* (Chap. 8). Berkeley: University of California Press.

Russell, S. T., Pollitt, A. M., Li, G., & Grossman, A. H. (2018). Chosen name use is linked to reduced depressive symptoms, suicidal ideation, and suicidal behavior among transgender youth. *Journal of Adolescent Health, 10,* 1016.

Sanders, A. R., Martin, E. R., Beecham, G. W., Guo, S., Dawood, K., Rieger, G., . . . Bailey, J. M. (2014). Genome-wide scan demonstrates significant linkage for male sexual orientation. *Psychological Medicine, 45*(7), 1379–1388.

Schmidt, G., & Schorsch, E. (1981). Psychosurgery of sexually deviant patients: Review and analysis of new empirical findings. *Archives of Sexual Behavior, 10*(3), 301–323.

Tran, B. K., O'Donnell, S. E., Balla, A., Adams, D. C., Grondin, L. S., & Tsai, M. H. (2017). Electroconvulsive therapy considerations for transgendered patients. *Journal of ECT, 33*(2), e14–e16.

5

Profiles in the Field

This chapter provides brief profiles spotlighting people who were trailblazers or are currently prominent or emerging leaders in the field. They include physicians, psychologists, and advocates.

HISTORICAL FIGURES

Harry Benjamin (1885–1986), Endocrinologist

Benjamin's original research interest was in finding a cure for tuberculosis, but his interest in ending the suffering of homosexuals and transgender people led to his becoming the leading expert on transgender transition in the mid-20th century. Benjamin knew Magnus Hirschfeld from their time in Berlin and worked with the police to protect sexual minority street people. After graduating in 1912 he came to the United States to pursue his original interest but found himself unable to return to Germany because of World War I. He opened a consulting practice in New York City but would spend every summer in San Francisco. After World War I, Benjamin would visit his colleagues in Germany and Europe including Magnus Hirschfeld.

After World War II, at the suggestion of Alfred Kinsey, probably the most prominent sexologist in the United States, Benjamin started to research and treat people who later would be called transitioning transgender people. His experience with transgender people lead him to reject the idea that they were motivated by sexual arousal as his friend, Magnus Hirschfeld, had initially believed but later recanted. He believed that his transitioning transgender patients were more interested in changing their bodies to match their congruent gender.

Benjamin started treating transitioning transgender patients with hormone therapy, since natural and synthetic sex hormones had become available. Transgender genital plastic surgery was available in Denmark but only to Danish citizens. The Danish referred patients who were U.S. citizens to Dr. Benjamin. Benjamin administered hormone therapy and found surgeons who would perform transgender genital plastic surgery, even though it was illegal at times in various states. He rejected psychotherapy as a "cure" for being transgender. These procedures were in stark contrast to many of those previously done on people who crossdressed or were homosexual, procedures that we now consider inhumane. He had several patients that became celebrities, notably Christine Jorgensen, who was born to Danish parents and met Benjamin after her surgeries in Denmark (Rudacille, 2005). Benjamin gave her hormone therapy and found a surgeon to complete her transgender genital plastic surgery.

Benjamin is most well known for his research on transitioning transgender people, which was summarized in the book *The Transsexual Phenomenon* (Benjamin, 1966). He formed the Gender Dysphoria Association for providers in 1966, which subsequently became the Harry Benjamin International Gender Dysphoria Association (HBIGDA) and now is known as the World Professional Association for Transgender Health (WPATH). This organization has published formal Standards of Care for providers since 1972.

Benjamin's research is further described in Chapter 11.

Stanley Biber (1923–2006), Physician and Surgeon

Dr. Stanley Biber was a military physician and OSS member who settled in Trinidad, CO, a small town on the road between Colorado Springs, CO, and Santa Fe, NM. After World War II, in 1948, he had gotten his medical degree at the University of Iowa. He performed all sorts of general surgery until one patient asked for transgender genital plastic surgery (TGPS) in

1969. He performed this surgery using diagrams from university gender clinics but gradually perfected TGPS for transwomen and transmen as his willingness to help transgender people became known. He continued to take care of local patients, delivering babies and setting broken bones. Trinidad gradually became known for TGPS and the town economy prospered from transgender medical tourism. The local inhabitants came to interact with and accept those who visited there, even if they were different. The United States finally had a reliable source for TGPS with Biber performing over 4,000 operations (Fox, 2006). He trained many surgeons on TGPS while continuing his local general surgery practice. He performed TGPS on Dr. Marci Bowers and taught her the technique. She now holds the active record for the number of TGPS operations.

Vern Bullough (1928–2006), Sexologist, and Bonnie Bullough (1927–1996), Sexologist

The Bulloughs were prolific researchers and writers on various sexology issues, including a landmark book summarizing transgender science as of 1993. Their activities bridged the gap between old-school researchers and newer researchers who had renewed interest in understanding being transgender. Vern held a PhD from the University of Chicago and held various academic posts at SUNY, Cal State Northridge, and Buffalo State College. He also held a bachelor's degree in nursing from Cal State Northridge. Bonnie received a master's in nursing from UCLA and her PhD in sociology in 1959.

Both Vern and Bonnie were champions of nursing involvement in sexology issues. Bonnie started one of the first master's programs in nursing, was a leader in the nurse practitioner field, and was a founder of the Society for the Scientific Study of Sexuality (SSSS). She held various academic positions in nursing. Vern was a president of the SSSS and was a founder of the American Association for the History of Nursing. Together the couple studied historical crossdressing, transgender transition, and the emergence of transgender support groups.

Vern organized several transgender research conferences that spanned the globe starting in 1966 in Northridge, CA, where he lived to Philadelphia, PA; Oxford, United Kingdom; and Perth, Australia, which established transgender science as a new field in academia. The Bulloughs facilitated the integration of transgender science into academic curricula.

Magnus Hirschfeld (1868–1935), Sexologist and Advocate

Magnus Hirschfeld was a German sexologist who studied and advocated for homosexuals and transgender people. He started one of the first advocacy organizations. He studied modern medicine as it was then emerging, earned a PhD degree, and became one of the first sexologists. Hirschfeld set up a practice near Berlin, Germany, and studied the homosexual subculture in both Berlin and Chicago, United States. He found transgender people to be suffering from cultural rejection. As a result, they had increased suicide rates and frequently were victims of violence. Being homosexual himself, he had personally experienced street violence. He joined groups of prominent scientists and humanitarians to advocate and lobby for the decriminalization of homosexuality and for women's rights.

In 1911, he published *The Transvestites,* a book on his case study research into the transgender phenomena. He worked with the Berlin police to end the harassment and arrest of transgender people (Stryker, 2008). One of his colleagues was Harry Benjamin (Stryker, 2008), who came to the United States in 1913.

During the post–World War I Weimar republic, he founded the Institute for Sexual Research in Berlin, which featured an exhaustive library and experts in various fields related to sexuality and gender. During this period, Hirschfeld conducted and/or arranged for the first transgender genital plastic surgeries and other procedures on Dora Richter and Lili Elbe. Although sex hormones had been discovered in the previous century, they were not synthesized until the 1930s, so some of the attempted operations involved ovary transplants.

In 1932, he left Germany on a world tour. Realizing that the political climate in Germany was hostile, he traveled to New York where he met with Harry Benjamin. The trip was the first leg of a world tour that would end his life. In 1933, the Reich destroyed the institute and burned its library. Although Hirschfeld lived in France for a time, he would never return to his native Germany and died in Nice in 1935.

Hirschfeld originated the theory of "sexual intermediaries" that feature psychological inclinations and behaviors. He believed that innate gender was biological in nature and that culture should adapt its rules and laws to human biology. Although the root words had originated in Italian and French (Zagria, 2018), he popularized the term **transvestite** in German and English, a term that has incorrectly acquired the connotation that being transgender is associated with sexual arousal, so it has become a transgender taboo word.

His research is further discussed in Chapter 11.

Milton Diamond (1934–), Biopsychologist

Milton Diamond is a professor emeritus of anatomy and reproductive biology at the University of Hawaii. He is a researcher and advocate for transgender and intersex people. Diamond received his PhD in psychology and anatomy from the University of Kansas. He became the president of the International Academy of Sex Research and the SSSS. His early work involved the effects of prenatal sex hormones on sexual behavior in infrahuman species (Diamond, 1960).

Diamond believes that neither transgender nor intersex conditions are pathological and should not be treated as disorders. He advocated that intersex children should not receive genital plastic surgery until they can reasonably give informed consent. He was in conflict with John Money over whether intersex children could be given genital plastic surgery at birth and assigned arbitrarily to a gender behavior category.

Money believed that congruent gender behavior was malleable and seemed to have found a perfect test case in the person of David Reimer, who suffered a circumcision accident as an infant and received genital plastic surgery and sex hormones. What made the case more interesting was that David was an identical twin whose behavior could also be observed and found to be masculine. David was raised as a girl, Brenda, but his gender behavior was in conflict with his assigned feminine gender, indicating that there was a biological predisposition that had not been considered. Money covered up his results with David and indicated that all was going well, but Diamond tracked down the adult David and found that he had adopted a masculine gender and had married and adopted children. David committed suicide at the age of 34 with indications that his assignment to the feminine gender contributed to his depression. The case was documented in a book that became a *New York Times* bestseller: *As Nature Made Him: The Boy That Was Raised as a Girl* (Colapinto, 2000).

Diamond has continued his research and published an article containing retrospective data on identical twins in which one twin was transgender (Diamond, 2013). In this study, about one-third of the twin pairs were both transitioning transgender, although this may have been an underestimate because the physicians surveyed were not required to collect data on twins of their patients.

John Money (1921–2006), Psychologist

John Money is primarily known for his repurposing of the word "gender" from language grammars and for his theory that, if young enough, all children could adapt to either gender behavior category with supporting surgeries, hormones, and appropriate parental supervision. He is also known for his theory of "lovemaps." Money was from New Zealand and received master's degrees in psychology and education from Victoria

University of Wellington. He later received his PhD from Harvard in 1952. He became a professor of pediatrics and psychology at Johns Hopkins University in 1951.

The idea to use the word gender came from the need to separate sex from gender, as Money could not tell the child's actual sex from external genitalia at a young age. The study of genetics had not developed, and has not yet developed, to the point where it could be definitively used to determine sex, so the common procedure still is for physicians to inspect external genitalia at birth and make a determination based on anatomy. Nevertheless, Money needed a way of describing his recommendations to parents about how to raise their intersex children. Money used the term gender role in contradistinction to sex.

He oversaw the David Reimer case in which he tried to demonstrate that David, who had received penis damage during circumcision, could be raised as a girl. In his later career, Money admitted that David Reimer had not adapted to his presumed new gender but insisted that this one case did not disprove his theory about gender role adaptation.

Money published research and a book on "lovemaps" (Money, 1986), which sought to explain how people developed their sexual preferences. According to Money, a lovemap is formed based on early learning with elaboration of detail in later life.

Money supported research on genital plastic surgery and transgender genital plastic surgery, which had been further developed at Johns Hopkins Hospital. Money was a founder of the Pediatric Gender Clinic as well as participating in the Sexual Behaviors Unit, which researched transgender genital plastic surgery. Evidence pertaining to both of these types of procedures resulted in improvements to both procedures. From 1965 to 1979, Johns Hopkins led the way in developing transgender genital plastic surgery in the United States. But under new management in 1979, research was discontinued. Techniques for transgender genital plastic surgery were already practiced outside of the clinic, so the Johns Hopkins and other gender centers were discontinued for a time. In 2017, Johns Hopkins reopened its gender clinics as have numerous other university research hospitals and medical centers.

Virginia Prince (1912–2009), Advocate and Researcher

Prince received a PhD in pharmacology in 1939 from the University of California, San Francisco, and spent much of her life there after a divorce. She was a founder of the first transgender support group, which became the Society for the Second Self in 1972. One objective of this heterosexual, nontransitioning group was to encourage marriages to continue. She published newsletters (*Transvestia*), how-to books (Prince, 1980, and advocacy books (Prince, 1960).

Although Virginia Prince is primarily known as an advocate for transgender people, she also was involved in large-scale research surveys to characterize transgender people in terms of demographics, childhood, sex and gender behavior, and marriage. With Peter Bentler at UCLA (1972), she conducted a survey of 504 transwomen, and later with Richard Docter at Cal State Northridge she conducted a study of 1,032 transwomen (Docter & Prince, 1997). The latter study showed that most had married (83%) and 60 percent were still married at the time of the survey. Compared with the results of the Bentler survey, 45 percent, as opposed to the previous 25 percent, had sought counseling and 5 percent were more inclined to transition. The percentage considering going full-time had also increased. Prince also conducted research on transmen (Bentler & Prince, 1969).

Lou Sullivan (1951–1991), Advocate

Lou Sullivan was an advocate for transmen and for people to be considered for TGPS regardless of sexual orientation. He founded FTM International, one of the first organizations to support transmen. Sullivan was denied transgender genital plastic surgery several times because his sexual orientation was to be attracted to males. At the time, although most lead providers believed that heterosexuality should not be a barrier to TGPS, some of their associates still held the impression that a female had to be sexually oriented toward other females in order to transition.

Sullivan started an advocacy campaign to allow homosexuals to obtain transgender genital plastic surgery. His advocacy began in his hometown of Milwaukee, Wisconsin, with articles entitled "A Transvestite Answers a Feminist" and "Looking Towards Trans Liberation," which were widely distributed in the community. He became the editor of the influential *Gateway* newsletter of the Gateway Gender Alliance in San Francisco. He wrote a biography about Jack Bee Garland, an early transman (Sullivan, 1990) and wrote pamphlets providing information to transmen. He lobbied both the American Psychiatric Association and WPATH to eliminate sexual orientation as a criterion for transition. In this campaign he was supported by the psychologist Lin Fraser.

Shortly after obtaining TGPS in 1986, Sullivan was diagnosed with HIV/AIDS, and he died in 1991.

CONTEMPORARY FIGURES

Walter Bockting (ca. 1963–), Psychologist

Dr. Bockting is an expert in the assessment and treatment of transgender people. He received his PhD from Vrije University, Amsterdam, in 1998 (DCP) and 1998 (PhD) and is a fellow of the Society for the Scientific Study of Sexuality (SSSS). He next directed transgender health services for 20 years at the Program in Human Sexuality at the University of Minnesota. Bockting is currently a professor of medical psychology in Psychiatry and Nursing at Columbia University where he is a co-director of the LGBT Health Initiative Division of Gender and Sexuality. He is a past president of WPATH, the editor of the *International Journal of Transgenderism,* and a coauthor of the WPATH Standards of Care, Version 7. He is on the

Three Unsung Female Transgender Providers and Advocates

While in the 1980s most of the advocacy was being conducted on the West or East Coasts of the United States, there was one trans advocate, **Dallas Denny,** who made inroads into the South. She is a transwoman who received her academic degrees in Tennessee but moved to Atlanta. There she organized the American Education Gender Information Service Support (AEGIS) group and became a prolific writer and editor. Her newsletters, *Chrysalis Journal* and *Tapestry Journal,* provided a beacon of hope and information. She was a founder of the Southern Comfort Conference, which brought thousands of people to Atlanta, increasing transgender visibility. She received the highest transgender awards—the Trinity Award, the Virginia Prince Award, and the Fantasia Fair Pioneer Award.

Virginia Erhardt quietly went her way helping transgender people and their spouses/partners manage their relationships. From what she learned, she provides know-how to other providers. Since most transgender people live in secret but 50 percent do get married, she was concerned with the welfare of probably the largest trans demographic. She frequently led the Significant-Other track of the Southern Comfort Conference. Virginia was a practitioner of the affirmative approach for transgender adults. She contributed articles to *Transgender Tapestry* and *Transgender Community News* and was a columnist for *Southern Voice.*

It took a lot of professional courage but **Lin Fraser** advocated to allow transgender people to transition and receive TGPS without regard to their sexual orientation. She did this initially to help one of her patients, Louis Sullivan, a pioneering transman. They worked together to change policy in spite of entrenched resistance. The traditional view was that one had to be a homosexual pre-transition and a heterosexual post-transition. Lin also saw the need for provider education and started the Global Education Initiative when she was WPATH president.

editorial boards of the *Journal of Homosexuality*, the *Archives of Sexual Behavior*, and the *International Journal of Sexual Health*. A portion of his research has been sponsored by the American Foundation for AIDS Research and the National Institutes of Health. His research interests include gender development, transgender health, sexuality and the Internet, and HIV prevention.

Marci Bowers (1958–), OB-GYN and Surgeon

Marci Bowers is an obstetrician-gynecologist and surgeon who specializes in transgender genital plastic surgery. She currently practices in Burlingame, California. She received her medical degree from the University of Minnesota in 1986. Before moving to Trinidad, CO, to work with Stanley Biber on TGPS, she had a successful OB-GYN practice in Seattle, WA. Today, she is one of the world's leading TGPS surgeons, having helped more than 1,500 patients with transition since she began practicing. Bowers has made many media appearances to inform the public about transgender transition and to advocate for transgender procedures. She currently is a surgeon and guest professor at the Icahn School of Medicine at Mount Sinai in New York City where she assisted in the funding and accreditation of their surgical program. Dr. Bowers made the initial donation to a surgical fellowship at Mount Sinai in the Center for Transgender Medicine and Surgery in 2017. Open to fully trained plastic surgeons, the surgical fellowship is a 12-month program with exposure to the full range of gender confirmation surgical procedures, including chest wall, facial feminization, and genital procedures. She is a member of the board of directors at GLAAD and the Transgender Law Center and provides expertise for advocacy and policy initiatives for transgender people. She provides restorative procedures pro bono to those who have suffered female genital mutilation.

George Brown (1958–), Psychiatrist

George Brown has led the way for research on transgender U.S. military personnel and veterans with over 150 publications. Brown is a professor of psychiatry at East Tennessee State University in the Department of Psychiatry and Behavioral Sciences. While at ETSU he has had joint appointments with the Mountain Home Veterans Affairs Hospital. He is also the associate chairman for Veterans Affairs. He was chief of psychiatry at the VA for 16 years before being promoted to conduct health disparities research at the VA Central Office in Washington, DC. He served in the USAF on active duty as a psychiatrist, dealing with active duty transgender servicemen. Dr. Brown is a graduate of the University of Rochester School of Medicine and took his residency at Wright State University. He was on the faculty of the University of Texas Health Science Center before coming to East Tennessee in 1994.

Brown has contributed to 24 book chapters on transgender science. In particular, he has performed research on why transgender people are attracted to the military and assessed the suicide risk for transgender veterans receiving care in the Veterans Administration. Currently he is involved as a key expert witness for lawsuits involving transgender troops who want to stay in U.S. military service.

Brown was recently presented with the Lifetime Distinguished Scientific Achievement Award by the World Professional Association for Transgender Health. The award recognizes Brown for making important contributions to advancing the knowledge and quality of care in transgender health through the research he has conducted over his entire career. He served three terms on the WPATH Board of Directors and was a secretary-treasurer. He also is a distinguished Fellow of the American Psychiatric Association.

Peggy Cohen-Kettenis (ca. 1943–), Medical Psychologist

Dr. Cohen-Kettenis received her doctoral degree at the University of Utrecht in 1968. She spent 12 years at the University of Utrecht in the psychology department and the Department of Child and Adolescent Psychology. She then moved to the VU University Medical Center in the Department of Medical Psychology where she was named emerita in 2013 and where she continues to conduct research. She is a member of WPATH and a member of the World Health Organization working group on the classification of sexual disorders and sexual health. Dr. Cohen-Kettenis is a former member of the Board of Directors of WPATH and was the sub–working group chair on the DSM-5 committee.

Dr. Cohen-Kettenis is a pioneer in assessing and treating transgender youth. She and her colleagues developed protocols for the use of puberty blockers to relieve acute distress and suffering caused by secondary sex characteristic development. Blocking puberty provides time for transkids to make a balanced decision about natural puberty and/or transgender transition at age 16. The protocols recommend supporting transgender individuals in their congruent gender behavior category with the possibility of performing interventions that will help make the body of the individual more compatible with their gender.

Eli Coleman (1948–), Sexologist

Eli Coleman is a professor in the Family Medicine and Community Health Department at the University of Minnesota where he directs the

Program in Human Sexuality. He received his PhD from the University of Minnesota. He has published research on being transgender, sexual orientation, the coming-out process, and sexual dysfunction. He is a past president of WPATH, the World Association for Sexual Health, and was the founding editor of the *WPATH International Journal of Transgenderism*. Dr. Coleman was the leader of the formulation of the WPATH Standards of Care version 7 (Coleman et al., 2017) and is currently leading the development of version 8.

Griet De Cuypere (ca. 1965–), Medical Doctor and Advocate

Dr. De Cuypere studied at the University of Ghent, Belgium, and currently works in the Department of Sexology and Gender Problems, Ghent University Hospital, Belgium.

She twice served on the WPATH board and was the WPATH secretary from 2005 to 2007. She conducted research on transgender heritability and studied outcomes of TGPS in transmen. She has published over 60 articles on transgender science. Dr. De Cuypere contributed to the revision of SOC 6 based on consensus recommendations incorporated into SOC 7 and served as an advisor to the WHO for ICD-11.

Dallas Denny (1949–), Psychologist and Advocate

Dallas Denny is an award-winning psychologist and advocate for the transgender community as an educator, writer, and activist. She received what are considered the top two awards for transgender service: the Virginia Prince Lifetime Achievement Award and the Trinity Award.

Dallas Denny received a BS from Middle Tennessee State University in 1974 and an MA in psychology from the University of Tennessee, Knoxville, in 1979 as well as a PhD in special education from Vanderbilt University. She was a licensed psychologist in Tennessee. Until 2009, she provided psychological services near Atlanta for Decatur, DeKalb County, Georgia, and was adviser to the mayor of neighboring Atlanta.

Denny started an advocacy organization called American Education Gender Information Service. She was a founder of the Southern Comfort Conference in Atlanta and directed Fantasia Fair, the world's longest running transgender conference.

She is a prolific writer and speaker, having contributed to newsletters, textbooks, and journal articles as well as numerous transgender conferences. She was a contributor and editor of the *Chrysalis Journal* and *Transgender Tapestry Journal*. Denny has written over 20 book chapters and research papers on transgender advice and policy. She wrote six books including *Gender Dysphoria: A Guide to Research* (Denny, 1994). She is a frequent keynote and workshop speaker at conferences and meetings.

She started the National Transgender Library and Archive, which now resides in the Labadie Collection of the University of Michigan in Ann Arbor, MI.

Virginia Erhardt (1942–), Psychologist

Virginia Erhardt is a PhD clinical psychologist who specializes in understanding how to deal with relationships involving LGBT people. She has intensely studied couples who stay together after one member declares that they are transgender. She practiced in Decatur, GA but now lives in Eastsound, WA. She is a member of the American Association of Sex Educators, Counselors and Therapists (AASECT) and WPATH.

Dr. Erhardt has written books on transgender relationships (*Head over Heels,* 2006) and lesbian relationships (*Journey Towards Intimacy: A Handbook for Lesbian Couples,* 1977). She has contributed articles to *Transgender Tapestry* and *Transgender Community News.* She was also a columnist for the *Southern Voice* newspaper for three years. For many years, she led the SOFFA track at the Southern Comfort Conference. She has appeared on television as an expert on married couples who stay together during transgender transition.

Randi Ettner (1952–), Psychologist

Randi Ettner is a psychologist who works with transgender people using the "emotional freedom" technique to remove psychologically limiting beliefs, fears, and memories of trauma. She received her undergraduate degree from Indiana University, her master's degree from Roosevelt University, and her PhD degree from Northwestern University in 1979. Dr. Ettner is a diplomate in clinical evaluation, trauma, and post-traumatic stress disorder. She has twice served on the WPATH Board of Directors and has led committees working on transgender prisoner rights.

She has published three books on being transgender: most recently on transgender medical care—*Principles of Transgender Medicine & Surgery* (Ettner, Monstrey, & Coleman, 2016), transgender experiences—*Confessions of a Gender Defender: A Psychologist's Reflections on Life Among the Transgendered* (Ettner, 1996), and on effective counseling for transgender people and their loved ones—*Gender Loving Care* (Ettner, 1999).

As an advocate, she has helped get antidiscrimination laws passed and provided testimony on transgender workplace rights and prisoner rights.

Lin Fraser (1956–), Psychologist

Lin Fraser has been a leader in transgender care and has advocated to allow transition and TGPS regardless of sexual orientation. She received her bachelor's degree in psychology in 1967 from Duke University, her MA in counseling from San Francisco State University in 1975, and a doctorate in counseling psychology from the University of San Francisco.

She is a former president of WPATH and the founding member and co-chair of the WPATH Global Education Initiative, which seeks to train providers on transgender care through CEU courses. She is a member of the American Psychological Association and the California Association of Marriage and Family Therapists. Dr. Fraser has participated in development of the WPATH Standards of Care process for WPATH and has been on the editorial board of the WPATH *International Journal of Transgenderism* since 2006.

Jamison Green (1948–), Advocate and Lawyer

Jamison Green is a leader in advocacy for transgender health, civil rights, and social safety. He led an initiative with Fortune 500 companies to eliminate transgender exclusions from insurance policies. He received his BA and MFA at the University of Oregon, and he was awarded a PhD in law from Manchester Metropolitan University, Manchester, United Kingdom. He was on the adjunct faculty of the California Institute of Integral Studies where he taught Gender and Society in the PhD in Human Sexuality Program.

He has been a president, board member, and communications director for WPATH; has served on the board of the Transgender Law and Policy Institute; and was the leader of the FTM International organization.

Green has published numerous articles, contributed book chapters, and published his own book—*Becoming a Visible Man* (Green, 2004), which was awarded best book by the Center for Lesbian and Gay Studies and was a finalist in the Lambda Literary Awards in 2004. He is a coauthor of the WPATH Standards of Care, version 7.

Mara Keisling (1959–), Advocate and Researcher

Mara Keisling is the founder (2003) and current executive director of the National Center for Transgender Equality. She received her undergraduate degree in social science from Pennsylvania State University and did graduate work in government at Harvard University.

Before moving from Pennsylvania to Washington, DC, she served on the board of the LGBTQ youth group Common Roads, and she was on the steering committee of the Statewide Pennsylvania Rights Coalition. Once moving to Washington, she conducted social marketing and opinion research in the public health area. She was an adjunct professor at George Mason University and Marymount University, teaching courses in government.

As leader of the National Center for Transgender Equality (NCTE), she has partnered with other organizations to achieve advances in transgender equality. She championed the inclusion of gender nondiscrimination in federal employment nondiscrimination bills. She helped build a partnership of organizations called the UnitedENDA coalition. Under her direction, NCTE developed the first trans-inclusive federal legislation, the Matthew Shepard Act; facilitated changes in State Department rules for changing sex markers on passports; and organized the first congressional hearing on being transgender. NCTE partnered with the National Gay and Lesbian Task Force to conduct a large-scale national transgender survey and issue the report—*Injustice at Every Turn* (Grant et al., 2011). NCTE also reported on the results of *The 2015 National Transgender Survey* in 2016 (James et al., 2016).

Gail Knudson (1975–), Psychiatrist

Gail Knudson is a clinical professor in the Department of Psychiatry at the University of British Columbia Medical School. She attended the University of Alberta, Dalhousie University, and the University of British Columbia (UBC) before becoming a clinical professor at UBC and consulting psychiatrist at the UBC Centre for Sexual Medicine in 2000.

She served as president of WPATH from 2016 to 2018 and fostered the development of WPATH Policy Statements, the Global Education Initiative, and a certification process for providers on transgender care. WPATH policy statements have been issued on such topics as transgender service in the military, rapid onset gender dysphoria, and requiring surgery to obtain personal identification documents.

She has authored over 30 research reports including the WPATH SOC version 7. Topics of other papers include review of TGPS (Berli, Knudson, & Schechter, 2017) and transitioning transgender fertility maintenance options (Knudson & De Sutter, 2017).

Arlene Istar Lev (ca. 1958–), Social Worker

Arlene Istar Lev is a clinical social worker and independent scholar whose work encompasses topics in gender, sexual orientation, and sexuality as well as LGBTQ family dynamics. Lev developed the Transgender Emergence Model as the process that transgender people go through to realize their congruent gender. She received her bachelor's degree at Binghamton University in 1979 and her master's of social work degree from State University of New York at Albany (SUNY-Albany) in 1986. She has been a lecturer at SUNY-Albany School of Social Welfare and adjunct professor and lecturer at several colleges in the northeastern United States.

Lev is the author of an important book about transgender people—*Transgender Emergence* (Lev, 2004). This book was chosen for an award by Division 44 of the American Psychological Association and the Society for Sex Therapy and Research. She has written over 10 chapters and 20 journal articles in various books and journals on LGBTQ treatment. She is a co-author of the popular book *The Gender Quest Workbook* for teenagers (Testa, Coolhart, Peta, & Lev, 2015). She has also published *The Complete Lesbian and Gay Parenting Guide* (2004) to support GLB families.

Lev is on the board of the American Family Therapy Academy and serves on the editorial board of the WPATH *International Journal of Transgenderism*. She participated in the development of the WPATH SOC, version 7.

Joan Roughgarden (1946–), Evolutionary Biologist

Joan Roughgarden challenged Darwin's sexual selection theory and in doing so changed our ideas of sex and gender diversity to oppose sex and gender stereotyping in our culture. Dr. Roughgarden received her BS degree in biology and BA degree in philosophy from the University of Rochester in 1968. She received her PhD in biology in 1971. She was an assistant professor of biology at the University of Massachusetts and later became a full professor at Stanford University. After retiring in 2012, she became an adjunct professor at the Hawaii Institute of Marine Biology.

She has authored several books and over 180 scientific articles, but she is primarily known in the transgender community for her book *Evolution's Rainbow* (2004). In this book and her writings, she challenges Darwinian theories of sexual selection, which result in stereotyped notions of sex and gender. These stereotypes are harmful to transgender acceptance but also to females who are stereotyped. She subsequently developed a replacement for the sexual selection theory.

Joshua Safer (ca. 1964–), Endocrinologist

Joshua Safer is the executive director of the Center for Transgender Medicine and Surgery at the Icahn School of Medicine at Mount Sinai in New York City. He is an expert on transgender hormone treatment procedures. Prior to this position he was the director of the Center for Transgender Medicine and Surgery at Boston University Medical School. He received his medical degree from the University of Wisconsin and completed both an internal medicine residency at Mount Sinai Beth Israel and an endocrinology fellowship at Beth Israel Deaconess Medical Center in Boston.

Safer is currently the president of the United States Professional Association for Transgender Health (USPATH), serves on several WPATH activities including the Global Education Initiative and the Standards of Care revision, and was scientific co-chair for a WPATH international meeting. He also served as a Transgender Medicine Guidelines Drafting Group member for the International Olympic Committee.

Safer has authored or coauthored 71 papers in peer-reviewed journals, including many critical reviews, textbook chapters, and case reports in endocrinology and transgender medicine. He wrote a series of online articles/tutorials on transgender care on the Endocrine Web for providers.

Vin Tangpricha (ca. 1971–), Endocrinologist

Vin Tangpricha is a professor of endocrinology at Emory University and the current president of WPATH. He received his bachelor's degree in 1992 at Case Western Reserve in biology and anthropology. Dr. Tangpricha later graduated with his medical degree from Tufts Medical School. He completed his residency and PhD in molecular medicine and residency at Boston University, and joined Emory in 2004. He provides care for transgender patients as well as those with vitamin D deficiency, osteoporosis, and cystic fibrosis.

Tangpricha is a member of the American College of Endocrinology, the Board of Directors of the American Association of Clinical Endocrinologists, and was a board member and president-elect for WPATH.

He has published over 200 peer-reviewed research articles, reviews, and book chapters. He serves on several national and international committees related to his clinical and research work. He also was a coauthor of the Endocrine Society guidelines for the medical care of transgender people.

Dr. Tangpricha was chosen as one of the top endocrinologists by *U.S. News and World Report* and received the Outstanding Service Award for the Promotion of Endocrine Health of an Underserved Population from the American Association of Clinical Endocrinologists.

EMERGING FIGURES

Madeline Deutsch (1972–), Physician and Public Health Researcher

Maddie Deutsch is an associate professor of clinical family and community medicine and is the director of UCSF Transgender Care, the clinical branch of the UCSF Center of Excellence for Transgender Health. She graduated from SUNY Binghamton University in computer science in 1994, Hudson Valley Community College in 1995 (paramedic certificate), SUNY Purchase Premedical Studies in 1996, Rosalind Franklin University School of Medicine (MD degree) in 2001, and graduated from UCLA (MPH) in community health sciences in 2015. She was appointed an associate professor at UCSF in 2009 in the Transgender Care Navigation Program.

Dr. Deutsch is the principal investigator in a study of methods for collection of gender data in a clinical setting, and a co-principal investigator in a California HIV/AIDS program to study HIV pre-exposure prophylaxis (PrEP) in transgender populations.

She is on the Board of Directors of the U.S. Professional Association for Transgender Health (USPATH) and is the lead author for the "Primary Care" chapter in the upcoming eighth revision of the World Professional Association for Transgender Health (WPATH) Standards of Care.

She has over 25 research publications. Her research interests include transgender treatment (Deutsch, Bhakri, & Kubicek, 2015; Feldman et al., 2016), transgender electronic health record processes (Deutsch & Buchholz, 2015), and prevention and care for transgender people with regard to HIV/AIDS (Poteat et al., 2014). Dr. Deutsch is the editor of the online *Guidelines for the Primary and Gender-Affirming Care of Transgender and Gender Nonbinary People* (Deutsch, 2016). She is a member of the editorial boards for the journals *LGBT Health*, *Transgender Health*, and the *International Journal of Transgenderism*.

Miroslave Djordjevic (1965–), Surgeon

Miroslave Djordjevic is a leader in TGPS for transmen and a professor of urology and surgery at the University of Belgrade, School of Medicine, Serbia. He and his colleagues have made Belgrade a medico-tourism and teaching center for transgender surgeries based on quality of expertise. Dr. Djordievic received his MD degree and finished his residency at the Belgrade School of Medicine where he now teaches and trained under Sava Perovic, an acknowledged expert in urologic surgery. He also is a member of the Center for Transgender Medicine and Surgery, Mount Sinai, New York City for international instruction. He has traveled all over the world to help people needing reconstructive surgery, in particular with the organization INTERPLAST. He is a member of numerous surgical societies as well as WPATH, and he has received awards and honors from the European Society for Sexual Medicine, the European Association of Urology, and the German Urological Association.

He has over 90 publications on various topics, especially TGPS techniques for transmen as well as surgery for intersex conditions and reconstructive surgery of the penis. He has edited or served on the editorial board of major urology journals, and he has given over 45 invited lectures and presentations around the world.

Diane Ehrensaft (1946–), Psychologist

Diane Ehrensaft is a psychologist who studies and treats transgender children. She is an advocate of affirmative care for transgender children, which features careful observation of the gender behavior of children. Diane Ehrensaft received both her undergraduate and PhD degrees from the University of Michigan. She is an adjunct associate professor at UCSF in the Pediatrics Department, which she combines with her private practice. She is on the Board of Directors for Gender Spectrum and a member of WPATH.

Ehrensaft has written two highly influential books to help providers, parents, and teachers understand and deal with transgender children using affirmative approaches. These two books are *Gender Made, Gender Born* (Ehrensaft, 2011) and *The Gender Creative Child* (Ehrensaft, 2016). In the former book, Ehrensaft provides information and tools to optimally raise transgender children. In the latter, she deals with the spectrum of gender behaviors in transgender children as well as explaining gender fluidity. In addition to these books, she also has written over 50 articles, reports, and presentations.

She has won several awards and fellowships including an Award for Outstanding Service from the Section on Childhood and Adolescence, Division of Psychoanalysis, American Psychological Association in 2013.

Kristina Olson (1981–), Psychologist

Kristina Olson is an award-winning psychologist who studies transgender children. She received her undergraduate degree from Washington University and PhD from Harvard University in 2008. She was an assistant professor at Yale until she moved to the Department of Psychology at the University of Washington in 2013.

Olson received the Janet Taylor Spence Award from the Association for Psychological Science in 2013 for her early career achievements, and the Sage Young Scholars Award in 2014. She received the coveted Alan Waterman Award from the National Science Foundation because of her early career research, and in 2018 she became a MacArthur "Genius" Fellow.

Currently, Olson directs the TransYouth Project, which is the largest longitudinal study of transgender children. The objective of this research is to improve understanding of human gender development. The project's recent findings indicated that transgender youth are not confused about their congruent gender identity and are not pretending or seeking attention from it (Olson, Forbes, & Belzer, 2011; Olson, Key, & Eaton, 2015). Transkids score the same as cisgender children on social gender knowledge. Subsequent findings have indicated that they do not suffer adverse mental health outcomes but that supportive parents and families are critical to their mental health.

Johanna Olson-Kennedy (1969–), Physician

Johanna Olson-Kennedy is an expert in care for transgender youth and is board certified in both pediatrics and adolescent medicine. She is a pioneer in providing medical intervention for transgender youth including the affirmative approach with puberty suppression. As assistant professor, she is the leader of the Center for Transyouth Health and Development at Children's Hospital Los Angeles, the largest transgender youth center in the United States. She is also an associate professor of clinical pediatrics at the Keck School of Medicine, University of Southern California. She obtained her MD from the Chicago School of Medicine and completed a residency and fellowship at Children's Hospital of Orange County.

Dr. Olson-Kennedy is a member of the board of USPATH, the U.S. affiliate of WPATH. She is a member of WPATH, the Society for Pediatric Research, and the Society for Adolescent Health and Medicine.

She currently leads a longitudinal clinical research study to evaluate the impact of puberty suppression in transgender youth. This includes detection of potential physiological side effects, bone development, growth, and cognition. Another aspect of this study is to evaluate HT for gender transition in later stages of puberty development. The study network includes four academic institutions with gender clinics in the United States. She has numerous publications including a prominent review of transyouth treatment (Olson, Forbes, & Belzer, 2011).

Dr. Olson-Kennedy has appeared frequently on national media and provided presentations to providers, parents, and other communities in the United States about the needs of transgender youth.

REFERENCES

Benjamin, H. (1966). *The transsexual phenomenon.* http://www.mut23.de/texte/Harry%20Benjamin%20-%20The%20Transsexual%20Phenomenon.pdf

Bentler, P. M., & Prince, C. (1969). Personality characteristics of male transvestites. *Journal of Abnormal Psychology, 74*(2), 40–43.

Berli, J. U., Knudson, G., & Schechter, L. (2017). Gender confirmation surgery and terminology in transgender health. *Journal of the American Medical Association Surgery, 152*(11), 1091.

Colapinto, J. (2000). *As nature made him: The boy who was raised as a girl.* New York: HarperCollins.

Coleman, E., et al. (2017). *Standards of care for the health of transsexual, transgender and gender nonconforming people.* Chicago: World Professional Association for Transgender Health. https://wpath.org/publications/soc (Confirmed December 27, 2018.)

Denny, D. (1994). *Gender dysphoria: A guide to research.* New York: Garland.

Deutsch, M. (2016). *Guidelines for the primary and gender-affirming care of transgender and gender nonbinary people.* Center of Excellence for Transgender Health, Department of Family & Community Medicine, University of California, San Francisco. https://www.sccgov.org/sites/bhd/info/Documents/LGBTQ%20Resources/ucsf-guidelines-for-the-primary-and-gender-affirming-care-of-transgender-and-gender-nonbinary-people-6-17-16.pdf

Deutsch, M. B., Bhakri, V., & Kubicek, K. (2015). Effects of cross-sex hormone treatment on transgender women and men. *Obstetrics and Gynecology, 125*(3), 605–610.

Deutsch, M. B., & Buchholz, D. (2015). Electronic health records and transgender patients—practical recommendations for the collection of gender identity data. *Journal of General Internal Medicine, 30*(6), 843–847.

Diamond, M. (1960). Comparative and structural effects of androgen injected into pregnant and non-pregnant guinea pigs. *Anatomical Record, 137,* 34.

Diamond, M. (2013). Transsexuality among twins: Identity concordance, transition, rearing and orientation. *International Journal of Transgenderism, 14,* 24–38.

Docter, R. F., & Prince, V. (1997). Transvestism: A survey of 1032 cross-dressers. *Archives of Sexual Behavior, 26*(6), 589–605.

Ehrensaft, D. (2011). *Gender made, gender born.* New York: Experiment Press.

Ehrensaft, D. (2016). *The gender creative child.* New York: Experiment Press.

Erhardt, V. (1977). *Journey toward intimacy: A handbook for lesbian couples.* New York: Couples Enrichment Institute.

Erhardt, V. (2006). *Head over heels: Wives who stay with cross-dressers and transsexuals.* Abingdon-on-Thames: Routledge.

Ettner, R. (1996). *Confessions of a gender defender: A psychologist's reflections on life among the transgendered.* Chicago: Spectrum Press.

Ettner, R. (1999). *Gender loving care: A guide to counseling gender-variant clients.* New York: W. W. Norton.

Ettner, R., Monstrey, S., & Coleman, E. (2016). *Principles of transgender medicine and surgery.* Abingdon-on-Thames: Routledge.

Feldman, J., Brown, G. R., Deutsch, M. B., Hembree, W., Meyer, W., Meyer-Bahlburg, H. F. L., . . . Safer, J. D. (2016). Priorities for transgender medical and healthcare research. *Current Opinion in Endocrinology, Diabetes and Obesity, 23*(2), 180–187.

Fox, M. (2006, January). Stanley H. Biber, 82, surgeon among first to do sex change operations (obituary). *New York Times.* https://www.nytimes.com/2006/01/21/us/stanley-h-biber-82-surgeon-among-first-to-do-sex-changes-dies.html

Grant, J. M., Mottet, L. A., Tanis, J., Harrison, J., Herman, J. L., & Keisling, M. (2011). *Injustice at every turn: A report of the national transgender discrimination survey.* National Center for Transgender Equality and National Gay and Lesbian Task Force.

Green, J. (2004). *Becoming a visible man.* Nashville: Vanderbilt University Press.

Hirschfeld, M. (1991). *Transvestites: The erotic drive to cross-dress* (M. A. Lombardi, Trans.). Amherst: Prometheus Books. (Original work published 1911.)

James, S. E., Herman, J. L., Rankin, S., Keisling, M., Mottet, L., & Anafi, M. (2016). *Report of the 2015 U.S. Transgender Survey.* Washington, DC: National Center for Transgender Equality.

Knudson, G., & De Sutter, P. (2017). Fertility options in transgender and gender diverse adolescents. *Acta Obstetrica Gynecologica Scandanavia, 96*(10), 1269–1272.

Lev, A. I. (2004). *The complete lesbian and gay parenting guide.* New York: Penguin Group.

Lev, A. I. (2004). *Transgender emergence: Therapeutic guidelines for working with gender-variant people and their families.* New York: Haworth.

Money, J. (1986). *Lovemaps: Clinical concepts of sexual/erotic health and pathology, paraphilia, and gender transposition in childhood, adolescence, and maturity.* New York: Prometheus Books.

Olson, J., Forbes., C., & Belzer, M. (2011). Management of the transgender adolescent. *Archives of Pediatrics & Adolescent Medicine, 165*(2), 171–176.

Olson, K. R., Key, A. C., & Eaton, N. R. (2015). Gender cognition in transgender children. *Psychological Science,* 26(4), 467–474.

Poteat, T., et al. (2014). HIV risk and preventive interventions in transgender women sex workers. *The Lancet, 385,* 9964.

Prince, V. (1960) The transvestite and his wife. San Francisco: Charles Prince.

Prince, V. (1980). *How to be a woman though male.* San Francisco: Chevalier Publications.

Prince, V., & Bentler, P. M. (1972). Survey of 504 cases of transvestism. *Psychological Reports, 31*(3), 903–917.

Roughgarden, J. (2004). *Evolution's rainbow: Diversity, gender and sexuality in nature and people.* Berkeley: University of California Press.

Rudacille, D. (2005). *The riddle of gender* (p. 83). New York: Pantheon.

Stryker, S. (2008). *Transgender history* (p. 39). Berkeley, CA: Seal Press.

Sullivan, L. (1990). *From female to male: The life of Jack Bee Garland.* Boston: Alyson Books.

Testa, R. J., Coolhart, D., Peta, J., & Lev, A. I. (2015). *The gender quest workbook: A guide for teens and young adults exploring gender identity.* Oakland, CA: New Harbinger Publications, Instant Help.

Zagria. (2018). A gender variance who's who. https://zagria.blogspot.com/2009/03/did-magnus-hirschfeld-coin-word.html#.XB_I4S2ZPzI

PART 2

Practice

6

Applications in the Field: Clientele, Presentation, and Screening

PROVIDER SERVICES FOR TRANSGENDER PEOPLE

Most providers will come into contact with transgender people whose chief complaints have nothing at all to do with being transgender. Being transgender is not rare; estimates are at least .7–1.0 percent of the population are transgender. Those providers need to know about being transgender in order to establish a provider-patient relationship that fulfills the medical or mental health needs of the patient. Just as providers learn to speak other languages and understand about patient subcultures to communicate with their patients and gain rapport, providers need to understand the basics of being transgender and try to understand transgender language and expectations. These providers need to guard against assumptions that all chief complaints are related to being transgender. It has even been reported that there is a recent trend for providers to engage in the "transgender broken arm" syndrome (O'Hara, 2015; Theodosiou, 2018).

This provider syndrome includes misdiagnosis, overtreatment, and overtesting because of curiosity about being transgender or the fallacious assumption that all complaints by transgender people require consultations with mental health providers. These reports prompted the Royal College of Psychiatrists to issue a public statement warning providers about these tendencies (Royal College of Psychiatrists, 2018).

Some providers will treat transgender people for chief complaints related to their being transgender. These complaints feature cultural and family rejection as well as wanting to modify their bodies through transgender transition. Transition involves making their bodies more compatible with what the culture expects of a person in their congruent gender behavior category. These providers need to master the knowledge of transgender treatments in their specialty and know the WPATH Standards of Care (WPATH, 2011) as well as guidelines from mental health and medical professional organizations. These include the Endocrine Society (Hembree et al., 2017), the American Psychological Association (American Psychological Association, 2015), UCSF Center of Excellence for Transgender Health (Deutsch, 2016), UCSF Health Considerations for Gender Non-conforming Children and Transgender Adolescents (Olson-Kennedy, Rosenthal, Hastings, & Wesp, 2018), and others as needed.

WPATH recommends that a provider who chooses to perform transgender procedures should also work with experienced transgender providers to gain expertise, which may take several months. Adequate experience with surgical and other procedures may take longer. Although the numbers are growing, there are very few providers who have the requisite experience. Transgender treatment is not an officially recognized specialty in the medical and mental health domains, although most knowledgeable transgender people learn from their peers as to who are the most skilled and trusted providers.

Providers need to understand that privacy of transgender people is paramount. Many transgender people rightly believe that their careers, family relations, and lives would be in danger if the information that they are transgender or receiving transgender treatment were to be revealed. Approximately 80–90 percent of transgender people are in the closet, meaning that their transgender status is known only to themselves or trusted family and/or friends. In the past, transgender people have often refrained from giving information on their transgender status to providers, even though this may interfere with interpretation of test results and diagnosis. This is particularly true in the case of transgender transition hormone therapy (HT), which influences physiological systems. But in the past several years, this tendency has been reversed and most transgender people now come out to providers and respond to surveys (Cahill et al.,

2014; Grant et al., 2011; Haider et al., 2017; Ruben, Blosnich, Dichter, Luscri, & Shipherd, 2017). The statistics are that 28 percent said that they were out to all their providers, another 38 percent said that they were out to most providers, and 33 percent said that they were out to some providers (Grant et al., 2011; Ruben et al., 2017).

Providers must still be careful to preserve the privacy of patients from their families who may not know that they are transgender.

Providers must not assume that transgender people are ignorant of transgender science or treatment; many are quite knowledgeable and well informed. Many transgender people, over 50 percent, report that they had to educate their providers on aspects of being transgender (Grant et al., 2011; Ruben et al., 2017). Information on being transgender is now plentiful on the Internet and elsewhere, and word travels quickly through transgender groups and networks. Of course, information from other than provider sources may be inaccurate, and it is still the responsibility of the provider to recommend the best course of action.

Education and training on being transgender is still lacking for providers. Medical and nursing schools are starting to cover transgender treatment in professional school curricula but progress is slow (Dubin et al., 2018). In some schools, initiatives have come from medical students themselves (Grosz et al., 2017) and in other schools, electives for medical students have involved direct care for transgender people (Park & Safer, 2018). WPATH and other organizations offer short courses and certifications for professional development, but these are not intended to be used as legal qualifications.

Feedback from transgender surveys indicates that all is not well between providers and transgender patients. A recent survey found that 33 percent of transgender people experienced negative provider encounters including harassment, being mocked, slurred, laughed at, pointed at, or taunted, or being refused care because they were transgender (Grant et al., 2011). A Williams Institute survey reported that 70 percent of transgender people reported harassment or maltreatment including refusal to touch them, abusive language, or blaming the patient for being transgender. In the same survey, 27 percent of transgender people reported that they were denied health care due to being transgender (Herman, Flores, Brown, Wilson, & Conron, 2017). In another survey transgender patients reported gender insensitivity, displays of discomfort, denied services, substandard care, verbal abuse, forced care, and being denied restroom use (Kosenko, Rintamaki, Raney, & Maness, 2013). Rejection by providers and provider organizations results in hesitancy for transgender people to obtain professional care, and they often opt for dangerous self-treatment (Rotondi, Bauer, Scanlon, Kaay, & Traver, 2013) such as do-it-yourself hormone therapy (HT).

DEMOGRAPHICS OF TRANSGENDER PEOPLE

There are transgender people in almost all demographic categories, and being transgender is not rare. Two of the four causal factors are biological and not due to learning or culture-genetic behavior predisposition and epigenetics unblocking. Considering these biological factors, a wide demographic spread is understandable. Precise demographic information is lacking because governments are reticent to collect it due to cultural rejection of being transgender. For example, collection of data about transgender status was recently deleted from the 2020 U.S. Census and the National Survey of Older Americans (Cahill et al., 2014). Another complicating factor is that most transgender people still live in secrecy or partial secrecy and do not want to publicly admit their transgender status on surveys.

Because being transgender is not a disease state, the term population frequency is used in this book instead of the term prevalence, which has pathological connotations for some people. The term population frequency is intended to be mathematically equivalent. Estimates from gender clinics of population frequencies in the early 20th century were extremely low since they only counted those who presented at hospital or university clinics.

The best recent estimates of transgender demographics in the United States come from estimation models based on counting transgender people in support groups, throughput of providers who perform transgender genital plastic surgery, and analysis of data collected by the CDC Behavioral Risk Fact Surveillance System (BRSS). The BRSS was not intended for this purpose, and not all states allow collection of transgender status information. Analysis requires use of demographic data from those states that do allow transgender status information to be collected and projected to other states on their demographic bases.

A lower bound estimate of population frequency of being transgender for transwomen is at least 1 percent, for transitioning transwomen at .1 percent, and those receiving TGPS at .025 percent (Conway, 2001–2002; Olyslager & Conway, 2007). These estimates were based on an engineering estimation model with data from support groups on those providers who serve transitioning transgender people.

There are two primary teams that have analyzed the BRSS data streams with regard to transgender demographics. One is centered at the Williams Institute at UCLA and the other consists of a team of OB-GYN providers from the University of Michigan.

Williams Institute results indicate that the population frequency for being transgender now stand at .5–.7% of the population with results for the data in the 13–24 age group being .7 percent (Herman et al., 2017).

Survey estimates for transmen is .3 percent (Flores, Herman, Gates, & Brown, 2016). The results of these statistical estimates from the BRSS have gradually increased as being transgender becomes more tolerated and accepted. Using these estimates, the overall population of the United States includes at least 1.4 million transgender people (Flores et al., 2016).

The Williams team also analyzed age population statistics for transgender people, which follow the same general pattern as the population at large, with 64 percent of transgender people being adults whereas 63 percent of the population are adult (Herman et al., 2017). The frequencies of being transgender are slightly higher in younger age groups and slightly lower in the 65 and older group. Estimates for the 13–17 age group, which is the critical group for treatment of transgender youth, indicate that .7 percent of the population or at least 150,000 children are transgender. The numbers of people seeking transgender treatments has also greatly accelerated in the past several years.

Analysis by the Michigan team using the CDC Risk Survey data was released somewhat later than the Williams team analysis. This team found that transgender people were not significantly different from nontransgender people in regard to marital status, employment, rural living, and age (Crissman, 2014). From their analysis, transgender people were somewhat more likely (13 percent more) to be people of color and 11 percent more likely to live in extreme poverty. Transgender people were less likely (21 percent) to have started college. Transwomen were somewhat more likely (14 percent) to live in rural areas.

There are additional survey estimates of demographics in Europe and elsewhere. Their results vary with the questions asked but follow the same trends (for a summary see Bevan, 2017). With regard to transitioning transgender people, estimates from surveys indicate that the frequency of transitioning transwomen is .1 percent (Conway, 2001–2002) and for transmen at .07 percent (Horton, 2008).

Recent surveys of high school students found that 1.3 percent of both transgirls and transboys reported being transgender (Eisenberg et al., 2017). However, this survey was done in San Francisco where one might expect that the population is more likely to self-report being transgender.

Large deficits in health care among transgender people were found in a major online survey conducted by the National Center for Transgender Equality and the National Gay and Lesbian Task force (Grant et al., 2011). The survey of transgender people indicated:

> Health outcomes for all categories of respondents show the appalling effects of social and economic marginalization, including much higher rates of HIV infection, smoking, drug and alcohol use and suicide attempts than the general population.

Refusal of care: 19% of our sample reported being refused medical care due to their transgender or gender nonconforming status, with even higher numbers among people of color in the survey.

Uninformed doctors: 50% of the sample reported having to teach their medical providers about transgender care.

High HIV rates: Respondents reported over four times the national average of HIV infection, with rates higher among transgender people of color.

Postponed care: Survey participants reported that when they were sick or injured, many postponed medical care due to discrimination (28%) or inability to afford it (48%). (Grant et al., 2011, pp. 6–7)

TRANSGENDER ETIQUETTE

Etiquette establishes expectations for behavior in social situations. Transgender people have different expectations from other patients as to how they want to be treated. Providers need to know about their expectations in order to effectively communicate and gain rapport so they can establish and maintain a modern provider-patient relationship (Bevan, 2017). Discussion and shared decision making can be disrupted by speech or behavior that causes anger or withdrawal by the transgender patient.

Providers may have initial negative reactions to transgender patients because of their upbringing and experience, but providers must overcome these feelings in order to do a professional job. Providers cannot risk doing harm to even the most difficult patients in these situations. They should assume that the patient's intent is genuine and the potential for harm is real. Simply using the patient's chosen name goes beyond mere courtesy or etiquette, because studies have shown that use of the correct name reduces depression and suicide attempts (Russell, Pollitt, Li, & Grossman, 2018).

There are over a dozen points of etiquette that should be observed for transgender people, which are given in sequential order of the typical encounter:

1. Transgender etiquette begins with asking what the person wants to be called, despite any legal or previous record name. This should be accomplished as early as possible in encounters, with the first person who greets the person. This is usually an appointment coordinator or receptionist. This information should be added to the patient's file and relayed to anyone in the practice who will have contact with the patient. If a provider or their staff makes a mistake, they should apologize and begin by using the correct name. Sometimes the patient may have to make a correction, which necessitates an apology, but pains should to be taken to avoid future mistakes.

2. Next, the provider or their staff should ask the person's preferred pronouns and form of address. Form of address might include name and

honorifics as in Miss, Mrs., Ms., or Mx. This applies not only to transgender people but also people who reject automatic use of conventional masculine or feminine pronouns. Again, this information should be shared immediately with others in the practice who will come into contact with patients.

There are at least a dozen gender-neutral pronoun systems. An up-to-date list of these is available at https://uwm.edu/lgbtrc/support/gender-pronouns/ (University of Wisconsin, 2019). They are often hard to remember, so, if not sure, one can always revert to calling the patient by their preferred name. A good fallback, and one of the most common gender-free preferred pronoun systems, is the third person plural (they, them, theirs), which is sanctioned by the *New York Times*, the American Dialect Society, and the *Washington Post* and has been common since the 14th century. If a provider or their staff makes a mistake, apologize and begin by using the correct pronoun and the chosen name.

3. Intake forms and questionnaires should provide a range of options for declaring both sex and gender separately. Transgender people have particular problems with instruments that mix sex and gender. It is incorrect to ask for gender and only provide options that refer to sex, and vice versa. Sometimes forms confuse being transgender with sexual orientation; they should be separate questions if declaration of sexual orientation is necessary.

Forms should use a two-step process for obtaining sex and gender (Tate, Ledbetter, & Youssef, 2017). Adjustments to electronic health records (EHR) or work-arounds may be required (Cahill & Makadon, 2013.) Such forms should include preferred name, preferred pronouns (she/her/hers, he/him/his, other), sex assigned at birth (male, female, other, decline to answer), congruent gender category (woman/girl, man/boy, gender neutral, gender fluid, other, decline to answer), and may ask for sexual orientation (heterosexual/straight, gay, lesbian, asexual, other, decline to answer). Next to the "other" response fields, the form should provide space for write-in answers.

4. Mistakes in address and pronouns are termed **misgendering**. Transgender people regard deliberate misgendering as an insult, but most will forgive an initial mistake if an apology is offered. If a transgender person believes that a person is deliberately misgendering them, they are likely to get angry, upset, and later depressed. This reaction will obviously negatively impact the patient-provider relationship.

5. In the southern United States and elsewhere, there is a tendency to call people "Sir" if their presentation is clearly not feminine. Most natal females do not like to be called "Ma'am" because they believe this to be a signal of looking old. Calling a transwoman "Sir" is another form of misgendering.

6. Transgender people are sensitive to the words sex and gender. **Sex** pertains to sex assigned at birth (male/female), usually based on external

organs of sexual reproduction, and **gender** refers to gender behavior categories. This is actually the original scientific meaning (Money, Hampson, & Hampson, 1955) for the word "gender" in this context, although sex and gender have become confounded in ordinary speech. This includes writing about transgender people, even in scientific journals or articles. There are transgender scientists, providers, and lay people who read scientific journals and articles and will judge the authors' performance accordingly.

Transgender people and providers often use the terms **gender identity** and **gender dysphoria**, which have been repurposed from pathology and given new meanings. In doing so, they are really talking about their congruent gender behavior category. They are not using it to indicate psychiatric pathology. When they use these terms, they are simply indicating the gender that they practice and a group to which they belong.

7. Transgender people reject the idea that they engage in transgender behavior as a **lifestyle choice**, and this term should not be used. Many will say that they just "knew" or "recognized" which gender category fit them the best, and did so at an early age. Lifestyle choice is a term used by anti-transgender hatemongers and so has a bad connotation among transgender people.

8. There are several pejorative words that should never be used to refer to transgender patients. They include **it**, **he-she**, **shim**, and **tranny**. Transgender people associate these words with transgender pornography and street language. They are used by some to imply that sexual arousal is the motivation for being transgender. The word "tranny" has been rehabilitated at least twice and may be again. Some transgender people came of age when it was a term of endearment and may still use it, but providers should not use it unless things change yet again in the future.

9. Unless it is germane to a chief complaint, symptom, or exam, transgender people should not be asked if they are **pre-op** or **post-op**, the "op" referring to transgender genital plastic surgery or "bottom" surgery. Most transgender people will simply refuse to answer, since they consider it private. Only about 15–25 percent of transitioning transgender people ever get the "op," but this is likely to increase in the future. Passable transwomen are frequently asked about menarche, their menstrual cycle, or whether they are pregnant, which may confuse interviewers, but most transitioning transgender people find that humorous. Likewise, some transwomen complete pelvic exams without providers realizing that they have received transgender genital plastic surgery (vaginoplasty). Providers should be able to tell that the person is transgender from the information on their intake forms and confirm transgender status before asking about reproduction or giving such exams.

10. Transgender people should always be called by their preferred name. To use previous names, including birth and legal names, makes

transgender people upset, and using these old names is known as **dead naming**. Many transgender people have worked hard to change their legal or given names, and it is disconcerting when providers use these old names.

11. Transgender is to be used as an adjective, never a noun as in **transgenders** or a verb as in **transgendered**. Transgender people may take these terms to be insulting.

12. Use the words **transwoman, transman, transgirl**, and **transboy**. The way to remember which to use is that the last parts of the words refer to presentation. Do not use **transgenderism, transsexual, transsexualism, MTF** or **FTM, TG** or **TS**. Younger transgender people, in particular, take offense at these terms. They prefer to use **transgender** and **transitioning transgender person** or **transgender transition** instead. This book adheres to these conventions.

13. Scientific writers and journalists should use the Associated Press (AP), *Washington Post*, GLAAD, or Transgender Media Watch (UK) style guides to determine how to write about transgender people including which terms and pronouns to use. The guides essentially say that a writer should use the pronouns associated with the person's declared gender behavior category, and if no declaration is available, then use the gender category that they live in. If that information is not available, then use the third-person plural for "they, their, them."

WHEN THE CHIEF COMPLAINT IS UNRELATED TO BEING TRANSGENDER

Transgender people are like other people; they get broken arms, have marital problems, become sad due to grieving, and have other mental health or medical problems that are unrelated to being transgender but nevertheless may require treatment. Transgender etiquette as described earlier should be followed by all providers in order to develop and maintain the provider-patient relationship.

Transgender people may sometimes withhold information in medical history development. There are some physical indicators of being transgender that might be observed. Transwomen, particularly those taking hormones and/or blockers, may have less hair on their bodies compared with natal males. Transwomen may shave their hands, arms, and legs in order to look more like natal females. Those taking hormones may have lost hair in those and other body locations. One of the drugs that transwomen take, finasteride (propecia), is also used to reduce hair growth in those with hirsutism because it blocks the conversion of testosterone to dihydrotestosterone. This drug is also used to treat male pattern balding. In the case of transmen, they may have more facial and other hair than natal males in order to obscure feminine facial features. This is possible because of the testosterone they take. Those suspected of being transgender should not be forced to admit their status, but these indicators might be useful in recognizing transgender people in diagnosis and treatment of nongender complaints.

Transgender people are prone to suffer from:

- Physical injury due to violence motivated by cultural rejection.
- Psychological injury, especially reactive depression, because of cultural rejection and keeping their transgender behavior secret.
- High rates of attempted suicide, particularly among young people.
- Do-it-yourself hormonal treatment, which may influence the results of blood tests and may cause abnormal blood clotting from certain estrogens and polycythemia (high red blood cell count) due to erythropoiesis stimulation by testosterone.
- Higher sexually transmitted infection rates due to rejection by family and community, leading to homelessness and participation in drug sales and prostitution.

Physical injury is particularly common for those transgender people who are homeless and/or may be engaged in illegal street economies, but all transgender people must be aware of potential attacks. Bullying in school and other venues is common for transgender children. None of this is excusable and providers should advocate against it.

Psychological injury can be caused by physical or verbal abuse through bullying, violence, and insult. Because post-traumatic stress episodes may be triggered by inappropriate interactions, it is yet another reason why following appropriate transgender etiquette is important. If these post-traumatic episodes result in distress or functional impairment of social and occupational behavior, then transgender people may be diagnosed with post-traumatic stress disorder (PTSD).

Psychological injury can also be the result of transgender secrecy. Many transgender people keep their transgender behavior a secret from family, friends, and social contacts for long periods of time. The effects of secrecy include a high mental workload that interferes with other brain activities and produces isolation, loneliness, and depression (Kelly, 2002). These effects, in turn, may also cause physical self-harm including attempted suicide.

There are two potential side effects of taking unprescribed drugs for transgender transition of which all providers must be aware. *The first side effect is especially dangerous.* Transwomen who are taking estradiol may have a higher incidence of thrombosis in the deep veins (DVT) and lungs. This problem has been greatly decreased with the replacement of **ethinyl**

estradiol by **estradiol valerate** in supervised hormone therapy. However, ethinyl estradiol is still used in birth control pills, so it is readily available. Birth control pills are commonly used in nonsupervised HT. The risk of clotting goes up if the transgender person smokes, and transgender people typically have higher smoking rates. Those transwomen taking estradiol should know the symptoms of DVT and pulmonary clotting.

The other potential side effect is that transmen who take testosterone may develop excess red blood cells, which may influence the results of blood tests. Polycythemia (high red blood cell count) is due to stimulation of red blood cell production (erythropoiesis) by testosterone. This condition can easily be treated in transition when it occurs during supervised and monitored hormone therapy but can cause misinterpretation of blood tests results if unreported.

The provider should still use standard procedures for such things as intake/triage information procedures, assessing pain and acute illness, and a survey of body systems to form a medical history. But with transgender patients the provider should take particular care to ask/confirm what medications they are taking, if any, for transition. Transgender people sometimes use self-treatment for transition, and there are countries in the world that do not require prescriptions for hormones or hormone-blocking drugs. Some hormone treatment drugs are widely available because they are prescribed for nontransition purposes, such as birth control (estradiol, progesterone), high blood pressure (spironolactone), hirsutism (finasteride/propecia), and low testosterone (testosterone). A particular reason for asking about these hormones/drugs is that they may affect diagnostic tests.

Providers should not assume that every transgender person has been exposed to sexually transmitted infections (STI), but for those transgender people "on the street" the provider should be alert for symptoms. Some free street clinics provide hormone therapy injections yoked with regular STI testing to try to reduce the rates of infection. Unless exposed to STI, there is no reason why transgender people should not be able to donate blood, but some blood banks have not updated their policies.

In order to change their bodies, transmen sometimes bind their chests if they have not had a mastectomy; transwomen sometimes bind (tuck) their external genitals. Transmen sometimes enhance their external genitalia, a procedure known as "packing," and may wear packing devices in their shorts. These procedures can sometimes surprise providers and may lead to injury.

People who are unsure if they may need transgender treatment should be first counseled by a qualified mental health provider with experience in treating transgender people. But they also may present to all types of providers—surgeons, family medical providers, emergency providers, or endocrinology providers—without such expertise. Only those experienced with transgender treatment should try to meet transgender needs; all others should refer the patient to a qualified and experienced provider. Transgender organizations, such as PFLAG, support groups, and WPATH will know who is appropriate in the area.

WHEN THE CHIEF COMPLAINT IS RELATED TO TRANSGENDER-SPECIFIC CONCERNS

While this and the previous section pertain to all providers, the following sections of this chapter and Chapter 7 pertain primarily to those who provide transgender services and procedures according to the chief/presenting complaint.

Transgender Adults

Providers and staff who treat transgender people should establish a positive environment in waiting rooms and examination rooms that meets the needs of transgender people. Publications that transgender people might find offensive should not be present. Staff should be trained as to how to deal with transgender people through continuing education, in-service, or other educational opportunities. Preferred name and pronouns should be obtained/confirmed by staff as early as possible and the information should be shared with those who will come into contact with the transgender person.

Patients who are unsure whether they need transgender procedures should be first counseled by a qualified mental health provider with experience in treating transgender people. Providers should perform standard interview procedures for exploring the patient's chief complaint and try to identify phenomena and illnesses that might be co-occurring. Providers should take a history of previous problems, person/family history, and medical systems. Several scales have been developed that are intended to characterize transgender status (Bandini et al., 2013; Becker et al., 2016; Deogracias et al., 2007; Lindgren & Pauly, 1975), but they have only face validity and have not been validated for large populations. Being transgender may affect how a person experiences co-occurring mental health conditions, or such a condition may complicate being transgender. For example, being transgender may exacerbate an existing eating disorder (Ålgars, Alanko, Santtila, & Sandnabba, 2012).

Chromosome testing (karyotype) is not generally performed on transgender patients because evidence indicates that almost none show chromosomal abnormalities (Auer, Fuss, Stalla, & Athanasoulia, 2013; Khandelwal, Agarwal, & Jiloha, 2010).

Transgender people usually present as quiet and concerned with their gender or with social problems. They typically are depressed and anxious due to cultural or family rejection. As described earlier, they may have co-occurring mental problems, some of which may require diagnosis and treatment. Since being transgender is not pathological, it does not count toward "comorbidity." The term comorbidity should not be used with being transgender. Providers should apply the principles of affirmative care, since there is no "cure" for being transgender, although transgender transition may be needed to reduce suffering. Patients should be encouraged to express transgender behavior as long as it is done in safe environments. **Change efforts**, sometimes called **reparative** or **conversion "therapies,"** have not been found to be effective but rather to cause psychological and/or physical harm in sexual orientation change efforts. Since being transgender is not pathological, the correct term is "change efforts" because therapy applies only to pathological conditions. **Gender change efforts** are discouraged by professional mental health and medical associations and WPATH guidelines. In at least 13 U.S. states and several countries they are illegal.

Mental health professionals should provide counseling treatment for social problems as described in Chapter 7. Patient management should also include recommendations for obtaining needed clothing and other items for cross-gender presentation and avenues for safe expression of transgender behavior. Some will cross present periodically, while others will live full-time. Only those who have social problems or those who want to transition usually see a mental health professional.

Of particular concern is marital therapy in which one client is transgender. Part of the motivation for marriage may have been to obtain a "cure" for being transgender. Discovery of clothing or makeup indicating that the person is transgender may come as a shock. The nontransgender client in such situations may be angry that they were not told about the other person being transgender before marriage or doubt their motives for marriage. They may start to doubt their own sexual orientation and fear loss of status in the community. They may go through the classic stages of grief because of perceived "loss" of a spouse. The couple should be referred to a mental health professional who has experience in this area. While many couples split up, some do not. With the increased acceptance of being transgender, more couples are now finding a way to stay together (Erhardt, 2006).

Medical and other procedures for transgender adults are covered in the next chapter.

Transgender Children

Affirmative protocols for children have been developed by clinicians in the United States and elsewhere (Guss, Shumer, & Katz-Wise, 2015;

Olson-Kennedy et al., 2018) based on adult experience and the established use of puberty-blocking drugs in the Netherlands (de Vries et al., 2014).

These protocols are supported by WPATH and professional society guidelines. They involve a team of highly specialized mental health and medical professionals for each patient, working closely with parents and guardians. Research in this area has only recently been started in the past several years (see Chapters 7 and 10).

Transgender children present as quiet, introverted, withdrawn, ill at ease, concerned about their gender (but not about sex), and sometimes depressed. Transkids enjoy normal childhood activities (Chiland, 2003; Lothstein, 1979). Transgender children are sometimes mistaken for prehomosexual children (Gottschalk, 2003). Prehomosexual male children present as effeminate and sexually aggressive toward same-sex children. They are concerned with sex, not gender per se (Davenport, 1972; Zuger, 1984). They also disdain rough-and-tumble play and competitive group sports (Zucker & Bradley, 1995). Prospective studies confirm that such children become homosexual as adults (Li, Kung, & Hines, 2017; Steensma, 2012). Prospective and retrospective studies both indicate that prehomosexual children crossdress (Bailey & Zucker, 1995).

Retrospective studies of transitioning transgender natal male adults reveal that, as children, they were not effeminate, nor did they exhibit the other behaviors associated with prehomosexual male children (Chiland, 2003; Lothstein, 1979). Note that this does not constitute a "differential diagnosis" because neither being transgender nor being homosexual are pathological.

There have been reports in clinical populations of a co-occurrence of being transgender and being on the autism spectrum (de Vries, Noens, Cohen-Kettenis, van Berckelaer-Onnes, & Doreleijers, 2010) in children and adolescents. Whether this is due to some common causative mechanism or whether it is due to people on the autism spectrum being insensitive to potential rejection of being transgender has not been determined. Experts have developed a consensus on how to proceed with treatment in cases of such co-occurrences (Strang et al., 2016). In such cases, treatment for both autism and being transgender should overlap, while improvement in communications by autistic children will help them to express their thoughts about being transgender.

Mental health professionals specializing in transgender children should evaluate the children with regard to social problems they might be encountering and offer counseling. They also may need to educate patients, parents, or guardians about being transgender and provide reassurance.

Some children may not want medical treatment within the affirmative approach, but may need counseling as described in Chapter 7. There are several proximal concerns that motivate transgender children to pursue hormone blockers and transition.

Some transchildren will want affirmative medical treatments because of several factors. First, they may be fearful about puberty changing their bodies. Of particular salience is stopping breast growth for transboys and preventing their voice from changing for transgirls. Second, they may be concerned about social rejection and bullying at school or elsewhere, hoping that by living in their congruent gender full-time they can reduce these problems. Third, they may be concerned that they are unable to wear the clothing of their congruent gender because of their body shape. And fourth, they may be thinking of suicide because they cannot conceive of living with a mismatch between their assigned gender (based on sex at birth) versus their congruent gender. Current studies indicate that at least 32–43 percent of transgender people eventually attempt suicide, and the rate among transgender youth is 31 percent (Clements-Nolle, Marx, & Katz, 2008; Bauer, Scheim, Pyne, Travers, & Hammond, 2015; Liu & Mustanski, 2012; Mustanski & Liu, 2013). These statistics do not reflect many who successfully commit suicide without revealing that they are transgender. Parental acceptance is a major factor in reducing suicide attempts (Ryan, Russell, Huebner, Diaz, & Sanchez, 2010).

Before they start medical treatment in the affirmative approach, transgender children should be evaluated to ensure that their claim to be transgender is (1) insistent, (2) consistent, and (3) persistent. Procedures for affirmative treatment of transgender children are discussed in the next chapter.

REFERENCES

Ålgars, M., Alanko, K., Santtila, P., & Sandnabba, N. K. (2012). Disordered eating and gender identity disorder: A qualitative study. *Eating Disorders, 20*(4), 300–311.

American Psychological Association. (2015). Guidelines for psychological practice with transgender and gender nonconforming people. *American Psychologist, 70*(9), 832–864.

Auer, M. K., Fuss, J., Stalla, G. K., & Athanasoulia, P. (2013). Twenty years of endocrinologic treatment in transsexualism: Analyzing the role of chromosomal analysis and hormonal profiling in the diagnostic work-up. *Fertility and Sterility, 22*, 1103–1110.

Bailey, J., & Zucker, K. (1995). Childhood sex-typed behavior and sexual orientation: A conceptual analysis and quantitative review. *Developmental Psychology, 31*(1), 43–55.

Bandini, E., Fisher, A. D., Castellini, G., Lo Sauro, C., Lelli, L., et al. (2013). Gender identity disorder and eating disorders: Similarities and differences in terms of body uneasiness. *Journal of Sexual Medicine, 10*, 1012–1023.

Bauer, G. R., Scheim, A. I., Pyne, J., Travers, R., & Hammond, R. (2015, June). Intervenable factors associated with suicide risk in transgender persons: A respondent driven sampling study in Ontario, Canada. *Biomed Central Public Health, 15*, 525.

Becker, I., Nieder, T. O., Cerwenka, S., Briken, P., Kreukels, B. P., Cohen-Kettenis, P. T., . . . Richter-Appelt, H. (2016, April). Body image in young gender dysphoric adults: A European multi-center study. *Archives of Sexual Behavior, 45*(3), 559–574.

Bevan, T. (2017). *Being transgender* (pp. 165–170). Santa Barbara, CA: Praeger.

Cahill, S., & Makadon, H. (2013). Sexual orientation and gender identity data collection in clinical settings and in electronic health records: A key to ending LGBT health disparities. *LGBT Health, 1*(1), 33–41.

Cahill, S., Singal, R., Grasso, C., King, D., Mayer, K., Baker, K., & Makadon, H. (2014). Do ask, do tell: High levels of acceptability by patients of routine collection of sexual orientation and gender identity data in four diverse American community health centers. *PLOS One, 9*(9), 107–104.

Chiland, C. (2003). *Transsexualism: Illusion and reality.* New York: SAGE 55.

Clements-Nolle, K., Marx, R., & Katz, M. (2008, October). Attempted suicide among transgender persons: The influence of gender-based discrimination and victimization. *Journal of Homosexuality, 51*(3), 53–69.

Conway, L. (2001–2002). How frequently does transsexualism occur? http://www.lynnconway.com

Crissman, H. P., Berger, M. B., Graham, L. F., & Dalton, V. K. (2014). Transgender demographics: A household probability sample of US adults. *American Journal of Public Health, 107*(2), 213–215. *J Public Health* (2017, February), *107*(2), 213–215. https://doi.org/10.2105/AJPH.2016.303571. Epub 2016. December 20, 2016.

Davenport, C. (1972, January). Homosexuality: Its origins, early recognition and prevention. *Clinical Pediatrics, 1,* 7–10.

Deogracias, J. J., Johnson, L. L., Meyer-Bahlburg, H. F., Kessler, S. J., Schober, J. M., & Zucker, K. J. (2007). The gender identity/gender dysphoria questionnaire for adolescents and adults. *Journal of Sex Research, 44*(4), 370–379.

Deutsch, M. (Ed.). (2016). *Guidelines for the primary and gender-affirming care of transgender and gender nonbinary people* (2nd ed.). Center of Excellence for Transgender Health. Department of Family and Community Medicine, University of California, San Francisco. https://www.sccgov.org/sites/bhd/info/Documents/LGBTQ%20Resources/ucsf-guidelines-for-the-primary-and-gender-affirming-care-of-transgender-and-gender-nonbinary-people-6-17-16.pdf

de Vries, A. L., McGuire, J. K., Steensma, T. D., Wagenaar, E. C., Doreleijers, T. A., & Cohen-Kettenis, P. T. (2014). Young adult psychological outcome after puberty suppression and gender reassignment. *Pediatrics, 134*(4), 696–704.

de Vries, A. L. C., Noens, I. L. J., Cohen-Kettenis, P. T., van Berckelaer-Onnes, I. A., & Doreleijers, T. A. (2010). Autism spectrum disorders in gender dysphoric children and adolescents. *Journal of Autism and Developmental Disorders, 40*(8), 930–936.

Dubin, S. N., Nolan, I. T., Streed, C. G., Jr., Greene, R. E., Radix, A. E., & Morrison, S. D. (2018, January). Transgender health care: Improving medical students' and residents' training and awareness. *Advanced Medical Education Practice, 2*(9), 377–391.

Eisenberg, M. E., Gower, A. L., McMorris, B. J., Rider, G. N., Shea, G., & Coleman, E. (2017). Risk and protective factors in the lives of transgender/gender-nonconforming adolescents. *Journal of Adolescent Health, 61*(4), 521–526.

Erhardt, V. (2006). *Head over heels: Wives who stay with cross-dressers and transsexuals.* New York: Routledge.

Flores, A. R., Herman, J. L., Gates, G. J., & Brown, T. N. T. (2016). *How many adults identify as transgender in the United States?* Los Angeles, CA: Williams Institute. https://williamsinstitute.law.ucla.edu/wp-content/uploads/How-Many-Adults-Identify-as-Transgender-in-the-United-States.pdf

Gottschalk, L. (2003). Same-sex sexuality and childhood gender non-conformity: A spurious connection. *Journal of Gender Studies, 12*(1), 35–50.

Grant, J. M., Mottet, L. A., Tanis, J., Harrison, J., Herman, J. L., & Keisling, M. (2011). *Injustice at every turn: A report of the National Transgender Discrimination Survey.* Washington: National Center for Transgender Equality and National Gay and Lesbian Task Force. https://transequality.org/sites/default/files/docs/resources/NTDS_Report.pdf

Grosz, A. M., Guiterrez, S., Lui, A. A., Chang, J. J., Cole-Kelly, K., & Ng, H. (2017). A student-led introduction to lesbian, gay, bisexual and transgender health for first-year medical students. *Family Medicine, 48*(1), 52–56.

Guss, C., Shumer, D., & Katz-Wise, S. (2015, August). Transgender and gender nonconforming adolescent care: Psychosocial and medical considerations. *Current Opinion in Pediatrics, 26*(4), 421–426.

Haider, A. H., Schneider, E. B., Kodadek, L. M., Adler, R. R., Ranjit, A., Torain, M. . . . et al. (2017). Emergency department query for patient-centered approaches to sexual orientation and gender identity: The EQUALITY study. *Journal of the American Medical Association Internal Medicine, 177*(6), 819–828.

Hembree, W. C., Cohen-Kettenis, P. T., Gooren, L., Hannema, S. E., Hassan, W. M., Meyer, W. J., . . . T'Sjoen, G. G. (2017, November). Endocrine Society guideline for endocrine treatment of gender-dysphoric/gender-incongruent persons: An Endocrine Society clinical practice guideline. *Journal of Endocrinology & Metabolism, 102,* 3869–3903. https://academic.oup.com/jcem/article/102/11/3869/4157558

Herman, J. L., Flores, A. R., Brown, T. N. T., Wilson, B. D. M., & Conron, K. J. (2017). *Age of individuals who identify as transgender in the United States.* Los Angeles, CA: Williams Institute.

Horton, M.A. (2008). The prevalence of SRS among US residents: Out and Equal Workplace Summit. http://www.tgender.net/taw/thbcost.html#prevalence, https://docplayer.net/21440139-The-incidence-and-prevalence-of-srs-among-us-residents.html

Kelly, A. E. (2002, January). *The psychology of secrets.* Springer Science and Business Media.

Khandelwal, A., Agarwal, A., & Jiloha, R. C. (2010). A 47,XXY female with gender identity disorder. *Archives of Sexual Behavior, 39,* 1021–1023.

Kosenko, K., Rintamaki, L., Raney, S., & Maness, K. (2013). Transgender patient perceptions of stigma in health care contexts. *Medical Care, 51,* 819–822.

Li, G., Kung, K. T., & Hines, M. (2017). Childhood gender-typed behavior and adolescent sexual orientation: A longitudinal population-based study. *Developmental Psychology, 53*(4), 764–777.

Lindgren, T. W., & Pauly, I. B. (1975). A body image scale for transsexuals. *Archives of Sexual Behavior, 4*, 639–656.

Liu, R. T., & Mustanski, B. (2012, March). Suicidal ideation and self-harm in lesbian, gay, bisexual, and transgender youth. *American Journal of Preventative Medicine, 42*(3), 221–228.

Lothstein, L. M. (1979). Psychodynamics and sociodynamics of gender-dysphoric states. *American Journal of Psychotherapy, 33*(2), 214–238.

Money, J., Hampson, J. G., & Hampson, J. L. (1955). Hermaphroditism: Recommendations concerning assignment of sex, change of sex and psychological management. *Bulletin of Johns Hopkins Hospital, 97*, 284–300.

Mustanski, B., & Liu, R. T. (2013). A longitudinal study of predictors of suicide among lesbian, gay, bisexual and transgender youth. *Archives of Sexual Behavior, 42*(3), 437–438.

O'Hara, M. E. (2015, August 6). "Trans broken arm syndrome" and the way our healthcare system fails trans people. *Daily Dot.* https://www.dailydot.com/irl/trans-broken-arm-syndrome-healthcare/

Olson-Kennedy, J., Rosenthal, S., Hastings, J., & Wesp, L. (2018). *Health considerations for gender non-conforming children and transgender adolescents: Increasing access to comprehensive, effective, and affirming healthcare services for trans communities.* University of California San Francisco, UCSF Medical Center. http://transhealth.ucsf.edu/trans?page=guidelines-youth

Olyslager, F., & Conway, L. (2007). *On the calculation of the prevalence of transsexualism.* Presentation at 2007 WPATH Symposium, Chicago, IL.

Park, J., & Safer, J. D. (2018). Clinical exposure to transgender medicine improves students' preparedness above levels seen with didactic teaching alone: A key addition to the Boston University model for teaching transgender healthcare. *Transgender Health, 3*(1).

Rotondi, N. K., Bauer G. R., Scanlon, K., Kaay, M., & Traver, R. (2013, October). Nonprescribed hormone use and self-performed surgeries: "Do-it-yourself" transitions in transgender communities in Ontario, Canada. *American Journal of Public Health, 103*(10), 1830–1836.

Royal College of Psychiatrists. (2018). Supporting transgender and gender-diverse people. Royal College of Psychiatrists Public Statement: PS02/18. https://www.rcpsych.ac.uk/pdf/PS02_18.pdf

Ruben, M. A., Blosnich, J. R., Dichter, M. E., Luscri, L., & Shipherd, J. C. (2017, September). Will veterans answer sexual orientation and gender identity questions? *Medical Care, 55*, S85–S89.

Russell, S. T., Pollitt, A. M., Li, G., & Grossman, A. H. (2018). Chosen name use is linked to reduced depressive symptoms, suicide ideation, and suicidal behavior among transgender youth. *Journal of Adolescent Health, 63*(4), 503–504.

Ryan, C., Russell, S. T., Huebner, D., Diaz, R., & Sanchez, J. (2010, November). Family acceptance in adolescence and the health of LGBT young adults. *Journal of Child and Adolescent Psychiatric Nursing, 23*(4), 205–213.

Strang, J. F., Meager, H., Kenworthy, L., deVries, A. L. C., Menvielle, E., Leibowitz, S., et al. (2016, October). Initial clinical guidelines for co-occurring autism spectrum disorder and gender dysphoria or incongruence in adolescents. *Journal of Clinical Child and Adolescent Psychology, 47*(1), 105–115.

Steensma, D., van der Ende, J., Frank C. Verhulst, F.C., Cohen-Kettenis, P.T.,(2012). Gender Variance in Childhood and Sexual Orientation in Adulthood: A Prospective Study. *Journal of Sexual Medicine, 10,* 11, 2723-2733.

Tate, C. C., Ledbetter, J. N., & Youssef, C. P. (2017, June). A two-question method for assessing gender categories in the social and medical sciences. *Journal of Sex Research, 50,* 171–173.

Theodosiou, L. (2018, March 28). There's no such thing as a transgender broken arm—trans people deserve fair, non-discriminatory access to services. *Pink News.*

WPATH. (2011). WPATH standards of care for the health of transsexual, transgender, and gender nonconforming people. WPATH. https://wpath.org/publications/soc

Zucker, K., & Bradley, S. (1995). *Gender identity disorder and psychosexual problems in children and adolescents.* New York: Guilford.

Zuger, B. (1984). Early effeminate behavior in boys: Outcome and significance for homosexuality. *Journal of Mental Diseases, 172*(2), 90–97.

7

Applications in the Field: Procedures, Side Effects, and Outcomes

Transgender people typically seek provider assistance because they are questioning about whether they are transgender, because they are having social problems due to their transgender behavior, or because they feel the need to transition. Mental health professionals, trained in dealing with transgender assessment and counseling, are the ones best qualified to deal with such questions. But a transgender person may approach any type of medical or mental health provider that they trust, even primary or family care doctors. These physicians can perform procedures, such as starting hormone therapy, as long as they have knowledge and experience with transgender transition and can obtain the informed consent of the patient. An objective of providers is to reduce the suffering of their patients, including transgender people, so all providers need to be sympathetic and help within the limits of their expertise. They should warn the inquirer that pursuing transition procedures without assistance from qualified providers carries substantial medical risk. Recent estimates indicate that about

22–49 percent of transgender people start hormone therapy on a do-it-yourself basis, particularly if access to health care is not available or is delayed (de Haan, Santos, Arayasirikul, & Raymond, 2015; Rotondi et al., 2013; Webberly & Webberly, 2018). Providers should encourage the transgender patient to find a mental health provider who is an expert in transgender assessment and counseling in order to lay the groundwork for potential TGPS if the patient is interested.

The largest group of transgender people, those that do not plan to transition, may need help because of social rejection of their behavior or because they suffer the pain of secrecy. Estimates are that about 10 percent of transgender people will seek transgender transition procedures, but only about 25 percent will elect to get TGPS (Conway, 2001–2002; Olyslager & Conway, 2007). Current actual percentages are increasing dramatically in government-run health care schemes or in surveys because of the improved tolerance and acceptance for being transgender.

The next four sections provide overviews of transgender treatment procedures for four demographic groups:

- Those transgender people with social problems due to cultural rejection or those who are questioning whether they are transgender. Most people in this group will not initially be interested in transitioning, but some eventually will.
- Those determined to be male at birth who seek to transition as transwomen as adults.
- Those determined to be female at birth who seek to transition as transmen as adults.
- Children and adolescents who are questioning or suffering rejection because of their transgender behavior and self-knowledge of their congruent gender.

The last group, children and adolescents, features those who may want to start treatment at an early age through social transition and puberty delay. Only those who meet the severe criteria of being insistent, persistent, and consistent in their transgender behavior, including verbal behavior, will be recommended for such procedures. Transgender children who do not follow this path may need continuing help as they mature and continue their transgender behavior in secret or in public.

ADULT NONTRANSITIONING TRANSGENDER PATIENTS

The chief complaint of this group is that they have social problems related to cultural rejection. Social problems may include accidental discovery by family members or others of the patient's transgender behavior, discomfort with keeping transgender behavior a secret, or marital discord involving with being transgender. The patient may be questioning whether they are transgender based on their own behavior and emotions, or, less often today, may be unaware of the concept of being transgender.

Procedures for this group start with counseling by qualified mental health professionals to briefly identify the chief complaint. The chief complaint typically will involve relationship issues. It may also involve questioning of congruent gender and sexual orientation. Understanding of the chief complaint should involve development of a history showing that the person has actually engaged in transgender behavior. This usually begins with an assessment of transgender status based on self-reports of behavior and verbal expressions of congruent gender. The provider may need to answer clarifying questions and provide education about definitions and the phenomenon of being transgender. At this point, many patients will need reassurance that they are not suffering from a disorder but that being transgender is a natural feature of biological gender diversity.

The mental health provider should determine if there are behavioral or medical phenomena related or unrelated to being transgender that co-occur with being transgender. Some of problems may need treatment or may interfere with treatment associated with the chief complaint. In many cases, these co-occurring phenomena will have treatment histories. For example, many transgender people suffer from reactive depression because of secrecy, isolation, despair, and loneliness related to keeping their congruent gender a secret. They may have been treated for such depression without informing providers about their transgender status. Transgender people typically become less depressed when their transgender behavior is addressed.

The mental health professional should develop a treatment plan for the chief complaint with the patient that may include consideration of:

- Benefits of continued counseling
- Relationship, marital, and family therapy
- Treatment of co-occurring and mental health phenomena and problems

Continued counseling may be indicated to address issues to establish congruent gender and sexual orientation through education and dialogue. Relationship, marital, and family therapy may be necessary to address social problems and conflicts. The provider may need to determine the order of treatment of co-occurring and mental health problems. In many cases, treatment with regard to transgender issues may alleviate some of these co-occurrences. Because of the recent increased numbers of transgender people presenting, there are not enough mental health providers who have experience with transgender procedures. This is particularly true in some local geographical areas.

Affirmative counseling should not discourage transgender behavior but instead ensure that it is conducted in safety. For patient management, this frequently means that the provider must stay in touch with sources of information to know which spaces and services are safe. The counselor should encourage exploration by the transgender person, which might include crosspresentation for longer and longer periods, such as at conventions or other gatherings. This allows the transgender person to experience what it might be like to go full-time. This may lead to consideration of whether the patient wants to transition and the benefits that it may bring.

In the past, research has focused on transitioning transgender people, to the exclusion of transgender people who do not intend to transition. However, this latter group makes up the vast majority of presenting transgender people. For this reason, future research is required to understand and address the needs of those who do not want to transition but still have social and, perhaps, medical issues that should be addressed. This is an area of emerging research that will be further explored in Chapter 12.

TRANSGENDER TRANSITION IN ADULTS

The chief complaint of some patients will involve transgender transition to modify their bodies to meet cultural expectations of their congruent gender. There are many procedures that might be involved in transgender transition. The basic principle of transgender transition is to perform those procedures that are more reversible before going on to those that are less reversible to be sure that continuance along the transition path is still desired. Beyond this principle, there is no requirement for particular transition procedures nor for a particular sequence. The WPATH Standards of Care are guidelines and meant to be flexible.

Transition is not a race to the top of a mountain with transgender genital plastic surgery (TGPS) being the goal. There are many misnomers for TGPS including gender confirmation surgery, sexual reassignment surgery, genital reconstruction surgery, or sex realignment surgery. All of these misnomers assume motivations or actions that are not in evidence or are inaccurate. Transitioning transgender people do not need confirmation of their gender; most have known since childhood. "Reconstruction" is usually reserved for fixing bodies after trauma, but there is usually no bodily trauma prior to surgery that needs correcting. Most of the "sexual reassignment" involved in transition is mediated by hormones or plastic surgery on other body parts. And there is no realignment involved because the person's new sex was never in alignment.

Transgender people are free to choose which procedures suit their situation best. As indicated by the ending of the word transition*ing*, transition never ends; there are always adjustments to be made in the future.

The chief complaint of a patient may involve transgender transition to modify their bodies to meet cultural expectations of their congruent gender. But automatically going to see a mental health professional may not be necessary. Competent medical providers can assess the situation and perform most procedures (e.g., breast enhancement, facial surgery, hormone therapy) with informed consent. However, many medical providers still require letters from mental health providers for various procedures for risk reduction. WPATH Standards of Care still requires letters from two mental health providers for TGPS by mental health "gatekeepers" and one letter for breast/chest surgery. The only purpose of this TGPS gatekeeping function is to ensure that the patient does not have mental health problems that might interfere with positive outcomes for a nearly irreversible procedure. Transition is highly individual and there is no "standard" path to follow.

MENTAL HEALTH ASSESSMENT

There are situations in which an initial mental health assessment is needed. Patients may be unsure that they are transgender. This is called **questioning** and is the "Q" in the LGBTQ initialism. Mental health providers can assist those who are unsure about whether they are transgender. Mental health professionals can also provide counseling, if needed, to help the patient deal with relationship and cultural rejection issues. In other situations, the patient may be confused about how to pursue transition procedures and mental health professionals can assist the patient in forming a transition plan. The provider and patient can develop a transition plan or at least identify the first intended steps in transition.

Mental health professionals should first assess such a patient by making a brief history of transgender presentation and verbal behavior about their gender. The goal is to reduce suffering through counseling and patient management. The counselor should be affirmative with regard to previous and current behavior and diagnoses. The provider should inquire regarding secrecy and which person(s) know about the behavior. The counselor then should address the person's questioning, transgender behavior, or transition plan issues. The patient may need information about being transgender or may need to confirm that the information they have received is correct. Questioning individuals may benefit by affirming, safe experience with transgender presentation.

The patient's motives for transgender transition should be discussed. Common desires are for improved authenticity, attractiveness, and quality of life. However, some patients express this in a negative way by referring to disgust with their body parts that do not fit with their congruent gender.

There are no reliable psychometric tests to help determine whether the patient is transgender or not. The ones that exist only have face validity and are not validated on actual patient populations. The same goes for the autism spectrum screening tests that some clinics require to investigate co-occurrences.

Events such as transgender conferences provide increased experience for questioning and transgender people to understand how they want to express themselves. Many years ago, it was required that a patient seeking transition undergo a **real-life test** (RLT) in which they had to demonstrate to providers that they could hold a job in their congruent gender and deal with family and cultural issues before transition. That requirement was relaxed to recommend a year of **real-life experience** (RLE) to be judged jointly by the patient and provider. There currently is no such requirement at all in the WPATH SOC; many transgender people already have come out when they present. Many now transition on the job.

Safety should be addressed. In particular, the patient should practice their congruent gender in safe situations. The counselor may need to provide patient management functions to direct the patient to safe locations for experiences. The patient may also need information on businesses that are safe to patronize, particularly in non-trans-friendly locales. The counselor should be sure that the patient is not self-medicating with sex hormones; if they are, the counselor should recommend an affirmative medical provider to monitor them.

The patient may need support for coming out to family and friends. It helps to rehearse what to say in advance of those situations and try to anticipate potential problems. With regard to transition planning, the patient should be able to consult a mental health provider to assess previous and future procedures.

The role of the mental health professional in gatekeeping with regard to a TGPS recommendation letter is to assess whether the patient has mental health problems that may interfere with a successful outcome of TGPS or breast/chest surgery. In many cases, mental health problems such as depression or suicidal thinking will be ameliorated by such surgeries.

It is good practice for medical and mental health providers to ensure that each transgender person has access to mental health counseling after surgery. TGPS and transition does not solve all of the problems of a transgender patient, and it is good for them to know that they can get postsurgical and post-transition counseling.

ADULT TRANSWOMAN TRANSITIONING PROCEDURES

Hormone Therapy

The objective of hormone therapy is to modify body parts that respond to sex hormones (Olson, 2012). Primary sex organs involved in reproduction have receptor sites for both estrogen and testosterone and can be transformed to various extents when exposed to a different predominant hormone. Examples are the breasts and genitalia. Secondary sex organs can also be transformed, such as the skin and hair. The brain and nervous system also are affected directly or because of neural plasticity. To a lesser extent, facial features may be affected. The transformation process can also be aided by drugs that interfere with sex hormone synthesis and/or conversion, such as the conversion of testosterone to **dihydrotestosterone** which is the most active of the androgens.

The correct term for this procedure is **hormone therapy** but it is sometimes incorrectly called **hormone replacement therapy**. Hormone replacement therapy properly refers to supplementation of natural hormones because of accident or because of surgical procedures to remove the gonads or other organs.

The basic principle of hormone therapy for transwomen is to reduce blood levels of testosterone and to increase estrogen blood levels to those of natal females. This is achieved by a combination of sex hormones and blocking drugs. Increasing the blood levels of estrogen affect receptors in the hypothalamus to block release of gonadotropin releasing factor. This, in turn, blocks the release of **LH** and **FSH** from the anterior pituitary that trigger the male gonads to manufacture and release testosterone. This feedback loop also responds to increased levels of progesterone or testosterone or anabolic steroids. Progesterone drugs such as **Prometrium** and **medroxyprogesterone** are also included in some HT regimes to help block gonadotropin releasing factor and encourage breast development.

The male gonads are not the only body organ that secretes testosterone. It is also secreted by the adrenal glands. The action of drugs such as **spironolactone** blocks synthesis and competes with testosterone at receptor sites to "mop" up remaining testosterone synthesis in the gonads or adrenal glands. **Finasteride** (propecia) also helps with the "mopping up" process because it blocks the conversion of testosterone to dihydrotestosterone, which reduces overall androgenic effectiveness.

The medical provider should obtain a baseline for testosterone, estrogen, and prolactin blood levels in addition to indicators of general health before beginning HT. They also should determine whether the patient is self-administering HT drugs.

The goal for HT is to drive down testosterone and increase estrogen in blood concentrations to normal female levels. Although testing technology is improving, there is often increased variability at low levels of testosterone in the results from many laboratories because of differences in test technology.

Providers may start with lower dosages, but the following is commonly used for HT in transwomen:

- Estradiol valerate: 4–6 mg/daily or 100–400 mcg by patch, 5–40 mcg biweekly IM or 1–4 mg daily sublingually
- Spironolactone (100–300 mg/daily)
- Finasteride (2.5–5 mg/daily)
- Prometrium (100–200 mg/daily) or medroxyprogesterone (5–10 mg/daily).

Other common dosages and routes of administration are shown in Table 7.1.

Note that **estradiol valerate** should be used and not **ethinyl estradiol.** The latter is believed responsible for increased deep vein thrombosis (**DVT**) and pulmonary clotting and embolism and is no longer used in HT. However, it is still available in birth control pills and other medications. Medical providers should be cautious about patients with histories of DVT or pulmonary clotting, but transition can continue without estradiol, with lower doses or other drugs. There are three drugs that block testosterone release through their action in the hypothalamus but are rarely used in adults; they can be used if the estradiol is contraindicated, such as for a history of DVT. **Goserlin, buserelin**, and **triptorelin** are sometimes used to block gonadotropin releasing factor instead of estradiol, but they are expensive and used only when other drugs are contraindicated. Some prescribe progesterone to minimize the dose of estrogen and thus minimize thrombosis risk (Tchaikovski & Rosing, 2010).

Some use **injectable estradiol valerate** or **estradiol patches** to avoid impacts on the liver. Because absorption through patches varies widely, the provider should carefully monitor blood levels. In the Netherlands and elsewhere, by policy, those over 65 years old are only provided with estradiol by patch.

Estradiol has two additional actions. In addition to blocking synthesis and formation of testosterone by its direct action on the tissue and direct action on the hypothalamus, estrogen increases the levels of sex hormone binding globulin, which binds to testosterone and inactivates it. Estrogen also is a stimulant to sexual interest in the absence of testosterone (Wibowo, Shellhammer, & Wassersug, 2011).

In addition to affecting testosterone, **spironolactone** is a potassium-sparing diuretic. So, patients often schedule administration during daylight hours to avoid sleep disturbance. The patient should keep hydrated to

Table 7.1 Transwoman HT Drugs

Drug	Route of Administration	Nominal Dosages	Interval	Protocol
Estradiol valerate	Oral	2–6 mg	Daily	SYPP; Gooren
Estradiol ethinyl		Not used		
Estradiol	Sublingual	1–4 mg	Daily	UCSF
Estradiol	Transdermal	100–400 mcg	Daily	UCSF; SYPP
Estradiol valerate	Intramuscular	5–20 mg	Biweekly	UCSF; SYPP
Estradiol valerate	Intramuscular	40 mg	Biweekly	Burnett (b)
Spironolactone	Oral	100–400 mg	Daily	UCSF
Ciproterone	Oral	100 mg	Daily	Gooren
Goserlin	Oral	UNK		
Buserelin	Oral	UNK		
Triptorelin	Oral	UNK		
Finasteride	Oral	2.5–5 mg	Daily	UCSF; SYPP
Dutasterone	Oral	UNK	Daily	UCSF; Burnett (b)
Methylprogesterone	Oral	5–10 mg	Daily	UCSF; Burnett (b)
Depo-medoxyprogesterone	Intramuscular	150 mg	3 months	SYPP; Olson
Prometrium	Oral	100–200 mg	Daily	UCSF; Burnett (b)
Depo-Provera progesterone	Intramuscular	150 mg	3 Months	UCSF; Burnett (b)

(*continued*)

Table 7.1 (continued)

Drug	Route of Administration	Nominal Dosages	Interval	Protocol
Viagra				
Depo Provera (illicit use)	Oral	UNK		UCSF; Burnett (a)
Depo Provera (illicit use)	IM	UNK		UCSF; Burnett (a)
				UCSF; Burnett (a)
Perlutal (illicit use)	Oral	UNK		UCSF; Burnett (a)
Perlutal (illicit use)	IM	UNK		UCSF; Burnett (a)
				UCSF; Burnett (a)
Phytoestrogens	Oral	UNK		UCSF; Burnett (a)

The information in this table comes from the Endocrine Society Guidelines (Hembree et al. 2009) with augmentation from WPATH and experience in treating homeless and poor transitioning transgender people:

- SYPP (Strengthening Youth Prevention Paradigms at Children's Hospital Los Angeles) (Olson, 2012)
- Gooren (Gooren, Giltay, & Bunck, 2008)
- UCSF (Urban Care Center San Francisco) (Davidson et al., 2006)
- Burnett (Burnett, 2011a; Burnett 2011b)

avoid **dehydration**. The patient also must guard against consuming too much potassium from sodium chloride substitutes or in food, otherwise **hyperkalemia** or **hypercalcemia** may result. **Cyproterone acetate** is widely used in Europe and has both blocking and progestin effects but is not approved for use by the U.S. Food and Drug Administration. This is because of adverse side effects on liver function, and because it is often combined with ethinyl estradiol, which is also not used in HT.

The efficacy and dosage regimen of **progesterone drugs** is not well established for breast development. Their use is intended in HT to stimulate growth of glandular (lobular) tissue in the breast whereas estrogens stimulate growth of ductal (stroma) tissue. Historically, medroxyprogesterone was given daily. More recently, some providers have seen better results with daily **micronized Prometrium**, while others prefer to cycle its administration to simulate the normal menstrual cycle for 10 days a month. Some prescribe progesterone to minimize the dose of estrogen and thus minimize thrombosis risk (Tchaikovski & Rosing, 2010). There is concern that the combination of estrogen and progesterone in menopausal medications might trigger breast cancer in natal women, but the studies did not show the effect in natal women who had been hysterectomized, who are more akin to transwomen (Stefanick et al., 2003).

Some estrogen and progesterone drugs (e.g., **Perlutal** combining estradiol enanthate and dihydroxyprogesterone acetophenide) have been deliberately synthesized to avoid legal restrictions. These drugs come mainly from Mexico and countries in South America (Burnett, 2011a). Little is known scientifically about the safety and effectiveness of these drugs.

Some patients self-medicate with phytoestrogens, which are derived from plant materials and have mild estrogenic effects. But the effective dose of these chemicals is believed to be toxic.

Initial monitoring of BUN, estrogen, testosterone, A1C, albumin, and potassium should be done at least every three months, tapering off to once a year. Prolactin levels should be observed only if symptoms (headache, vision changes, lactation) develop. The reason for mentioning this in the WPATH Guidelines is because of three cases of HT in which prolactinomas were found in transwomen. High doses of estrogen may provide an explanation, because high doses in rats produce prolactinomas (Xu et al., 2000), and in an industrial accident one person exposed to a high dose of estrogens had prolactinoma (Baron, Sowers, & Feinberg, 1983). If the patient is taking oral hormones, then liver enzymes should be measured to detect any impact on that organ. Finally, it was found that transwomen had lower bone density levels before starting HT (Wiepjes et al., 2018), so initial assessment may be prudent, particularly in older transwomen. However, bone mineral density does not appear to be affected by HT. So continued assessment is not necessary for HT monitoring but may be necessary because of age or other factors (Wiepjes et al., 2018).

Table 7.2 Transwoman HT Effects

Effect	Source
Decreased muscle mass/strength	ES; WPATH
Body fat redistribution to approximate female	ES; WPATH
Accretion of bone-mineral content	UCSF; Burnett
Softening of skin/dry skin	ES; WPATH
Thinning and slowed growth of body and facial hair	ES; WPATH
Decreased libido/difficulty reaching orgasm	CPATH
Male sexual dysfunction	ES; WPATH
Decreased spontaneous/morning erections	CPATH
Progressive reduction in testicular volume to 50%	CPATH
Nonpermanent testicular shrinkage	UCSF; Burnett
Infertility	SYPP
Tender breast buds within 3–6 months	CPATH
Breast and nipple growth through 2 years	CPATH
Permanent changes to nipple-areolae	CPATH
Heightened sense of touch	SYPP; Olson
Increased sense of smell	SYPP; Olson
Increased emotionality	SYPP; Olson
Will not raise voice pitch	UCSF; Burnett
Will not shrink Adam's apple	UCSF; Burnett
Will not cause regression of the beard	UCSF; Burnett

Bevan (2015) from the following sources:

- ES, Endocrine Society (Hembree et al., 2009)
- WPATH (WPATH, 2013)
- CPATH (Canadian Professional Association for Transgender Health, 2014)
- SYPP (Strengthening Youth Prevention Paradigms at Children's Hospital Los Angeles) (Olson, 2012)
- UCSF (Urban Care Center San Francisco) (Davidson et al., 2013)
- Burnett (Burnett, 2011a; Burnett, 2011b)

Transwomen on HT should perform breast examinations. After age 50, they should have mammograms every two years or after 5–10 years of HT (Deutsch, 2016).

The outcome of HT is generally good. HT reduces depression and anxiety (Gómez-Gil et al., 2012; Gorin-Lazard et al., 2012). A summary of its effects is shown in Table 7.2.

Patients report elevated mood and less depression, whether from hormone action on the body or from observing progress in transition. Breast

Table 7.3 Transwomen HT Risks

Risk	Risk Level per WPATH
Thrombosis	Likely increased risk
Cardiovascular disease	Likely increased risk with additional factors
Hypertension	Possible increased risk
Hyperprolactinemia or prolactinoma	Possible increased risk
Type 2 diabetes	Possible increased risk with additional risk factors
Gallstones	N/A
Elevated liver enzymes or liver disease	N/A
Weight gain	N/A
Hypertriglyceridemia	N/A

development varies widely, with at least half of patients getting breast implants after two years of HT when maximum breast growth is achieved. Hair growth is reduced but not eliminated.

The risks of transwoman HT from WPATH (WPATH, 2013) are shown in Table 7.3.

Side effects of HT in transwomen include dry skin, redistribution of fat similar to natal females, and reportedly, increased emotionality. As described previously, administration of ethinyl estradiol increases the risk of blood clotting, but estradiol valerate appears to have a reduced effect (Gooren et al., 2008). However, side effects of taking overdoses of estradiol valerate have been noted in do-it-yourselfers (Asscheman et al., 2011). Some providers minimize the risk of thrombosis by minimizing estrogen dosages and compensating with synthesis blockers (spironolactone) and progesterone.

Fertility Maintenance

Over several weeks, hormone therapy will reduce fertility of sperm and over years reduce erections and orgasms. For this reason, providers may order sperm to be frozen for later use. This may not be necessary for those who already have children. There are no reports regarding reversibility of sperm production, although theoretically it should be possible with reduction of female hormones and administration of testosterone.

If done early in HT, outcomes for this procedure should be the same as for natal males who bank their sperm. There are no side effects from this procedure, but sperm count will decline as HT progresses.

Electrolysis

Electrolysis is often used to remover unwanted hair in transwomen, particularly facial hair that is a remnant of being male. Although removal by laser may be accomplished if the patient has dark hair roots, in patients with light or gray hair laser removal is ineffective. Electrolysis involves insertion of a thin needle into the hair follicle and propagation of radio frequency and/or electrolytic electricity through the needle to coagulate the follicle. For each follicle, this may take two or more treatments, making this a tedious and painful procedure. Patients may use numbing creams or have dentists numb their upper lip to reduce the discomfort.

While facial electrolysis is standard for transwoman transition, unwanted hair is sometimes removed from other body areas. HT can reduce the need for electrolysis, particularly if finasteride is administered, although there are unsubstantiated reports of increased pain sensitivity due to HT.

Some TGPS surgeons insist on hair removal from the penis, scrotum, and peritoneum prior to the surgery, while others use operative procedures during surgery to reduce hair in/near the neovagina. The goal is to avoid growth of hair in the neovagina, which can accumulate, interfere with sexual relations, and cause inflammation and infection.

Electrolysis is effective but may take many hours to accomplish, even by a skilled operator. Each individual hair follicle may have to be treated two or more times. The danger of infection is minimal if sterile procedures are used. Transwomen typically have to return for yearly supplemental treatments once the initial treatment sessions are completed.

Breast Augmentation Surgery and Health

After two years of HT, which provides the maximum breast growth for an individual, about half of transwomen elect to have breast augmentation done. The procedures for these operations are similar to those on natal females, except transwomen typically require larger implants in proportion to their body size. After 7 to 10 years, many transwomen have these implants replaced. Some manufacturers recommend periodic MRI examinations.

Transwomen on HT should perform monthly breast examinations. After age 50, they should have mammograms every two years or after 10 years of HT (Deutsch, 2016). Having breast implants may complicate these examinations, but the complications are the same as for natal females with implants.

Outcomes for breast implants are good. Such implants facilitate dressing in feminine clothing by transwomen and improve their presentation. A frequent error, however, is to initially select a breast implant that is too small for formerly male bodies, necessitating a second operation.

Problems with breast implants are the same for transwomen as for natal females. The implant may be displaced or encapsulated by the breast tissue. Problems with the implant leaking have declined precipitously over the past 30 years with improved technology. There is a slight chance that nipple and skin innervation may not fully recover after the nerves have been stretched in the procedure.

FFS and Other Plastic Surgeries

Transwomen may elect to have several types of plastic surgeries to reduce masculine features and enhance feminine features. Most of the procedures are established on natal females but a few are unique to transwomen. Transwomen typically have longer foreheads and prominent super-ciliary arch boney structures above the eyes. Foreheads can be shortened using scalp advance and the super-ciliary arches ground down. Transwomen tend to have longer upper lips compared with natal females; these can be shortened. The Adam's apple can also be reduced in a "tracheal shave" operation. Other common operations are similar to those for natal women such as rhinoplasty, brow lift, and cheek and lip augmentation.

Outcomes are generally good and are similar to those for natal females. They allow transwomen to appear more authentic in their congruent gender.

Side effects are the same for natal females, although some procedures are particular to transwomen.

Transgender Genital Plastic Surgeries

Transwomen may undergo three types of transgender genital plastic surgeries:

- Vaginoplasty (neovagina)
- Vulvoplasty
- Orchiectomy

The early advocacy of Magnus Hirschfeld and Harry Benjamin was directed at development of a surgical procedure to form a neovagina in transwomen. Today, vaginoplasty is the most common type of TGPS surgery for transwomen. Tissue is recycled from the penis, scrotum, and other areas to form a neovagina. Testes are removed. There are several surgical procedures, depending on the source of the tissue. Some glans tissue and nervous connections to the glans (head) of the penis are preserved in a newly formed clitoris. The urethra is brought out to the surface as in natal women. Other features of female external genitalia are also created.

The neovagina requires considerable postoperative maintenance to retain its form and prevent prolapse. This involves dilation several times a day to start, with tapering dependent on progress. Outcomes are positive (Michel, Ansseau, Legros, Pitchot, & Mormont, 2002; Lawrence, 2003) with regret less than 1 percent (.5% in the most recent study; Davies, McIntyre, Richards, & Rypma, 2019). Transwomen are able to have vaginal intercourse and typically experience orgasm. Side effects typically involve the potential for infection or prolapse, and urinary tract infections (Gaither et al., 2018).

The second type of TGPS is relatively recent in origin. Vulvoplasty does not involve creation of a neovagina but does involve creation of a female vulva, which does not allow for vaginal penetration. Again, tissue from various sources may be used and the innervation of the neoclitoris is maintained from the penis. This type of TGPS is popular with those who do not want the responsibility of maintaining a neovagina or do not plan to have vaginal intercourse. So far, outcomes are positive for this type of TGPS and no unexpected side effects have been reported (Jiang, Witten, Berli, & Dugi, 2018).

The third type of TGPS is the orchiectomy, probably the oldest of the three procedures, used to remove the male testes. The surgical approach may be external or internal through fiberoptics, using an incision in the inguinal area. This operation is also used in the case of testicular cancer, so it is well practiced and understood. Transwomen benefit from this operation because they no longer have to take testosterone blockers and can take reduced doses of sex hormones. Outcomes for this type of TGPS are good. Side effects are minimal and well understood because of its use in treating testicular cancer. Either later vaginoplasty or vulvoplasty are possible after orchiectomy through the inguinal route.

A high degree of pelvic floor muscular development appears to be lacking in transwomen prior to TGPS surgeries, but progress is being made toward treating this condition with physical therapy Kegel exercises to improve function (Manrique et al., 2018).

Voice Therapy and Surgery

The objective of voice therapy for transwomen is to enable them to communicate in a manner that aligns with their congruent gender. Transwomen seeking help with their voices have typically gone through male puberty, which results in a tonal quality comparable to natal males. In particular, they differ in their speaking in fundamental frequency (pitch), tonal resonance, and other distinguishing voice characteristics such as melodic intonation (pitch variability). The fundamental frequency range for adult cisgender females is 175–277 Hz (musical notes F3–C4#) and for males is 100–165 Hz (G2–E3), but there is considerable overlap in achievable frequencies. Resonance refers to the frequency characteristics of the vocal tract and is related to physical dimensions.

HT for transwomen does not change the speaking fundamental frequency (pitch). Fortunately, voice training has been demonstrated to help make appropriate and desired changes to the voice. It appears that it is the interaction of fundamental frequency, resonance, frequency range, and frequency variation (intonation) that allows perception of a speaker as female (Dacakis, 2000). But how these physiological abilities are used in speech generation and perception are gendered as influenced by culture, learning, and preference.

It takes considerable practice and effort to achieve good results. Success is not dependent on pretraining voice characteristics but is dependent on practice. The outcome is generally good with the appropriate training program and sufficient practice. Transwomen can always revert back to speaking in their natural lower voice, if needed, although they usually prefer not to. Side effects of training include voice fatigue, which is perceived as a dry or sore throat. This can be addressed with proper adherence to a vocal hygiene program as specified by the speech training provider.

The objective of voice surgery is to make anatomical changes to speak more easily and in a typical fundamental frequency in the range of natal females. A number of pitch-altering surgeries are currently offered by providers. There are generally two types of procedures—creation of an anterior web of the vocal folds (cords) or pulling the vocal folds through a small "window" created in the thyroid cartilage. Both surgeries shorten the vibratory margins of the vocal folds, which raises the fundamental frequency. In addition, a procedure called "feminization laryngoplasty with thyrohyoid elevation" addresses both fundamental frequency and resonance (Thomas & Macmillan, 2013).

Voice therapy with a qualified speech-language provider is usually recommended prior to voice surgery and is always recommended following surgical procedures. Such surgeries are generally effective, but there is no review study that characterizes results, so many transwomen are uncertain of their outcomes. Side effects of these operations are generally hoarseness for some period of time, sometimes for periods of months.

Prevention of STI

Because transwomen may be having sex in different ways than before transition, they may need education on proper protection procedures.

Many will try out new ways of having sex as well as old ways with both male and female partners. Although statistics in this area are not very reliable, it is estimated that about 25 percent of transwomen previously attracted to females will become attracted to males (Lawrence, 2006). Some will remain attracted to females, and others will be asexual.

Education on the use of condoms and dental dams may be needed as well as learning about proper cleanliness for the neovagina. Sexually active transwomen should get the HPV vaccine, if possible. Although the conventional age limit for vaccination is 26, in 2018 the FDA approved use of a newer vaccine for women and men up to age 45. Sexual experience is a factor in obtaining the vaccine, since it will not protect against those viruses to which one has already been exposed. Transwomen who are at risk for HIV because of a particular partner or having multiple partners should definitely take prophylactic PrEP medication to prevent HIV infection. Outcomes of STI education and practices are good. Side effects are minimal.

Post-Transition/TGPS Counseling

Transition and TGPS will not solve all of the social and cultural rejection problems that transwomen have. For this reason, it is strongly recommended that transwomen have access to counseling even though they may have completed all of the procedures they intend to undergo. The social pressures of being transgender continue after transition and TGPS. Where the government or insurance companies control health care, this consideration needs to be observed. To do otherwise invites future medical suffering and costs for depression and other negative outcomes. Outcomes for counseling are good. No side effects are observed.

TRANSMEN ADULT TRANSITIONING PROCEDURES

Hormone Therapy

The objective of hormone therapy is to modify body parts that respond to sex hormones. Most primary sex organs involved in reproduction have receptor sites for both estrogen and testosterone and can be transformed. Secondary sex organs can also be transformed, such as the skin and hair. The brain and nervous system may also be affected because of direct action or neural plasticity.

The correct term for this procedure is **hormone therapy** but it was previously incorrectly called **hormone replacement therapy**. Hormone replacement therapy properly refers to supplementation of natural hormones because of accident or surgical procedures to remove the gonads.

The basic principle of hormone therapy for transmen is to reduce blood levels of estrogens and to increase testosterone blood levels to those of natal males. This is achieved by the administration of testosterone, which the body can convert to dihydrotestosterone, the more potent androgen. Increasing the blood levels of testosterone causes receptors in the hypothalamus to block release of gonadotropin releasing factor, which, in turn, blocks the release of **LH** and **FSH** from the anterior pituitary that trigger the female gonads to manufacture and release estrogens.

The medical provider should obtain a baseline for estrogen and testosterone blood levels in addition to indicators of liver enzymes and general health before beginning HT. The goal will be to drive up testosterone to the normal male range and decrease estrogen in blood concentrations. Although testing technology is improving, there is often increased variability at low levels of estrogens in the results from many laboratories. Providers also should determine whether the patient is self-administering HT drugs or if they suffer from **polycystic ovarian syndrome** (PCOS). Approximately 5–10 percent of females have PCOS, which results in increased production of testosterone (from the ovaries). Many transmen have elevated testosterone levels before starting HT, so it is important to get a baseline.

Although providers may start with lower dosages, the following is commonly used for HT in transwomen:

- Testosterone cypionate (50–100 mg IM biweekly) *or*
- Testosterone enathate (50–100 mg biweekly IM) *or*
- Testosterone propionate (100–200 mg IM biweekly)

Other drugs and routes of administration used in transman HT are shown in Table 7.4.

Most providers use injectable testosterone and some use **testosterone patches** (4–8 mg/daily), **testosterone gels** (1%, 50–100 mg/daily), and **testosterone cream** (50–100 mg/daily) to avoid adverse impacts on the liver. Subcutaneous injection has been gaining popularity over IM to avoid scarring. Because absorption through patches, gels, and creams varies widely, the provider should carefully monitor blood levels. In the Netherlands and elsewhere, those over 65 years old are provided only with patches. Oral **methyltestosterone** is no longer used due to the risk of liver damage.

Initial monitoring of blood estrogen and testosterone levels should be done at least every three months, tapering off to once a year. Liver enzymes should be measured to detect any impact on this organ, particularly if the patient is taking oral hormones.

Effects of transman HT are shown in Table 7.5. The effects of testosterone include lowering of voice fundamental frequency and redistribution of

Table 7.4 Transman HT Drugs

Drug	Route of Administration	Nominal Dosages	Interval	Note
Testosterone cypionate	IM	50–100 mg	2 weeks	Cottonseed oil
Testosterone enanthate	IM	200 mg	2 weeks	Sesame oil
Testosterone propionate	IM	100–200 mg	2 weeks	
Depo-testosterone	IM	50–200 mg	2 weeks	
Testosterone patch	TD	5 mg	Daily	
Testosterone gel 1%	TD	5 mg	Daily	
Testosterone 1.62%	TD	No published research		
Testosterone axillary	AX	No published research		
Methyltestosterone	Oral	Not used		
Finasteride	Oral			For male pattern baldness
Topical testosterone	Topical	Subtracted from T dose		For clitoris overenlargement

Information in this table comes from Endocrine Society Guidelines (Hembree et al., 2009) and Tom Waddell Health Center (Davidson et al., 2013).

Table 7.5 Transman HT Effects

Potential Risk	Source
Increased muscle mass	Tom Waddell Health Center
Increased muscle strength	Tom Waddell Health Center
Redistribution of fat	Tom Waddell Health Center
Beard/body hair growth	Endocrine Society
Permanent voice change	Tom Waddell Health Center
Permanent clitoral enlargement	Tom Waddell Health Center
Increased libido	Tom Waddell Health Center
Increased physical energy	Tom Waddell Health Center
Cessation of menses	Endocrine Society
Vaginal atrophy	Endocrine Society
Male pattern scalp hair loss	Endocrine Society
Protection against osteoporosis	Tom Waddell Health Center

fat similar to natal males. Muscle growth with exercise is facilitated. Hair growth increases and male facial hair growth becomes possible. This is beneficial because it hides feminine facial features, but those can also be addressed with facial masculine surgery.

The outcome of HT is generally good. Anxiety and depression are reduced and quality of life improves. Patients report elevated mood and less depression, whether from hormone action on the body or from observing progress in transition. Hair growth is greatly increased and male pattern baldness may be observed. HT for transmen is generally safe and effective (Wierckx et al., 2011).

Side effects of testosterone include redistribution of fat similar to natal males and, reportedly, increased aggressiveness. Risks from WPATH (2013) are shown in Table 7.6. Unlike estrogen, testosterone readily crosses the blood-brain barrier and can influence aggressiveness and increase libido. The greatest side effect with a health risk is increased red blood cell production and **polycythemia**, which can be treated by using a lower dose more frequently, phlebotomy, or blood donation. Using a lower dose more frequently also reduces the side effect of acne.

Fertility Maintenance

Within a few weeks after starting HT, female fertility will cease in transmen. However, transmen have successfully conceived and delivered children if testosterone HT is temporarily stopped. Nevertheless, some

Table 7.6 Transman HT Risks

Risks	Degree of Risk per WPATH
Increased red cells	Likely increased risk
Weight gain	Likely increased risk
Acne	Likely increased risk
Sleep apnea	Likely increased risk
Elevated liver enzymes	Possible risk
Hyperlipidemia	Possible risk
Cardiovascular disease	Possible risk with additional factors
Hypertension	Possible risk with additional factors
Type 2 diabetes	Possible risk with additional factors
Loss of bone density	No increased risk
Breast cancer	No increased risk
Cervical cancer	No increased risk
Ovarian cancer	No increased risk
Uterine cancer	No increased risk

transmen freeze their ova for later use with surrogate pregnancy. The procedure for harvesting gametes is exactly the same as with natal females. Outcomes will be as good as with natal females. Side effects may occur due to the harvesting operation but risks are the same as for nontrans females.

Chest Surgery

Transmen typically start out binding their breasts to look more masculine, but this is a dangerous practice. After going on HT, the next procedure that transitioning transmen usually undertake is to get mastectomies, which include chest reconstruction to bring the chest into anatomical conformance with natal male chests. The procedure is the same for mastectomies in natal women. WPATH SOC specifies that one letter from a mental health professional is required but surgeons vary on the number of letters, if any, they require. The surgery should include construction of a male-looking chest, but insurance companies sometimes balk at coverage, even though this is the goal of chest surgery for transmen. The outcomes are usually good. Temporary pain is the only usual side effect.

Facial Masculinization Surgery

Some transmen get facial masculinization surgery to improve their appearance, but many grow facial hair to cover feminine features.

Transgender Genital Plastic Surgeries

Many transmen have hysterectomies and salpingo-oophorectomies, but very few undergo TGPS. The goal is to construct a penis and external genitalia that look similar to that of natal males. Synthetic testes are implanted.

The two TGPS procedures that are used are **phalloplasty** and **metioplasty**. In phalloplasty, tissue is taken from other areas of the body to construct a neopenis. The urethra is rerouted through the clitoris. In metioplasty, the clitoris is enhanced from nearby tissue (Djordjevic et al., 2009). In metioplasty, the clitoris is augmented and the urethra is elongated and augmented. Both procedures usually involve scrotoplasty, construction of a scrotum with implants to resemble testes. Metioplasty is a simpler operation, but phalloplasty creates an organ that is capable of penetration. Electrolysis is often used to remove hair from the graft site(s). Although the outcome is usually good with regard to appearance, improved functionality is still needed. Mechanical and hydraulic means for erection has been tried but functionality is still a problem. Side effects are minimal. Procedures for penile transplants are starting to be developed for natal males who have been injured in combat, but these have not been tried in transmen.

Voice Therapy and Surgery

HT will lower the fundamental frequency of voices of transmen but it will not change resonance and other voice characteristics. Testosterone lengthens and thickens the vocal cords as in male puberty. Because transmen, particularly older transmen, do not go through the growth of normal male puberty, the cavities that affect the voice resonance do not increase in size. Voice quality may sound thin and weak compared to males who have gone through normal puberty. This phenomenon has been termed "entrapment." But physiological abilities used in speech generation and perception are gendered as they are influenced by culture, learning, and preference. Voice therapy is less common with transmen than transwomen, but outcomes are acceptable and side effects are minimal.

Prevention of STI

Because transmen may be having sex in different ways than before transition, they may need education on proper protection procedures. Many will try out new ways of having sex as well as old ways with both male and female partners. Although statistics in this area are not very reliable, it is estimated that about 35 percent of transwomen previously attracted to females will become attracted to males. Some will remain attracted to females, and others will be asexual. Sexually active transmen should get the HPV vaccine, if possible. Although the conventional age limit for vaccination is 26, in 2018 the FDA approved use of one vaccine up to age 45. Sexual experience is a factor in obtaining the vaccine, since it will not protect against those viruses to which the patient has already been exposed.

Education on the use of condoms and dental dams may be needed. Transmen who are at risk for HIV because of a particular partner or having multiple partners should get prophylactic PrEP medication to prevent HIV infection. Outcomes of STI education and practices are good. Side effects are minimal.

Post-Transition Counseling

Transition and TGPS will not solve all of the social and cultural rejection problems that transmen face. For this reason, it is strongly recommended that transmen have access to counseling even though they may have completed all of the transition procedures they intend to undergo. Where the government or insurance companies control health care, this consideration needs to be observed. To do otherwise invites future medical suffering and costs for depression and other negative outcomes. Outcomes for counseling are good. No side effects are observed.

TRANSGENDER CHILDREN AFFIRMATIVE TREATMENT

The affirmative treatment for transgender children advocates treatment as soon as it is recognized and confirmed that a child is consistent, insistent, and persistent in their congruent gender. At this point, social transition is started and blockers are administered at early signs of puberty (Tanner Stage 2). Blockers continue until age 16 when the child and the team of supportive parents (Simons, Schrager, Clark, Belzer, & Olson, 2013) and providers must decide whether the child should transition using sex hormone therapy (HT). This approach (Olson-Kennedy, Rosenthal, Hastings, & Wesp, 2018) emerged in the United States as an adaptation of the VU University Medical Center's "watchful waiting" approach. As currently implemented, along with blockers, the child may take low doses or receive topical administration of sex hormones in order to regulate bone growth and growth of external genitalia. The concern is that there should be sufficient external genitalia tissue to facilitate transgender genital plastic surgery, although new surgical techniques to "borrow" tissue from other locations are now established.

Assessment

The first step in the affirmative approach for a transchild is to form a team of providers to assess the candidate. The **support team** is initially composed of parents, mental health professionals, an endocrinologist, and the family medicine medical provider. Although the parents are responsible for final decisions, this team is there to advise them and the child. Each of the team members does an assessment in their specialty and no action is recommended until it is clear that the child is insistent, consistent, and persistent in their transgender behavior and verbal statements of congruent gender. At this stage, children are more interested in hormones and transition and parents in transition and acceptance (Lawlis, Donkin, Bates, Britto, & Conard, 2017).

Social Transition

Social transition involves the transgender child living in their congruent gender. This can be complicated by family, school, and social problems. The transgender support team can provide assistance. Sometimes there are legal problems, which must be solved to allow the child to engage in school and other activities. Families sometimes move their homes in conjunction with the start of social transition, so that the child can have a fresh start in their congruent gender in a new school and locality. Social transition results in reduced anxiety and depression and increased self-worth compared with controls and does not contribute to mental health problems (Durwood, McLaughlin, & Olson, 2017).

Puberty Blocking

The goal of puberty blocking is to delay the onset of irreversible anatomical effects of puberty. This allows the child and the team time to be sure about their congruent gender. Puberty blocking begins at age 7–11 depending on the start of puberty and ends at age 16, which provides five to nine years of delay before decisions must be made about treatment with sex hormones. This occurs at Tanner stage 2 with breast buds in natal female children and increased size of testes in natal male children.

The initiation of puberty blockers can be beneficial, even up to age 15, for some effect in minimizing the growth of the superciliary arches in males.

In the United States, the typical puberty-blocking drugs are gonadotropin analogs that overstimulate the cells in the anterior hypothalamus, which is responsible for mediating puberty. This overstimulation causes the receptors to be down-selected and the cells do not release gonadotropin releasing factor into the anterior pituitary where LH and FSH are produced. This halts sex hormone production from the gonads. In the United States, the drugs of choice are injected **leuprolide acetate** or implanted **histrelin**. These drugs have been used for many years to block precocious puberty and for other purposes. They cannot be used after age 16 or bone density development might be imperiled.

Monitoring of blood levels of testosterone, estradiol, FSH, and LH begin at 6–8 weeks after blocking begins and is conducted usually every three months using ultra-sensitive lab testing procedures. Although Endocrine Society guidelines discourage the administration of sex hormones before age 16 in other protocols, many providers start children on low doses to stimulate development and maintain bone density growth.

Sex Hormones and Start of Transition

Blockers must be terminated at age 16 to avoid adverse bone density effects. It is at this age that the team must decide whether to allow endogenous puberty to start or whether to switch over to administration of sex hormones as in adult HT and transition. In either case, the support team will provide assistance. TGPS can occur as early as age 18 with informed consent of the child and parents. HT at age 16–18 with subsequent TGPS results in young adults who function well psychologically, socially, and sexually (Cohen-Kettenis & van Goozen, 1997).

Outcomes and Side Effects

The outcome of the affirmative procedure described in the previous sections has generally been positive (Olson, Durwood, & McLaughlin, 2018), and a long-term study is underway to confirm or disconfirm some postulated side effects.

The major downside of this procedure is that the child is likely not to reproduce using their own gametes. This is because gamete production typically begins after puberty blocking begins. Another concern is that the blocking procedure may not allow the development of enough penile tissue to create a neovagina during TGPS; however, new methods for finding tissue for this purpose have been developed. Other potential side effects are reduced growth and reduced bone density, which are currently under study.

GENERAL HEALTH OUTCOMES AFTER TRANSITION IN ADULTS

Gooren et al. (2008) found that mortality for both transwomen and transmen was not different than for controls, but there was a 6–8 percent increase in mortality for transwomen who took ethinyl estradiol as opposed to estradiol valerate, mainly due to thrombosis. Asscheman et al. (2011) and Dhejne et al. (2011) found that mortality of transwomen was somewhat higher than for the population, but death was from causes unrelated to transition procedures. They included suicide, drug abuse, and HIV/AIDS.

Most transwomen report satisfaction with HT (Gomez-Gil et al., 2012), as do transmen (Constantino, Cerpolini, Morselli, Venturoli, & Merriggiola, 2013), and it has been found generally safe (Weinand & Safer, 2015).

Most transwomen report satisfaction after completing transition with TGPS despite continuing social and cultural rejection problems (Kuiper & Cohen-Kettenis, 1988; Lawrence, 2006). Overall, regret is less than 1 percent. Several studies have shown no regret at all (Krege, Bex, Lummen, & Rubben, 2001; Lawrence, 2003; Lobato et al., 2006; Weyers et al., 2009). Two showed a low incidence of regret (3.8%, 3.2%) (Landen, Walinder, Hambert, & Lundstrom, 1998). Studies indicate that counseling should be available post-op to patients. Regret for transition with TGPS occurs only rarely but is typically due to social pressures. In a recent study (Davies et al., 2019) researchers found regret only occurred at a rate of .47 percent and two-thirds of those who detransitioned (12 of 16) said that they would retransition in the future. Reasons given for detransitioning had to do with social pressure. Transmen who do regret TGPS sometimes report family rejection or death of both parents (Lindemalm, Korlin, & Uddenberg, 1987). Transmen report satisfaction with TGPS (Wierckx et al., 2011) although procedures are needed to improve functionality.

Transition does not solve all of the problems that transwomen and transmen face, so access to counseling is required.

APPENDIX: TRANSGENDER TREATMENT PROCEDURES

Strategy: Not a race to the top. Patient decisions on individual procedures and their order.

Counseling, Assessment, Gatekeeping: Counseling indicated if person is questioning. Gatekeeping letters needed for TGPS. Some doctors require letters for other procedures.

Hormone Therapy (Basic): Can be administered by trained family physician with patient's informed consent. Sex hormones block release of gonadotropin releasing factor from hypothalamus that releases LH and FSH from anterior pituitary to trigger sex hormone production by gonads. Direct action of administered sex hormones on tissues to change them. Spironolactone blocks testosterone synthesis and effects. Finasteride blocks conversion of testosterone to dihydrotestosterone (DHT).

Transwomen

- Estradiol valerate: 4–6 mg/daily or 100–400 mcg by patch, 5–40 mcg biweekly IM or 1–4 mg daily sublingually
- Spironolactone (100–300 mg/daily)
- Finasteride (2.5–5 mg/daily)
- Prometrium (100–200 mg/daily) or medroxyprogesterone (5–10 mg/daily)

Transmen

- Testosterone cypionate (50–100 mg IM biweekly) *or*
- Testosterone enathate (50–100 mg biweekly IM) *or*
- Testosterone propionate (100–200 mg IM biweekly)

Surgeries

Breast/Chest: Mastectomy in transmen; 50% of transwomen get augmentation

TGPS

Transwomen

Vaginoplasty or vulvoplasty

Orchiectomy

Transmen

Phaloplasty or metioplasty

Oophorectomy

Testicular implants

Facial: Feminization or masculinization

Voice

Transwomen need voice coaching to speak in female pitch range and resonance.

Transmen voice will deepen with testosterone.

Hair Removal

Transwomen: Facial hair removal and TGPS

Fertility Maintenance

If desired before HT

Transgender Children

Affirmative approach

Team of mental health, endocrinology, family medicine to guide treatment

Must be consistent, insistent, persistent in congruent gender

Social transition

Hormone blockers

Sex hormones

Decision on transgender transition at age 16

Potential Side Effects

- **Transwomen**: DVT, PE blood clots due to estradiol HT. Considerabley reduced with estradiol valerate versus ethinyl estradiol.
- **Transmen**: high red blood cell count due to testosterone HT

Outcomes

Outcomes of treatment generally good; regret minimal <1%

Counseling should be available post planned transition.

REFERENCES

Asscheman, H., Giltay, E. J., Megens, J. A., de Ronde, W. P., van Trotsenburg, M. A., & Gooren, L. J. (2011). A long-term follow-up study of mortality in transsexuals receiving treatment with cross-sex hormones. *European Journal of Endocrinology, 164*(4), 635–642.

Baron, S., Sowers, J., & Feinberg, M. (1983). Prolactinoma in a man following industrial exposure to estrogens. *Western Journal of Medicine, 138*, 720–722.

Bevan, T. (2015). *The psychobiology of transsexualism and transgenderism.* Santa Barbara, CA: Praeger.

Burnett, J. (2011a). *Harm reduction for treatment of M2F TS below the poverty level—four year follow-up.* Presented at the Southern Comfort Conference 2011, Atlanta, GA.

Burnett, J. (2011b). *Cross gender hormone treatment for GID.* Presented at the Southern Comfort Conference 2011, Atlanta, GA.

Canadian Professional Association for Transgender Health. (2014). E-course in transgender endocrine therapy. CPATH and AstraZeneca Canada, Inc. https://www.3blmedia.com/theCSRfeed/Free-e-Learning-Module-Endocrine-Therapy-Transgender-Patients

Cohen-Kettenis, P. T., & van Goozen, S. H. (1997). Sex reassignment of adolescent transsexuals: A follow-up study. *Journal of the American Academy of Child Adolescent Psychiatry, 36*(2), 263–271.

Constantino, A., Cerpolini, S., Morselli, P., Venturoli, S., & Merriggiola, M. (2013). A prospective study on sexual function and mood in female-to-male transsexuals during testosterone administration and after reassignment surgery. *Journal of Sex and Marital Therapy, 39*, 321–325.

Conway, L. (2001–2002). How frequently does transsexualism occur? http://www.lynnconway.com

Dacakis, G. (2000). Long-term maintenance of fundamental frequency increases in male-to-female transsexuals. *Voice, 4*, 549–556.

Davidson, A., et al. (2006). Protocols for hormone reassignment of gender. Tom Waddell Health Center Transgender Team. https://www.sfdph.org/dph/comupg/oservices/medSvs/hlthCtrs/TransGendprotocols122006.pdf

Davies, S., McIntyre, S., Richards, C., & Rypma, C. (2019, April). Rates of detransition and regret in NHS gender identity clinic. EPATH, 2019.

de Haan, G., Santos, G. M., Arayasirikul, S., & Raymond, H. F. (2015). Non-prescribed hormone use and barriers to care for transgender women in San Francisco. *LGBT Health, 2*(4), 313–323.

Deutsch, M. B. (2016). *Guidelines for primary and gender-affirming care of transgender and gender nonbinary people.* Center for Excellence in Transgender Health, University of California San Francisco. http://www.transhealth.ucsf.edu/trans?page=guidelines-home

Dhejne, C., Lichtenstein, P., Boman, M., Johansson, V., Langstrom, N., & Landen, M. (2011). Long-term follow-up of transsexual persons undergoing sex reassignment surgery: Cohort study in Sweden. *PLOS ONE, 6*, e16885.

Djordjevic, M. L., Stanojevic, D., Bizic, M., Kojovic, V., Majstorovic, M., Vujovic, S., . . . Perovic, S. V. (2009). Metoidioplasty as a single stage sex reassignment surgery in female transsexuals: Belgrade experience. *Journal of Sexual Medicine, 6*(5), 1306–1313.

Durwood, L., McLaughlin, K. A., & Olson, K. R. (2017). Mental health and self-worth in socially transitioned transgender youth. *Child & Adolescent Psychiatry, 56*(2), 116–123.

Gaither, T. W., Awad, M. A., Osterberg, E. C., Murphy, G. P., Romero, A., Bowers, M. L., & Breyer, B. N. (2018) Postoperative complications following primary penile inversion vaginoplasty among 330 male-to-female transgender patients. *Journal of Urology, 199*, 760–765.

Gómez-Gil, E., Zubiaurre-Elorza, L., Esteva, I., Guillamon, A., Godás, T., Cruz Almaraz, M., . . . Salamero, M. (2012). Hormone-treated transsexuals report less social distress, anxiety and depression. *Psychoneuroendocrinology, 37*(5), 662–670.

Gooren, L., Giltay, E., & Bunck, M. C. (2008). Long-term treatment of transsexuals with cross-sex hormones. *Journal of Clinical Endocrinology and Metabolism, 94*(1), 19–25.

Gorin-Lazard, A., et al. (2012). Is hormonal therapy associated with better quality of life in transsexuals? A cross-sectional study. *Journal of Sexual Medicine, 9*(2), 531–541.

Hembree, W. C., Cohen-Kettenis, P., Delemarre-van de Waal, H. A., Gooren, L. J., Meyer, W. L., Spack, N. P., . . . Montori, M. (2009). Endocrine treatment of transgender persons: An Endocrine Society clinical practice guideline. *Journal of Clinical Endocrinology and Metabolism, 94*, 3132–3154.

Jiang, D., Witten, J., Berli, J., & Dugi, D. (2018). Does depth matter? Factors affecting choice of vulvoplasty over vaginoplasty as gender-affirming genital surgery for transgender women. *Journal of Sexual Medicine, 15*(6), 902–906.

Krege, S., Bex, A., Lummen, G., & Rubben, H. (2001). Male-female transsexualism: A technique, results and long-term follow-up in 66 patients. *BJU International, 88*, 396–402.

Kuiper, B., & Cohen-Kettenis, P. (1988) Sex reassignment surgery: A study of 141 transsexuals. *Archives of Sexual Behavior, 17*, 439–457.

Landen, M., Walinder, J., Hambert, G., & Lundstrom, B. (1998). Factors predictive of regret in sex reassignment. *Acta Psychiatrica Scandinavica, 97*, 284–289.

Lawlis, S. M., Donkin, H. R., Bates, J. R., Britto, M. T., & Conard, L. A. E. (2017). Health concerns of transgender and gender nonconforming youth and their parents upon presentation to a transgender clinic. *Journal of Adolescent Health, 61*(5), 642–648.

Lawrence, A. (2003). Factors associated with satisfaction or regret following male-to-female sex reassignment surgery. *Archives of Sexual Behavior, 32*, 299–315.

Lawrence, A. (2006). Patient-reported complications and functional outcomes of male-to-female sex reassignment surgery. *Archives of Sexual Behavior, 35*, 717–727.

Lindemalm, G., Korlin, D., & Uddenberg, N. (1987). Prognostic factors vs. outcome in male-to-female transsexualism. A follow-up study of 14 cases. *Acta Psychiatrica Scandinavica, 75*, 268–274.

Lobato, M. I., et al. (2006). Follow-up of sex reassignment surgery in transsexuals: A Brazilian cohort. *Archives of Sexual Behavior, 35*, 711–715.

Manrique, O. J., Adabi, K., Huang, T. C., Jorge-Martinez, J., Meihofer, L. E., Brassard, P., & Galan, R. (2018). Assessment of pelvic floor anatomy for male-to-female vaginoplasty and the role of physical therapy on functional and patient-reported outcomes. *Annals of Plastic Surgery*. https://www.pubfacts.com/detail/30422842/Assessment-of-Pelvic-Floor-Anatomy-for-Male-to-Female-Vaginoplasty-and-the-Role-of-Physical-Therapy

Michel, A., Ansseau, M., Legros, J. J., Pitchot, W., & Mormont, C. (2002). The transsexual: What about the future? *European Psychiatry, 17*(6), 353–536.

Newfield, E., Hart, S., Dibble, S., & Kohler, L. (2006). Female-to-male transgender quality of life. *Quality of Life Research, 15*(9), 1447–1457.

Olson, J. (2012). *Treating transgender youth: Basics of cross-sex hormones*. Strengthening Youth Prevention Paradigms at Children's Hospital Los Angeles. http://lachildrenshospital.net/webinar/SYPP_webinar_Olson_10_10_12/lib/playback.html

Olson, K. R., Durwood, L., & McLaughlin, K. A. (2018). Mental health of transgender children who are supported in their identities. *Pediatrics, 142*(2), e20181436.

Olson-Kennedy, J., Rosenthal, S. M., Hastings, J., & Linda Wesp, L. (2018). *Health considerations for gender non-conforming children and transgender adoles-*

cents. Regents of the University of California. http://transhealth.ucsf.edu/trans?page=guidelines-youth

Olyslager, F., & Conway, L. (2007). *On the calculation of the prevalence of transsexualism*. Presentation at 2007 WPATH Symposium, Chicago, IL.

Rotondi, N. K., Bauer, G. R., Scanlon, K., Kaay, M., Travers, R., & Travers, A. (2013). Nonprescribed hormone use and self-performed surgeries: "Do-it-yourself" transitions in transgender communities in Ontario, Canada. *American Journal of Public Health, 103*(10), 1830–1836.

Simons, L., Schrager, S. M., Clark, L. F., Belzer, M., & Olson, J. (2013). Parental support and mental health among transgender adolescents. *Journal of Adolescent Health, 53*(6), 791–793.

Stefanick, M., Cochrane, B., Hsia, J., Barad, D., Liu, J., & Johnson, S. (2003). The WHI Postmenopausal Hormone Trials. *Annals of Epidemiology, 13,* S78–S86.

Tchaikovski, S. N., & Rosing, J. (2010). Mechanisms of estrogen-induced venous thromboembolism. *Thrombosis Research, 126,* 5-11.

Thomas, J. P., & Macmillan, C. (2013). Feminization laryngoplasty: Assessment of surgical pitch elevation. *Archives of Oto-Rhino-Laryngology, 270*(10), 2695–2700.

Webberly, H., & Webberly, M. J. (2018). Self-medication is common in patients who face long delays in accessing NHS services in the UK. *WPATH 2018 poster session*.

Weinand, J. D., & Safer, J. D. (2015). Hormone therapy in transgender adults is safe with provider supervision; A review of hormone therapy sequelae for transgender individuals. *Journal of Clinical & Translational Endocrinology, 2*(2), 55–60.

Weyers, S., Elaut, E., De Sutter, P., Gerris, J., T'Sjoen, G., Helens, G., et al. (2009). Long-term assessment of the physical, mental, and sexual health among transsexual women. *Journal of Sexual Medicine, 6,* 752–760.

Wibowo, E., Shellhammer, P., & Wassersug, R. (2011). Role of estrogen in normal male function: Clinical implications for patients with prostate cancer on androgen deprivation therapy. *Journal of Urology, 185,* 17–23.

Wiepjes, C. M., de Jongh, R. T., de Blok, C. J., Vlot, M. C., Lips, P., Twisk, J. W., & Heijer, M. (2018, December 7). Bone safety during the first ten years of gender-affirming hormonal treatment in transwomen and transmen. *Journal of Bone Mineral Research*. https://doi.org/10.1002/jbmr.3612 [Epub ahead of print].

Wierckx, K., et al. (2011). Quality of life and sexual health after sex reassignment surgery in transsexual men. *Journal of Sexual Medicine, 8,* 2279–3388.

World Professional Association for Transgender Health (WPATH). (2013). Standards of care. Version 7. https://wpath.org/publications/soc

Xu, R., Wu, X., Di, A., Xu, J., Pang, C., & Pang, S. (2000). Pituitary prolactin-secreting tumor formation: Recent developments. *Biological Signals and Receptors, 9,* 1–10.

8

Applications in the Field: Associated Treatments and Resources

Since providers are charged with reducing the suffering of their patients, they should be knowledgeable about patient management resources, external to treatment procedures, that improve patients' physical and mental health and resilience. Such outside resources can better their quality of life and resilience and help them avoid reactive depression, isolation, loneliness, and suicidal thinking.

Providers need to be aware of these resources to encourage the overall physical and mental health of transgender people. These include:

- Social support resources
- Marital and family therapy
- Health care resources
- Support for identity document changes
- Gender presentation support

- Advocacy for transgender rights
- Spirituality
- Housing
- Perineal exercise
- Employee assistance groups
- Augmentation of knowledge
- Building resilence

SOCIAL SUPPORT OPPORTUNITIES

It is vital for transgender people to build social support networks that can affirm their congruent gender and authentic selves. This is particularly true for elder transgender people, where it is a matter of survival (Witten, 2014), just as it is for all elders (Olaya et al., 2017). Realizing this need, transgender people have taken it upon themselves to organize various social support organizations and to encourage transgender people to build informal social contacts.

Support Groups

In Chapter 1, we referred to the formation of the Society for the Second Self, or Tri-Ess, by Virginia Prince in 1972 as part of transgender history. This was an initial effort at social support building. Membership in Tri-Ess was restricted to those assigned male at birth who were married and did not want to transition. However, less restrictive support groups grew up all across the United States, United Kingdom, Europe, and Australia. Although today transgender people can network through social media, one of the current functions of social media is to coordinate meetings and meetups outside of formal support groups.

Today, transgender support groups are alive and well in many places both at the local and national level. Support groups continue to be led by peers, but many mental health providers lead or participate in them to get to know local transgender people and to understand what local transgender people are currently doing and thinking. Such groups may also assist providers in knowing safe spaces for patient management. Providers also increase their visibility to attract new patients. Support groups are formed by hospitals, churches, and other organizations because they sense the need in the community. Some local churches foster support groups, even though their hierarchy may not approve of being transgender.

All it usually takes is for one transgender parent or family member to stand up for their transgender relative, family member, or friend and realize the need.

At the national level, PFLAG (https://pflag.org), which originally was an initialism for Parents, Families and Friends of Lesbians and Gays, now just uses the acronym "PFLAG" to indicate its dedication to the entire LGBTQ community. The organization was formed in New York City in 1973 and now has over 400 chapters in the United States. It is peer-led. The numbers of transgender children and parents have greatly increased in their membership, and local chapters can be found in most areas. PFLAG not only provides support group meetings for all ages, but also sponsors social events for LGBTQ children, tweens, and teenagers. The social networks formed in their meetings are extended by social media. It is common for transgender children to use social media to form networks based on meeting others at support group meetings. In addition to support group meetings, PFLAG also provides organization for LGBTQ advocacy.

Tri-ESS (https://www.tri-ess.org/docs/whatis.html) continues to operate with over 40 chapters in the United States and also is peer-led. Their main emphasis is on keeping adult married couples together although one spouse is transgender. Female spouses are encouraged to attend and participate. Each chapter has a monthly meeting with seasonal celebrations. As their founder, Virginia Prince, did, many distain the term transgender and instead prefer the term crossdresser. Tri-ESS has become somewhat less exclusive with former members who are transitioning or have been divorced still in contact with their home chapters.

Seniors can participate in local groups sponsored by SAGE (https://www.sageusa.org) for LGBT social contact and advocacy.

Because transgender people who are not out also participate, support groups try to maintain the privacy of those who are members and the confidentiality of discussions. This facilitates open discussion.

Adult Social Groups and Meetups

Adult transgender people use social media to organize social groups and meetups (https://www.meetup.com), which are typically open. They do not officially maintain secrecy or confidentiality, but most transgender people respect the identities of others in the group. They organize social events such as dinners, concerts, dance classes, and happy hours through Internet social media meetup facilities. These social groups tend to be a mixture of transgender people and transitioning transgender people. Overlaid on these groups are lesbian, gay, and other groups that accept transgender members. They stimulate friendships and informal gatherings of transgender people with others.

Internet Social Media

Transgender people have a long history of interaction on social media, even before the Internet was widely available. Social media allows interaction with anonymity when desired. Prior to the Internet, private dial-up bulletin boards and commercial networks allowed transgender people to connect. They also included locations for documents providing information of importance to transgender people including gender presentation assistance, news, and support group publications. Today, Internet social media provides additional bandwidth for images, videos, and live chat.

FAMILY AND MARITAL COUNSELING

Family acceptance is important for transgender people. It predicts greater self-esteem and general health. It also protects against depression, substance abuse, and suicidal ideation and behaviors (Ryan, Russell, Huebner, Diaz, & Sanchez, 2010). For these reasons it is important to encourage family and marital counseling that fosters family acceptance. The families and spouses of transgender people often need counseling to deal with social problems and cultural rejection because of a transgender member. For transgender people in the closet, families and spouses often are shocked by the revelation of being transgender. The spouse of a transgender person has thoughts about the authenticity of their own gender and sexuality when being transgender is revealed. For transitioning transgender people, it is often said that their families are forced to transition along with them.

When a transgender person comes out to them, family members and spouses go through the well-documented stages of grief—denial, anger, bargaining, depression, and acceptance. Their perception is that they have lost the person they thought they knew who is now a different person to them. This is especially true for parents who are used to dealing with a child of one gender, only to learn that their child is not really congruent with that gender. Some family members take radical action to disconnect from their transgender relatives. When parents disown or disconnect them, young transgender people may be forced to be homeless and live on the street. Other family members may initially reject a transgender person, but with patience, time, and counseling may come to accept them.

Counseling should take an affirmative approach; to do otherwise risks lack of cooperation from the transgender person. The goal should be to inform family members about being transgender, to accept who the transgender person really is, and to understand that being transgender is not a mental illness or immoral, just a product of human genetic diversity.

Because being transgender was kept in secret for so long, many family and marital therapists have little or no training or experience with transgender people. As more and more transpeople become visible, such providers are in the process of learning.

Some transgender people who are separated from their families because of rejection form new types of family units. They consist of friends and roommates grouped together into "families we choose," which helps provide the some of the social support they are missing from biological families (Hull & Ortyl, 2018).

HEALTH CARE RESOURCES

Providers may need to help transgender people deal with government or insurance problems that transgender people encounter due to discrimination. Discrimination discourages transgender people from seeking and getting health care. One study showed 22 percent of transgender people reported avoidance or postponement of needed medical care due to experienced discrimination (Mirza & Rooney, 2018).

Although the Affordable Care Act (ACA) in the United States banned discrimination, the implementation of this rule is, at this writing, tied up in court. Many health care administrators in hospitals and insurance companies still do not understand that the procedures explained in Chapter 7 and this chapter are necessary for transgender health. Experiences in the University of California system indicate that no savings in coverage costs can be gained by refusing transgender care, because the alternative is to pay for the costs of treating depression, substance abuse, and injuries suffered during suicide attempts (Zaker-Shahrak, Chio, Isaac, & Tescher, 2012). Studies summarizing a wide range of experience have found that transition-related health care benefits are low in cost, but provide substantial benefits for both employees and employers (Herman, 2013). Providers often have to write repeated justifications for transgender treatments to insurance companies because the companies do not understand the realities of transgender health care. Government control also causes problems because every transgender patient has individual needs, which cannot always be anticipated in regulations.

Because computer algorithms are used to screen insurance claims, sometimes a claim may be rejected because the algorithm is taught that only males or only females can get that particular treatment. The algorithm compares the patient's sex with the claim code. Such treatments may be denied unless the code "45" is put on the claim form, which tells the computer that this is not a mistake and to ignore this instruction about sex. Many providers and organizations do not know that they should do this. (The number 45 has no intrinsic meaning; it is just an arbitrary number.)

The ACA policy is that transwomen can get screening mammograms at no cost, just as other women can, but many radiology departments are only accustomed to performing mammograms on "males" when breast cancer is suspected. This male test is more elaborate than the screening test, but this is frequently confusing to radiology departments even if a male on HT enters with a doctor's order for a screening test.

The largest employer of transgender people in the United States and the world is the U.S. military. There are currently at least 15,000–20,000 transgender people in the U.S. military, the equivalent of an army division. Transwomen volunteer at a rate twice their peers and transmen at a rate three times their peers (Randall, 2012; Vanneman et al., 2015). Although policies keep shifting without consideration of scientific evidence about transgender people, their performance and dedication as soldiers has never been questioned. In 2016, when transgender people could serve openly for the first time, the military made a substantial effort to educate military providers through CEU courses and in-service training. The internal policy has been for internal providers to address transgender needs and to send transgender people outside the military for procedures that they could not perform internally. Undoubtedly, these providers are collecting data and conducting research studies, which could contribute to transgender health beyond the military, but none of these studies have ever been released.

There has been great progress in treating military veterans and active duty transgender people in the military, despite discriminatory and conflicting policy decisions by government. In the past, transgender veterans have received HT and certain surgeries, but at the time of writing are not allowed to get TGPS. There are now veteran LGBT care coordinators located at VA facilities, and there are active programs at over 28 VA facilities (Dietert, Dentice, & Keig, 2017). The VA provides support groups and counseling as well as medical treatment.

Some Planned Parenthood (https://www.plannedparenthood.org) locations now provide services for transgender hormone therapy, including hormones and HT drugs as well as blood monitoring services.

SUPPORT FOR IDENTIFICATION CHANGES

Providers will often be asked to assist transgender people in obtaining accurate personal identification. Policies in many states and countries require medical support letters indicating that the transgender person has taken steps to live in their congruent gender. Some require letters indicating that the person has had TGPS. Some require letters in support of name changes. The law and policy of each state and federal agency is somewhat different, which makes for a confusing situation.

Accurate identification is guaranteed by international law as a right. Yet, particularly in the United States, there is a patchwork system in which each state sets rules and policies for birth certificates, driver's licenses, and other forms of identification. Some states will not change identification to match the person's congruent gender or sex *at all.* This chaotic situation sets up cases in which a person's identification does not match their gender presentation, leading to unnecessary legal problems. To deal with this complexity, the NCTE has set up a website with identification requirements for all states and the U.S. federal government agencies (https://transequality.org/documents).

Many states and countries are in the process of revising their personal identification policies. The general trend in the United States is to liberalize identification policies to make it easier to change sex or gender markers. In some cases, this was forced by lawsuits. Some allow people to declare no sex or gender and have an "X" on their identification rather than an "M" or "F."

GENDER PRESENTATION SUPPORT

As part of patient management, providers should know how to direct transgender people to safe sources of clothing, hairstyling, and makeup to fit their congruent gender presentation. This is particularly true for transwomen.

The difficulty in finding safe sources has decreased because of online purchasing and delivery, but there are still situations in which a transwoman needs personal attention by a store salesperson for things like bra fittings and makeup selection to best match their coloring. Many national chain stores now have a policy of allowing transgender women to try on clothing and makeup in the store, but this is not always followed in their local stores. Transgender people often have to call ahead and get private service. With regard to bra fitting, some stores accept transgender people while others do not. Sometimes the best source for bra fitting is at a hospital that also serves women who have had breast operations but, again, the transgender person may need to call ahead to avoid embarrassment in the waiting room.

One of the things transmen often do is to take up bodybuilding to alter their bodies to look more masculine. This is aided by the testosterone they are taking in HT. However, finding a gym that will allow them to exercise may be a problem, and there is awkwardness in which locker room to use. Providers may need to obtain information from other patients on sources that can help new transmen with bodybuilding.

ADVOCACY FOR TRANSGENDER RIGHTS

Transgender rights are guaranteed by international law and ethics conventions, yet more needs to be done to implement and defend transgender rights in many countries, including the United States. Providers can help by supporting transgender people in lawsuits over identification, employment, restrooms, schooling, and other issues by sending letters of support that explain about being transgender. Organizations such as WPATH and the American Psychological Association advocate for transgender rights across the world, and there are local advocacy groups in many countries.

Whether providers realize it or not, they are community authority figures and experts whom people rely on for leadership. Leadership in the community is key to convincing and supporting parents not to reject their transgender children. Such rejection is a primary cause of the high numbers of homeless transgender youth. Too many community leaders do not understand the phenomenon of being transgender and sometimes stir up animosity at being transgender for political purposes. Providers need to set good examples. Providers should not allow transgender people to be verbally misgendered or denigrated by other people.

Providers should actively prepare for and seek transgender people as employees. All gender restrooms in provider facilities should be labeled outside as such with specification of the equipment available inside like urinals and toilets. Reach out to let the public know that LGBTQ people are accepted as patients and employees. Public affirmation of transgender people is of benefit to the knowledge of cisgender people.

SPIRITUALITY

Many individual churches provide support to transgender people in the spiritual context. Some are individual churches, but the major international church that supports transgender rights and accepts transgender people is the Unitarian Universalist Church (UUC, https://www.uua.org). This church has a remarkable record of advocating for civil rights and LGBT rights in America. The church is diverse in many ways including beliefs, minority participation, and political views. Some churches have undergone intensive education programs to become "Welcoming Churches" for LGBT people (Unitarian Universalist Association, 2018), but all UUC churches have adopted a policy of acceptance. Although they are smaller than the largest denominations, the Evangelical Lutheran Church in America, Presbyterian Church, and Episcopal (USA) churches are also accepting of transgender people. Some sects of the Jewish religion accept transgender people. In fact, the Jewish subculture historically allowed for several gender behavior categories. Some Methodist churches in the United States are accepting of transgender people but many foreign Methodist churches are not. This may result in a schism.

Other church denominations may seem to be accepting of transgender people, but providers and transgender people need to be aware that some churches entice them with acceptance, only to condemn their behavior once they have joined.

HOUSING

Many transgender people become homeless because of family, community, and cultural rejection. Several cities have developed not-for-profit housing initiatives for transgender people. For example, Atlanta has the Trans Housing Atlanta Program and Chicago has its Transgender Life Center. Such not-for-profits provide both short-term and long-term housing.

The Veterans Administration has active housing programs that cover transgender veterans. Their programs provide grants for local housing providers, vouchers for public housing, and management to prevent home loss.

PERINEAL EXERCISES

Perineal exercising is an emerging procedure for transitioning transwomen. Physical therapy nurses are obtaining good results with both pre-TGPS and post-TGPS exercise. Exercise builds the muscles that support the neovagina, the new, rerouted urethra, and the anal sphincter. The perineal muscles include the muscles extending from the vulva to the rectum, which can be exercised using the **Kegel** procedures. Reports overall are that exercise is good but overindulgence in pre-op exercise can interfere with urination immediately post-op. It is helpful for the patient to get coaching at the start of the exercise regimen.

EMPLOYEE RESOURCE GROUPS

LGBT employee resource groups exist in many companies and organizations to deal with employee isolation, difficult workplace climates, and inequitable benefits and policies (Githens & Aragon, 2009). Employers support these groups because they improve workplace effectiveness and morale. The organization Out and Equal (http://outandequal.org) helps train internal leaders of such resource groups and LGBT advocates to organizations.

PATIENT KNOWLEDGE

Providers can support the acquisition of knowledge on being transgender for their patients by providing references to books and publications. Informed people make better patients. However, there is plenty of misinformation available, so one of the tasks of providers is to provide the right information.

The Internet is usually the first source of information for transgender people and their **SOFFAs** (Significant Others, Friends, Family and Allies), but the accuracy of information on the Internet is uneven and usually the first search is misleading. Transgender youth rely on information on the Internet to preserve their privacy, but some inaccurate information can lead to further rejection and depression. For these reasons it is particularly important for providers and their professional organizations to provide accurate information on their websites. It is also incumbent on providers to teach transgender people and SOFFAs to be skeptical consumers of information found on the Internet (Evans et al., 2017).

A list of suggested readings is provided in the Resources section at the end of this book.

BUILDING RESILIENCE

Because transgender people are subjected to the stress of rejection, it is important for them to learn how to build stress resilience to ward off PTSD. Methods for building stress resilience have been researched and applied in the militaries of the United States, Israel, and other countries. There are several techniques and approaches that have been found useful (Meredith et al., 2011; Pietrzak et al., 2010; Wounded Warrior, 2019). Such approaches are now also being applied to prevent PTSD from sexual harassment/assault and to help minorities under stress, which includes transgender people.

The two primary techniques that transgender people can use to build resilience are (1) to learn the **relaxation response** and (2) to learn how to make a **positive interpretation of events**.

The relaxation response (Benson, 2001) should be practiced to enable a transgender person to voluntarily relax in the presence of stress. The relaxation response involves systematic relaxation of muscles with awareness to maintain some parasympathetic tonus in the face of seemingly overwhelming sympathetic response. The relaxation response can be learned through yoga, meditation, biofeedback, and certain Lamaze techniques. The relaxation response is not new; Zen and Samurai warriors practiced this response so that they could keep a cool head in battle. Athletes learn the response to control their arousal levels during competition because arousal levels that are too high can interfere with performance. Relaxation does not mean that one ignores the situation, but rather keeps a cool head, or one's poise, to deal with the situation. To be effective, the relaxation has to be practiced in the presence of increasingly intense stressful situations starting with very low stress.

Positive interpretation of events has to do with verbal reinterpretation to portray a stressful situation as nonstressful or humorous. The person is then free to think about how to solve the specific situation problems that they encounter. The language we use in our thoughts and verbalizations may provide triggers to negative emotional reactions, and negative emotions can be attached to situations to form conditioned reflexes. *The idea is that events only have the meanings that you give to them.* Assigning negative interpretations to events is sometimes termed "awfulizing," exaggerations of "the sky is falling" type. Negatives interfere with physical and mental performance. In athletics, one should not be depressed by falling behind in a competition; rather, it should be looked upon as an opportunity and as being relieved of pressure, having nothing to lose by trying. Transgender people who typically experience cultural rejection and misgendering should reinterpret those experiences as opportunities to teach other people about being transgender. "I do not agree with you, but if you are willing, I will teach you something useful that you do not know yet." Obviously one does not do this in the face of potential violence, but it can be practiced in everyday activities like going to the supermarket or shopping. Reinterpretation does not prevent higher brain functions from dealing with problems, but it does prevent, to some extent, more primitive emotions from interfering with higher functions.

Most importantly, positive reinterpretation interrupts the classical conditioning of the emotions associated with trauma to situational stimuli. This is the essence of PTSD in which later exposure to such trigger stimuli evoke the original trauma emotion. PTSD can be treated with counseling in which such emotional associations can be extinguished through discussion.

Social support helps deal with stress and builds resilience. This includes family, friends, support groups and medical providers, mental health counselors and organizational cohesion (Dickstein et al., 2010; Pietrzak et al., 2010).

REFERENCES

Benson, H. (2001). *The relaxation response.* New York: HarperCollins.

Chicago Housing: Transgender Life Center. http://chicago.gopride.com/news/article.cfm/articleid/44139769

Dickstein, B. D., McLean, C. P., Mintz, J., Conoscenti, L. M., Steenkamp, M. M., Benson, T. A., . . . Litz, B. T. (2010). Unit cohesion and PTSD symptom severity in Air Force medical personnel. *Military Medicine, 175*(7), 482–486.

Dietert, M., Dentice, D., & Keig, Z. (2017). Addressing the needs of transgender military veterans: Better access and more comprehensive care. *Transgender Health, 1*(2), 1, 35–44.

Evans, Y. N, Gridley, S. J., Crouch, J., Wang, A., Moreno, M. A., Ahrens, K., & Breland, D. J. (2017) Understanding online resource use by transgender youth and caregivers: A qualitative study. *Transgender Health, 2*(1), 129–139.

Githens, R. P., & Aragon, S. R. (2009). LGBT employee groups: Goals and organizational structures. *Advances in Developing Human Resources, 11*(1), 121–135. https://rodgithens.files.wordpress.com/2012/12/lgbt_ee_groups_2009.pdf

Herman, J. (2013). *Cost and benefits from providing transition-related healthcare coverage in employee health benefit plans.* Williams Institute. https://williamsinstitute.law.ucla.edu/wp-content/uploads/Herman-Cost-Benefit-of-Trans-Health-Benefits-Sept-2013.pdf

Hull, K. E., & Ortyl, T. A. (2018). Conventional and cutting-edge: Definitions of family in LGBT communities. *Sexuality Research and Social Policy.* https://link.springer.com/article/10.1007/s13178-018-0324-2

Meredith, L. S., Sherbourne, C. D., Gaillot, S. J., Hansell, L., Ritschard, H. V., Parker, A.M., & Wrenn, G. (2011). Promoting psychological resilience in the U.S. military. *Rand Health Quarterly, 1*(2), 2–184. https://www.rand.org/pubs/monographs/MG996.html

Mirza, S. A., & Rooney, C. (2018). *Discrimination prevents LGBTQ people from accessing health care.* Center for American Progress. https://www.americanprogress.org/issues/lgbt/news/2018/01/18/445130/discrimination-prevents-lg

Olaya, B., Domènech-Abella, J., Moneta, M. V., Lara, E., Caballero, F. F., Rico-Uribe, L. A., & Haro, J. M. (2017). All-cause mortality and multimorbidity in older adults: The role of social support and loneliness. *Gerontology, 1*(99), 120–126.

Pietrzak, R. H., Johnson, D. C., Goldstein, M. B., Malley, J. C., Rivers, A. J., Morgan, C. A., & Southwick, S. M. (2010). Psychosocial buffers of traumatic stress, depressive symptoms, and psychosocial difficulties in veterans of Operations Enduring Freedom and Iraqi Freedom: The role of resilience, unit support, and post deployment social support. *Journal of Affective Disorders, 120*(103), 188–192.

Randall, M. J. (2012) Gap analysis: Transition of health care from Department of Defense to Department of Veterans Affairs. *Military Medicine, 177,* 11–16.

Ryan, C., Russell, S. T., Huebner, D., Diaz, R., & Sanchez, J. (2010). Family acceptance in adolescence and the health of LGBT young adults. *Journal of Child Adolescent Psychiatric Nursing, 23*(4), 205–213.

Trans Housing Atlanta Program. http://transhousingatlanta.org/

Unitarian Universalist Association. (2018). Lesbian, gay, bisexual, transgender and queer ministries. https://www.uua.org/offices/staff/mgw/lgbtq-ministries

U.S. Veterans Administration Housing Programs. https://www.va.gov/HOMELESS/housing.asp

Vanneman, M. E., Harris, A. H. S., Chen, C., et al. (2015). Army active duty members' linkage to veterans health administration services after deployments to Iraq or Afghanistan and following separation. *Military Medicine, 189*, 1052–1058.

Witten, T. M. (2014). It's not all darkness: Robustness, resilience, and successful transgender aging. *LGBT Health, 1*(1), 24–33.

Wounded Warrior. (2019). Heal your mental wounds: Help for combat stress, PTSD and TBI. https://www.woundedwarriorproject.org/programs/combat-stress-recovery-program?msclkid=27620b3231941842925c57056f89aede&utm_source=bing&utm_medium=cpc&utm_campaign=SEM~WWP~NB~US~ALL~PTSD&utm_term=%2Bptsd%20%2Bprograms%20%2Bveterans&utm_content=Veterans_PTSD_Programs_MDBR

Zaker-Shahrak, A., Chio, L. W. C., Isaac, R., & Tescher, J. (2012). *Economic impact assessment: Gender nondiscrimination in health insurance*. Department of Insurance, State of California. REG-2011-00023. http://transgenderlawcenter.org/wp-content/uploads/2013/04/Economic-Impact-Assessment-Gender-Nondiscrimination-In-Health-Insurance.pdf

9

Case Studies: Understanding Their Struggle

To respect client privacy and protect client identities, the following concocted examples were developed using combinations of elements from actual case histories. Consistent with guidelines discussed in Chapter 6, pronouns should normally be determined by the declared or observed congruent gender of an individual. In this chapter, however, gender pronouns change throughout to reflect the case study person's gender assigned at birth and their later self-declared gender, giving the reader greater insight into the confusion and real struggle that exists when a person emerges as transgender.

TERI L.

Teri was declared to be male at birth in 1948 by his uncle who was a GP and a no-nonsense general practitioner. Her mother was an elementary

Elements of Transgender Case Histories

Emergence: Usually about ages four to seven, but at those ages they may just know something is a problem, something is not right with their gender identification.

Secrecy: Public emergence may be delayed/prevented by secrecy. Secrecy causes medical and mental health problems. It causes high mental workload, anxiety, depression, isolation, and physiological stress. Those who know the secret may also be affected.

Cure: There is no cure for being transgender and it is not pathological. A wide variety of treatments have been tried to "cure" it, but gender change efforts have been unsuccessful and some are dangerous.

Adult Treatment: Current accepted treatment is affirming care with counseling to deal with problems of rejection, marriage, and family. Crosspresentation is encouraged in safety to determine the desirability of transition. Most transgender people do not transition and live in secrecy.

Suicide: Depression and isolation lead to a suicide attempt rate of approximately 40 percent of transgender people. Chances of suicide can be reduced by acceptance and transition.

Hormone Therapy: Usually one of the first steps in transgender transition. The goal is to achieve the normal sex hormone blood levels of the opposite natal sex.

Treatment of Transgender Children: Current best practice is affirming care for those who are persistent, insistent, and consistent about their congruent gender and wanting treatment. Affirming treatment may involve administration of puberty-blocking drugs until age 16. At that point, they and their parents choose to begin transition or let natural puberty take effect.

Flight: In an effort to hope for a "cure," transgender people may engage in flight to faraway schools, into marriage, or into the military. A large percentage of transpeople get married and the rate of joining the military is twice the rate for nontransgender peers for transwomen and three times for transmen.

school teacher, and her father was a biologist for the state of Wyoming. Teri's parents had lived through the 1928 Depression and married in 1945 as World War II ended. Her father's family had been prosperous in a local city in construction, but moved to their country house to survive during the Depression. Teri's father had been a radio repairman but became a farmer, hunter, trapper, and fisherman to help his family during the downturn. During World War II, her father was declared medically ineligible to serve in the military, so he became a biologist for the state. Her father had had scarlet fever as a child and as a result, became infected with osteomyelitis causing one leg to be shorter than the other. Her mother had worked in the city but moved to the family's country house when she was married.

Although her parents were in love, they delayed marriage and pregnancy because of unsettled times and because her father was uncertain of his future because of his medical history. So, Teri became one of the post-war baby boomers. Teri grew up taller and stronger than her peers and had a normal medical childhood history. She was fascinated by electrical gadgets. One of her first toys was a record player, which she used to play Christmas music, including the Nutcracker Suite. She also listened to ballet music—*Sleeping Beauty* was her favorite. She was fascinated by electric trains, and every Christmas she asked for and got a new electric train accessory—log loader, cattle loader, switchman's hut. She and her father built the train set and played with it nonstop until the end of the Christmas season. Since her father had fixed radios in his first job, the attic was full of radio equipment, which helped in science fiction fantasy play. She had two teddy bears and access to her mother's dolls, but preferred the magic of music, electricity, and radio. She listened to radio programs every night and when television started in the 1950s, it had her rapt attention.

Teri's mother, an elementary school teacher, helped Teri to learn how to read by the age of 4. She graded papers and wrote lesson plans by night as she went back to work after her pregnancy. One day, Teri came up to her and said, "I am a girl, not a boy." Trying not to be shocked, in her best schoolteacher manner she carefully explained that Teri was born a male and males had certain responsibilities. They included doing well in school, playing sports, serving in the military, and raising a family. Teri's uncles had served in the military, although Teri's father had not because of his leg. That seemed to end the discussion.

Both parents' families took pity on their country cousins and passed on magazines to them—*Look, Life, National Geographic, Saturday Evening Post.* Although Teri could not understand all the words in the articles, there were plenty of illustrations and pictures of famous people in the news. Among these was an article about Christine Jorgensen, who was now a celebrity after taking hormones and receiving TGPS in Denmark where it was legal at the time. Teri immediately understood. She went back to her mother and again told her that she was a girl, not a boy. This time her mother told her that she was a fireball of activity and could not possibly be a girl. She showed her the article and said, "She changed from a boy to a girl!"

Her mother had to admit that it was possible but told Teri that if she became a girl now, she would end up in the state mental institution because she would be diagnosed as insane, unable to play or see her family or friends again, and they would shock her and operate on her. Her mother's advice was to keep it a secret and someday when she was an adult, she could decide for herself about changing.

Teri presented to several mental health providers as a 45-year-old male, asking for help in transgender transition. The first mental health professional tried Freudian psychoanalysis; the second tried cognitive therapy. Neither was successful. Neither mental health professional had knowledge and experience with transgender people, as this was before professional school or CEU courses were offered. The third mental health professional had experience with LGBT patients, developed a history, and recommended a low dose HT to an endocrinologist. Instead of a low dose, the endocrinologist started with full doses of estradiol, medroxyprogesterone, and spironolactone. The patient's mood improved, but she became panicky because her breasts started to grow within a few weeks. She stopped taking the hormones. When her mental health professional found out, she told Teri to go back to the endocrinologist where she got a stern lecture about taking the drugs she been had prescribed and was started on lower doses of HT medications. Teri continued on HT and eventually worked up to full dosages.

That was three years ago. Today Teri is presenting to her mental health professional to get a transgender genital plastic surgery "gatekeeping" letter.

JAN H.

Jan was declared female at birth in 2003 in a small rural town in Missouri. As a child, Jan showed signs of being a tomboy, engaging with her older brother in rough and tumble play, playing soccer and other sports. She presented in masculine clothing and resisted wearing dresses and skirts. His parents thought that she was a tomboy and would just "grow out of it." They had seen examples in their family of female children who changed their behavior in later life.

At age nine, Jan showed the early physical signs of puberty. Her parents told her what to expect. But as she developed breast buds, her behavior began to change and she became sullen, brooding, depressed, and unable to get through the day. Her schoolwork suffered and she had violent outbursts, attacking other children and her parents. Her parents took her to see their family doctor, who concluded that she was a normal girl who was experiencing the early effects of puberty.

Jan confided in several of her friends, who told her that she might be transgender and to check out information on the Internet. They already knew of one transgender boy in their high school. What Jan read on the Internet convinced her to seek out the transboy on social media. They had several long chats and found a way to meet after basketball practices at the local YMCA. The older transboy told her that if she thought that she was trans, she should go to the gender clinic in Kansas City. They could help her by stopping puberty until she had time to think. But she would have to convince her family and her family doctor to do it, which would not be easy because they probably did not know about being transgender. When she got to the clinic, she had to be consistent, insistent, and persistent to get puberty blockers to meet the criteria that the doctors and shrinks used at the clinic. In this way, she could decide later about her gender.

She tried to convince her parents that she should go to the clinic, without success. Her family doctor was not convinced either, but he did say that if she was concerned about her hormones, she should see the endocrinologist in a neighboring town. She begged her parents to go see the endocrinologist and they grudgingly agreed. The endocrinologist had been to a CEU course on treating transgender people but had no direct experience with treating transgender children. He did recommend that she go to the Kansas City clinic.

Jan and her family went to the gender clinic to see the team of medical doctors, endocrinologists, and social workers. Jan was so knowledgeable that they were skeptical at first, but after several visits they were convinced that social transition was appropriate. After a year, they recommended that she start taking blockers. Her parents could not afford the implants and the shots were a financial stretch, but one of their family members went to Kansas City often and could take her for the shots. The clinic established a Skype connection with the family to keep in touch.

Jan's mood immediately picked up. Since she had been presenting in the masculine gender category anyway, no social transition was required. She now augments her blocking drugs with low doses of testosterone to ensure proper bone growth.

Jan and her family now have six years of time to decide whether to allow female puberty to occur or to start transitioning to male. Jan has experienced some bullying at school but her friends there have closed ranks to stop the bullies. Although Jan may not be able to compete in high school athletics because of taking hormones, she has joined an amateur running club that encourages runners to compete against themselves by establishing "personal bests." She hopes to go to a college that has "mixed-sex" competition that conforms to NCAA rules.

MICHAEL N.

Michael was assigned male at birth, but since age four felt that she was living in the wrong body. She told no one about these feelings and began to experiment with crossdressing at age six. Crossdressing was shameful to her, but he felt compelled to do it in private. At first, crossdressing gave her a rush of sexual excitement, but by age 12 all she felt was a sense of relaxation and peace. She kept his crossdressing a secret, which required lying about his activities. She isolated himself from friends and family in order to maintain secrecy and keep his lies straight.

She managed to get a job but fell into depression when his parents died in an automobile crash. She found himself all alone and just managed to get through the day. Michael presented as masculine during the day and at work, and presented as a woman at night. She started going to gay bars and met some gay men, but she was turned off by them. He felt more comfortable with the lesbians she met there, but they were not interested in her sexually or romantically. His depression grew worse.

The shame grew more intense and so did her depression. She wished he could be normal but did not know how.

She began to have thoughts of suicide and planned it out in great detail so that no one would know that she had been a crossdresser. She boxed up his feminine clothing and took it to Goodwill. She threw out her makeup and purged her social media and email accounts. She realized that even though she erased his online presence, the social media giants and his ISP would still have copies, but she figured that no one would try to get these records if he left no traces in her personal life. She started monthly cash withdrawals from his accounts but they were not large amounts each time. She mailed them anonymously as donations to transgender charities.

Last spring at the age of 25, late at night so no one else would be hurt, she climbed into her car, drove onto the Interstate, and crashed the car into a bridge abutment, becoming one of the suicides that no one could attribute to being transgender. The police and her parents attributed the accident to black ice.

GEORGE Y.

George was determined to be male at birth. As a child, he was active and happy and found that he had a good boy soprano voice, which was in demand for Christmas cantatas and church recitals. He was selected to sing a patriotic song at eighth-grade graduation, but there was something going wrong with his voice; it would occasionally crack. His parents tried singing lessons and even had his throat painted with silver nitrate in case he had strep throat. He made it through eighth grade graduation, but two weeks later he became a baritone.

He had read about puberty in his science and health books but always thought it was something far away. He had seen a growth of hair on his genitals and tried to cut it off, but thought that puberty was not going to happen to him.

But the voice change put him into panic. He became increasingly confused over sex and gender. He was attracted to girls but suddenly realized that he wanted to behave as a girl. She enjoyed taking his male body out for a spin in athletics and bodybuilding, but somehow it was not part of her.

She was expected to take girls out on dates, but was overwhelmed by the thoughts of what his date must be thinking. It was hard enough playing the role of the boy, but she also played the role of the girl in her mind at the same time. She considered that he might be a lesbian, but at age 14 she realized that he did not know any lesbians.

George went to college and got married to a female classmate. After graduation, they started a business together, but did not get started on a family for seven years. After the birth of their second child, George went to two Halloween dress-up parties as a woman. She felt as if she was floating on air and knew it was for her, whatever it was. Unbeknownst to her wife, she started to go to transgender support groups where she could express her congruent gender.

After two years of support groups, she told her wife about her secret in an effort to save their marriage, which she saw as falling apart. Her wife was outraged and threw him out of the house for a time. George finally decided that life was too short to not transition. She hoped that her wife would stay with her. George started hormone therapy and in a few months, having sex with her wife became impossible. It was then that they started to divorce. Her wife was angry at her because she had taken away her husband, and she went through the stages of grief.

After two years, George got breast implants and four months later she got both facial feminization surgery and TGPS from the same surgeon.

George, now Georgina, changed her name and started her own business. She now says that she is happy and spends much of her time meeting prospective clients and attending transgender meetups. She even started her own weekly professional transwoman luncheon meetings.

RHODES T.

Rhodes was judged to be a male at birth, but told her parents that she wanted to wear girls' clothing, not boys' clothes, at age five. They refused to talk about it and forbade her from presenting in her congruent gender. At age nine, when she was old enough to be left alone by her parents in her house, she continued to crossdress in secret. While they were gone, she wore her mother's clothing and took careful mental notes as to where it came from in her mother's closet. Not just clothing, but shoes and lipstick. Perfume would have been detected.

Her church put on an annual musical show to raise money for the missionaries in the South Pacific. She was cast as a male dancer, which was not her first choice of roles, but it entitled her to wear full makeup for the dress rehearsal and four performances. It was delightful; she could see herself in the mirror and smell the lipstick and makeup. The Sunday school teachers would put makeup on the students and cackled with delight over Rhodes looking like a girl. She learned her dance role well—too well. She was asked to do a solo. No one was sure whether she was a girl or boy as she moved with flowing grace across the stage.

Rhodes's father wanted his boy to play football and coached him, even before high school. His foreman had been a single-wing center. This was soon to be a dying art in football as the split-T took over. And it was an art: leading the ball by sending the ball in advance of runners; calling blocking formations and assignments at the line, and sometimes pulling ahead of runners. By the time Rhodes got to high school, he had mastered this skill, to the joy of his coaches and the admiration of his peers. Little did they know that when Rhodes went home he would put on his mother's discarded stockings and lie in bed, pretending to be studying.

Rhodes was smart enough in math and science that after the launch of Sputnik—the first satellite successfully put into space—he was drafted by his teachers to represent the school at a National Foundation Summer Camp. He spent eight weeks learning about nuclear physics and early computer science, but he was most fascinated by the game of soccer when someone told him that girls played soccer, too. Almost every night there would be a game and it was played until dark. He thought of himself as a girl playing in the game. His football coach was pleased that he was in shape, but she was pleased that she had learned a new sport—one that girls could play.

Rhodes went off to an all-male college where he played football, volunteered for military training to avoid Vietnam, and got into the jock fraternity. Opportunities were scarce to crossdress, so he hit upon a plan. She would pull the hood down over his head, put on lipstick and walk around campus where people could see him and not detect that he was a male. If he got panicky, he would simply wipe off the lipstick.

During college, he studied abnormal psychology hoping to learn more about his self-perceived shameful behavior. But no information on the topic was in the lectures. No information was in the textbooks. The college library card catalog listed several books on transsexuals, but they were nowhere to be found in the shelves. People had either stolen them or the giggling librarians kept them under the counter to prevent theft.

At graduation, she learned that the U.S. military no longer needed him and his reserve commitment was erased. He was interested in psychology, so he went on to psychology graduate school. The Cold War was still on, so there were scholarships and many paying teaching assistantships in graduate schools. He moved back into the graduate dormitories, but this time she had a single room and plenty of time to crossdress. Again, he sought out information on crossdressing and found only a single book—*Conundrum* by Jan Morris, a famous Welsh travel writer and transsexual. Jan Morris also took female hormones with prescriptions from Harry Benjamin. Rhodes was totally turned off by the description Morris gave of going to Casablanca to get TGPS. Following the law, Morris had to divorce his wife. Rhodes decided that he wanted none of those things. They would ruin his life and his career.

Rhodes got a job helping the military design computer systems. Most software engineers did not understand users, but Rhodes managed to bridge the gap between users and designers, so was in demand.

Rhodes was bothered by his need to crossdress and wanted to be "normal." Maybe if she got married and loved someone she would be cured. She had long since stopped getting sexually aroused by crossdressing, so she wanted sex as well. Rhodes got married to his college sweetheart and had two children, but his crossdressing continued. He kept a spare suitcase in the garage full of feminine clothing and makeup, which she would take with him on his consulting trips to fix computer systems in other states and make them usable. The pattern was the same; she would do his work and go immediately back to his hotel room to crossdress.

But she eventually wanted to go outside of his hotel room and decided to go to a support group near his firm's headquarters. It required a personal vetting interview to find out where the meeting was located. The first time he went to the support group it was in masculine clothing. She found all the people there to be friendly and encouraging. The next meeting, she had a feminine presentation, which she felt was inadequate, but got encouragement from the group to come back. She became a regular.

One day, Rhodes's wife found the suitcase in the garage. Thinking it was just some discarded clothing, she looked at the sizes and realized that she had no feminine relatives anywhere near those sizes. When Rhodes came home she wanted to know whether that was his suitcase and what he was doing with those clothes and the makeup. Rhodes loved her too much to lie, so she told her the truth. She became angry and would not talk to him for two days. At the end of that time, she told her about his crossdressing history; that it was just a hobby and that he had not used it to have sex with anyone. He would get tested for STI, to prove that he was safe. The results were negative and by that time his wife had done some research online. She had found a support group for couples that allowed males to crossdress, but observe the rules of heterosexuality and faithfulness to the spouse.

They currently are still in this couples support group, which has monthly meetings and galas. Rhodes's wife compares notes with the other spouses and helps to plan the meetings.

Rhodes believes that being a crossdresser is different from being transgender, although he cannot explain why. The only thing that he can point to is that he does not crossdress full-time, although he admits he enjoys it.

MARY M.

Mary knew that he was transgender at age four. He had been born female but as soon as he learned about gender categories, he knew that the masculine category fit him better. Mary's family was poor and he did not want to make matters worse by telling them that he was transgender. Mary was a decent student and her high school had an exercise room with weight machines and free weights. She found a female buddy who exercised with him and got into bodybuilding. She could not put on muscle like the male football players, but he did more reps to compensate. The football players tolerated him and had respect for her work.

Mary got interested in the field part of track and field. She learned how to throw the shot, discus, and hammer. Soon, he was a district champion in each event. Although he had a couple of junior college athletic scholarship offers, when he became a senior she decided that she should go into the military in order to earn money for college. His father and older sister had been in the military and had fought in Vietnam and Desert Storm. His father had been drafted and decided not to stay in, and his sister had been medically discharged for some mysterious reason. She would not say.

Mary enlisted and went off to boot camp where he did well in strength and agility tests and okay in running endurance. He did so-so in shooting, but got high marks for leadership. Her intake IQ tests said that she was intelligent enough to become a medic, so off she went to medic school at San Antonio where she continued her bodybuilding. He got her medic certification and her civilian EMT certification there, so she had a marketable skill when he would get out. Her strength helped him because several of the final exam practicums required carrying dummies that weighed the same as real people on stretchers through obstacle courses and over rugged terrain.

When the regulations were changed to allow transgender people in the military, he felt that he did not have to hide anymore. Her whole medical battalion received training as to how to treat transgender people, and her coworkers were all accepting. He learned fast and was a model soldier. Transgender people could now get counseling and medical treatment. At first he was hesitant to come out to the medical people, but found them supportive. He learned that transgender people volunteer for the military at a rate two to five times that of their peers.

She deployed to Afghanistan where he rescued and treated soldiers in several engagements. He came back with service medals and commendations.

When he returned stateside, he became a medic instructor at one of the predeployment refresher training locations, because he knew what the outgoing medics would face. He had several interviews with social workers and finally decided that he would transition. He knew all about it from his medical training and from online reading in the medic school library.

He started HT and found that bodybuilding became much easier. Her mood was more positive and she found work more interesting. He changed her name to David and got his birth certificate and driver's license changed with a new name and sex marker. He was thinking about starting paramedic training at the local hospital, so that he would have an even better skill set to earn his way through college. But first he wanted to get breast surgery to masculinize himself. The military was willing to give her the operation, but then a transgender ban in the military was announced and its implementation delayed, leaving the surgery in limbo.

He felt that he had been deceived. He had come out in good faith to his unit and the medical authorities and now was being punished for it. If he was thrown out, he would lose his money for college and go back into poverty, like his parents. Here he was, a model soldier being treated this way. He called her older sister who had left the military. She confessed that she had been forced to leave the military before its liberalization policy because he too was transgender.

LUTHER/LUCRETIA B.

Luther was born male. When she was seven, she essentially told her parents that she was transgender. They refused to believe it. Being transgender is a delusion, they said; they had heard radio broadcasts to that effect and two widely known medical doctors agreed. They implied that being transgender was a mental disorder.

Luther insisted that she was transgender, but his parents punished him for even bringing up the topic. They spanked her and grounded him each time she tried to talk to them about it. They caught her trying on his mother's clothing, spanked her and put him in the corner for an hour. Luther was sullen, would not talk, and when prodded would get aggressive.

Luther was taken to a psychiatrist who diagnosed him as depressed and sent her to a mental hospital to determine the appropriate medication. Conditions at the mental institution were a little better than being at home; at least they did not punish Luther. The psychiatrists examined him and said that she appeared to be transgender but they should use the "watchful waiting approach" as it would take some time to be sure. Luther said that her femme name was Lucretia. They did not have the expertise to deal with transgender children and referred her parents to a local gender clinic. Her parents did not accept this conclusion and wanted her committed. The doctors said that she did not meet the criteria for commitment. They prescribed antidepressant drugs for her and sent her home.

At age 11, Lucretia slashed his wrist with a butcher knife from the kitchen. Her parents put on a tourniquet and took her to the emergency room, where she had surgery to repair the damage. The parents tried to hush up the episode, saying that it was just an accident. But in an abundance of caution, the ER doctor called for a psych consult. As she was recovering in the hospital, Luther told the consulting psychologist everything was all right and that it had been an accident. She did not want to hurt her parents. Her parents took her home and cleared her room of anything with which she could harm herself, as well as anything that could be construed as feminine. They watched her behavior every moment when she was out of his room and not at school. Gradually, they relaxed the restrictions, believing that she had "grown out" of it by age 14. Luther was allowed to go to school and the YMCA for basketball practice by herself.

One Saturday, Lucretia did not go to basketball practice but instead went to a transgender support group that she had found online. Lucretia told them about the rejection from her parents and her experiences in mental hospitals. She said that she was likely to try suicide again. The support group members encouraged her not to do it; they said that they wanted her to come back alive and well. One of the participants was a clinical psychologist and, in the state where they lived, she was required to report to the authorities anyone threatening to hurt themselves or others. Lily returned home. The state child protective agents came the next day to investigate.

The parents said it was all a misunderstanding and that Lucretia was getting treatment from the local psychiatric clinic. Afterward, Luther received the worst beating of her life. This time, before they could put her back in the psychiatric clinic, she managed to run away from home. She still had the card of the clinical psychologist who had reported her intention to commit suicide and called her, saying that she was homeless and intended to commit suicide. The police were summoned.

Lucretia was sent back to the psychiatric hospital and this time was involuntarily committed for two weeks until the doctors could evaluate her suicidal ideation. They concluded that she had been abused by her parents but was not likely to commit self-harm. They recommended that she go to the gender clinic. Child protective services found a foster home for her.

Although Lucretia loves her parents, she refuses to live with them and wants to transition. She has filed a petition for emancipation from her parents, who will not give her permission to transition.

JON/MARJORIE AND EDWARD/MARTINE B.

Jon and Edward were born male three years apart in Philadelphia. When the oldest was seven and the youngest four, their parents decided to divorce. After heated divorce proceedings, the court awarded custody of the older child to the father and the younger child to the mother because of his tender age. The father eventually moved away to the South because he had found carpentry work there. His son, Jon, was apprenticed as an electrician and managed to build his own business. Jon had had misgivings about his gender in childhood, but never came out as transgender. Now he was too busy with his business and his new wife to even think about being transgender.

Meanwhile, brother Edward grew up and became a pharmacist. The work was somewhat boring but steady as he joined a large supermarket chain as a pharmacist. His mother continued to work as a social worker in Philadelphia.

The two brothers were not encouraged to interact with one another because of their parents' continuing animosity, but they exchanged Christmas cards and became Facebook friends.

Jon and Edward's mother died in a car accident, and both siblings and their father were briefly reunited at the funeral. They put all of her things into storage, planning to sort them out someday. Because Edward felt a huge loss, it got him thinking about the lack of meaning in his life. He wanted to be nurturing and help people, which was why he had become a pharmacist in the first place. He had also taken care of his mother, but now she was gone. He suddenly realized that he felt like a woman, not a man, and began to express himself with more feminine clothing and manner, which he enjoyed. Underneath his white pharmacist coat he could wear anything he wanted, but stopped short of skirts. His mother was gone, so she was not around to be shamed, and his father and brother were far away in Georgia. He could not tell whether this meant that he was gay or transgender at first, but eventually realized that he must be transgender. He started to use birth control pills and his mood was immediately lifted. The backlog of birth control pills at his pharmacy was huge, so no one noticed. So, he started do-it-yourself HT. And he liked it. He did not tell anyone.

Meanwhile, Edward broke up with his wife because she had discovered his cache of feminine clothing and makeup, which he kept in his work truck. Edward had been secretly crossdressing since 14 and eventually got his own place where he was free to dress as he wished. His mother walked in on him but did not care about his crossdressing as long as Edward did not get into trouble. Edward started HT with an endocrinologist and loved it. Gradually, she no longer felt sexually aroused from crossdressing but kept doing it because he enjoyed it.

Elsewhere, Jon's knowledge of hormone therapy was flawed and he was not being monitored by qualified medical authorities. He was taking ethinyl estradiol. One day at work, he developed a clot—pulmonary thrombosis. The EMTs rushed him to the hospital and saved his life. Jon's father and brother rushed to see him and the cat was out of the bag. Jon admitted what he had been doing because he thought he was transgender, and Edward told him that he was transgender. So, Marjorie and Martine came out to one another. The doctors told them that it was not uncommon for a close relative of a transgender person to also be transgender.

Later, as they were trying to dispose of their mother's things, in a box full of medicines they found one labeled diethylstilbestrol. They didn't think much about it and threw it out.

WALTER S.

Walter was judged to be male at birth. He grew up in the masculine gender behavior category, but when he was seven years old, he decided that neither masculine nor feminine gender categories suited him. As others had done at his school, at the age of 8 they described themselves as "genderqueer." They wore a combination of masculine and feminine clothing and experimented with makeup, hair color, and jewelry.

His parents thought it was just a phase. Their child, however, still claimed to be genderqueer. Walter had read all about puberty and knew that it had started; they did not want their voice to get deeper and did not want hair development. They were panicky because they did not want to be forced to go through male puberty. Fortunately, Walter lived in a city with a gender clinic. They got his parents to take them there to ask for help.

The gender clinic judged that Walter was consistent, insistent, and persistent in his fear of going through male puberty. The doctors at the gender clinic decided to put Walter on puberty-blocking drugs to give them time to make up their mind about which gender category was best for them. Walter's parents were well off, so they could afford puberty-blocking implants, each of which would last for one to two years.

Walter received the first implant and felt better. The doctors still had to give them low doses of sex hormones in order to regulate bone growth, and in case Walter might want TGPS for transwomen someday, so that he would have adequate genital tissue.

Walter has had four implants and is now 16, when they must decide which gender behavior category fits the best. If they go off of the blockers, he will go through male puberty and assume the masculine gender behavior category. Alternatively, they could start transwoman HT to prepare Walter for potential female TGPS. They learned that although genderqueer children are only about 10 percent of the transgender children being treated with this affirmative approach, the numbers are increasing.

CHRIS Z.

Chris was female at birth. She grew up normally, but in her teenage years she sensed that she was attracted to females. In elementary school, all of her friends were girls. She was good at soccer and outdoor sports. She hung out exclusively with girls in junior high and high school, wearing the lesbian badge, which consisted of flannel shirts and black jeans. She did like the males who would take her on motorcycle rides and eventually she learned from them about how to ride and how to take care of the motorcycles. She found other girls who also were interested in motorcycles and when she got to high school, got both her car and motorcycle license. When she went away to college, it was on a motorcycle. She considered herself to be a soft butch lesbian.

She did not like her college roommate. The roommate was into boys, spending huge amounts of time on fashion, makeup, and flirting. She showed no sign of being open to a lesbian relationship. Chris joined the local lesbian student group and found that she liked many of the girls there. One in particular caught her eye. She was very intelligent and took an interest in Chris. They hung out together in the dorms, student center, and in the quad. They took long motorcycle rides together and went to outdoor parks to drink.

One night, Chris told her roommate to get lost for the evening and Chris and her new friend had sex together. It was the first time for both to have lesbian sex, so there was some fumbling around at first but they did manage to satisfy themselves. From then on, they were a couple and shunned advances from other lesbians. Chris found herself being more assertive and her girlfriend liked it. Chris was on her way to become a stud lesbian.

After graduation, Chris and her girlfriend stayed together and eventually got married when it became legal in California. Through a male that they knew, Chris's wife got pregnant twice and they started to raise a family. Chris became a soccer coach and her wife became a software engineer. But Chris began to feel that she was more than a stud lesbian and began to think she was transgender. She had not been certain when she was younger but now recognized that her congruent gender was masculine.

Chris told her wife and they had several long talks together. They decided that they loved each other and that if Chris transitioned, it would not change much. They would have to find new ways of having sex but that had always been fun. And they dearly loved their children and wanted to take care of them.

Chris went to a support group and found a mental health professional who had extensive experience with transmen. He was hesitant at first but decided to start HT with a recommendation from his counselor to see an endocrinologist with experience with transmen. Taking shots every two weeks took a lot of time out of his soccer practice schedule, but he eventually learned how to do them himself and his wife learned as well. Chris began to grow hair everywhere, especially facial hair. The hair covered his feminine features, so no facial feminization surgery was necessary. His wife actually liked the hair growth.

The next step was mastectomy. Chris had been binding for two years until he got up enough nerve to ask for one. His wife decided she would miss playing with his breasts but she understood.

At this point Chris had to decide about soccer coaching. He had coached mostly girls' teams but decided that he should start coaching boys' teams because his voice was deepening.

He made the switch just as his mastectomy was healing. The plastic surgery allowed him to go shirtless when needed. The mastectomy surgery qualified him in his home state to have his birth certificate changed. Next, he got a passport with an "M" on it. He also got the sex marker changed on his driver's license and Social Security. He never had to change his name because the name Chris can be used for both men and women.

Chris is considering TGPS for transmen, but he has decided to wait until the operation and/or transplant procedures improve.

10

Obstacles and Controversies

There are gaps in our scientific knowledge about being transgender. This is because in the United States and elsewhere, funding for scientific research is focused on diseases. Being transgender is not a disease, and since research on it is sometimes regarded as politically incorrect, frivolous, self-evident, or all three, important research goes unfunded. Hence, there are some controversies and obstacles that remain. There are some unresolved ideas about transgender treatment that are now controversial within the research and provider communities. They are mainly unresolved because the scientific method has not been applied to them to clearly define them as scientific theories and operationalize them for evidence collection. In too many such issues, the controversies have been fought with argument by authority rather than argument by scientific evidence. Some authorities, influenced by their unsubstantiated beliefs or by religious conviction, try to portray being transgender from the point of view of heterosexism, meaning that only sex and sexual arousal exists, not gender. And since there have been extensive cultural efforts to bring sex under control, controlling being transgender falls under these efforts.

Since transgender people have become more visible, they have become political targets, with authoritarian populists using transgender matters as wedge issues in political campaigns. Some of these issues include the use of restrooms and locker rooms, whether being transgender is contagious, whether it is triggered by Internet information, and transgender regret. Some want reparative therapy to be permitted, although experience with reparative therapy in gay/lesbian people with regard to homosexuality has been found to be ineffective and injurious.

CONTROVERSIES

Sex and Gender

There are two continuing controversies over the terms sex and gender. The first has to do with whether the term gender is necessary or appropriate; the second has to do with whether transgender transition actually changes sex. Although sex and gender are commonly conflated in public discourse, the discussion here is over their scientific definitions.

The first controversy revolves around whether sex organs are different from culturally defined behaviors. Sex organs are clearly biological and gender behaviors are culturally defined. We know that gender categories are culturally defined because they vary from place to place, culture to culture, and time to time and are often arbitrary, although they may make unsubstantiated assumptions about biology based on cultural beliefs. When subjected to scientific inquiry, many of these cultural beliefs are refuted or shown to be unsupported by evidence.

John Money repurposed the word "gender" to refer to culturally defined gender roles or categories (Money, Hampson, & Hampson, 1955). He did so because he was dealing with intersex children. Parents of these children needed guidance on how to raise their children in either the masculine or feminine gender role. This was a time when genital plastic surgery was common on newborn intersex children to bring them into alignment with culturally influenced sex categories. Although such surgeries have declined in frequency, they still go on and are still legal in many places despite female genital antimutilation laws. In the repurposing of the word gender, Money was distinguishing it from visible external genital organs because, at the time, there was no other definition of cultural behavior categories. Milton Diamond was a severe critic of Money for supporting genital plastic surgery in infants and for believing that gender could be changed through child rearing, but even he believes that sex and gender should be treated as separate phenomena (Diamond, 2002).

Cultural gender categories should be distinguished from biological gender behavior predispositions, which determine the initial emotional reactions of a person to various gender behaviors. Although gender behavior predisposition may correlate with sex, it is clearly independent and dissociable from sex as a biological phenomenon. We know that transgender people exist who report and behave in a way that demonstrates that their gender predisposition does not fit with their assigned gender behavior category according to cisgender cultural rules. And we know that if one identical twin is transgender, then the other will be as well at about a 50 percent rate, although *they both have the same sex.*

Some want to subsume gender behavior as sex-type behavior (McHugh & Mayer, 2016) because of their religious and philosophical beliefs, but this is not supported by definition or by scientific evidence. John Money was dealing with newborn children who were far from being sexually active or capable of reproduction when he gave gender its current definition. Money had no way of knowing the children's sex or gender predisposition at that age, which is why treatment of intersex children has changed. In many cases, intersex children are now allowed to grow up without genital plastic surgery to at least their teenage years, when they are able to declare their sex or congruent gender. The evidence that organs are different from behavior is clear. One refers to biological gross external anatomy and the other refers to cultural, abstract ideas of how societies should be structured.

Sex is usually determined at birth by inspection of the gross anatomy of external genitalia as an indicator of the organs of reproduction. Although later it may be determined that other sex organs are different or nonfunctional, this determination is the one commonly used. For example, females who have had hysterectomies are still referred to as females, and males who have had removal of their testicles because of cancer are still referred to as males.

Some maintain that sex can only be determined by genes and chromosomes (they have yet to discover the epigenome) but deterministic science is far from being able to predict the structure and function of the organs of reproduction including external genitalia. It is well *after* a person's sex has been determined by inspection of external genitalia at birth that defects in sexual reproduction are detected that can be traced back to genes and chromosomes. This is because there is wide variability in genes and chromosomes. People do not just have XX or XY chromosomes; there are a host of variations with more than two sex chromosomes in some people. The presence of a Y chromosome does not always indicate that the person will have male sex organs at birth. The recipe for sex organs is to be found mainly on nonsex chromosomes that form the body structure. Genes that determine various traits may vary from cell to cell. A person gets cells with DNA from their mother, from preceding siblings, and from bone marrow transplants. The brain appears to be a safe haven for such cells because the brain has defenses against the body's immune system, which would attack these foreign cells (Cogle et al., 2004). All female XX people are mosaics, meaning that the active X chromosome genes vary from cell to cell. This is because only one of the corresponding X genes can be expressed due to X-inactivation. Many people are mosaics, having more than one genome in the cells of their bodies. This is most apparent in such phenomena as genetic *heterochromia iridum* in which the two eyes are of different colors.

Do transgender people change sex during transgender transition? Certainly, many of their primary and secondary sex organs change because they have receptors for both estrogen and testosterone. Stimulation of the appropriate receptors occurs during HT to change anatomy. HT results in obvious changes in breast and genital tissue, but it also changes anatomy and functioning of the nervous system due to neural plasticity or directly on the brain (see Chapter 7). TGPS and other surgeries change anatomy. So the question really is: how many sex organs have to change in order for a person to be considered to have changed their sex? It is a variation of the *sorites* or "heap" philosophical paradox of semantics. Given the wide variation of anatomy and function of the sex organs of cisgender people, it is clear that one can change sex organs to be within that range.

Sexual Arousal, Fetishism, and Autogynephilia

The idea that sexual arousal is the motivation of transwomen to crossdress and crosspresent has resulted in pathologization of transgender people and the association of transwomen with sexual arousal in the public eye. Magnus Hirschfeld observed sexual arousal in his transgender patients, which started the hypothesis that being transgender was motivated by sexual arousal. Hirschfeld later recanted this belief. The sexualization of behaviors was continued by Freud, who asserted that unconscious sexual drives motivated many behaviors. When the DSM-I was issued in 1952, and in subsequent DSM versions, many behaviors were considered pathological because they were thought to be associated with sexual arousal.

Blanchard (2005) asserted a typology of transwomen that included two categories: a category for older transwomen attracted to females (heterosexual) who had **autogynephilia**, and younger transwomen attracted to males (homosexual). The supposed motivation in the first group in crosspresentation was to experience "love of oneself as a woman." This is often implied by its proponents to be a "paraphilia" or "fetish." A pathological diagnosis of paraphilia would require a diagnosis of disability or distress, which most transwomen do not have.

Autogynephila notions do not rise to the level of scientific theories for several reasons. First, autogynephilia has been defined in at least six different ways. It is not clear what the proponents mean by the idea. It is variously defined as "arousal by thought," "fantasy of having intercourse with a woman," "arousal with the thought of being a woman," "the thought of acquiring a woman's body," "wanting to become what women love," and "romantic, having attachment-based elements." There are no biological references; for instance, there is biological evidence that oxytocin is involved in pair-bonding in animals, but this and other potential biological mechanisms are not mentioned in the formulation of autogynephilia.

There is little doubt that sexual arousal accompanies initial crossdressing by transwomen, but this rapidly decreases. The novelty of new stimuli contributes to this arousal, but also transwomen learn sexual arousal through classical or Pavlovian conditioning. Both the novelty and the learned sexual arousal decline with exposure. Transwomen report that they continue to crossdress, not because of sexual arousal, but because it relaxes them and makes them feel authentic (Buhrich, 1978; Hirschfeld, 1910; Levitt & Ippolito, 2014). We know that novelty stimulates sexual arousal from the work of Frank Beach (Ford & Beach, 1952) and from the "Coolidge effect" in which sex refractory times of male dogs were reduced by exposure to a new female dog in heat. We know that sexual arousal obeys the laws of classical conditioning from many studies in both male (Hoffman, Janssen, & Turner, 2004; Janssen, Everaerd, Spiering, & Janssen, 2010; Lalumiere & Quinsey, 1998) and female humans (Both, Brauer, & Laan 2001; Both et al., 2008; Hoffman, 2012; Hoffman et al., 2004) and animals (Koksal et al., 2004). Because the laws of classical conditioning also indicate that exposure to the stimuli that have been associated with an unconditioned stimulus will weaken and extinguish the reflex, we should expect transwomen to experience reduced arousal from repeated crossdressing. In fact, the experience of crossdressing should hasten extinction because it complies with the principle of **flooding desensitization**, which therapists use to desensitize phobias and anxiety (Levis & Castelda, 2007).

During puberty, natal males are easily triggered to sexual arousal and typically use stimulus materials involving feminine clothing and presentation for pleasure. During this period, they acquire classically conditioned arousal reflexes. This may account for Blanchard's categorization of older transwomen into the autogynephilia typology. They have simply had more time and opportunity to acquire conditioned sexual arousal reflexes to females than to males.

There are two lines of evidence cited in support of autogynephilia. The first concerns the use of a **phaloplethysmograph** to measure penile blood volume. In the one experiment cited, crossdressing stories were presented after abstinence from crossdressing for six months. The data indicated that the crossdressers were sexually excited by the stories, which the authors took as proof that the older transwomen had autogynephilia (Blanchard, Racansky, & Steiner, 1986). What was really demonstrated in this study was yet another principle of classical conditioning known as "spontaneous recovery," in which if a conditioned stimulus is not presented over time, the conditioned reflex will recover from extinction, although it will be weaker.

The other line of evidence often cited involves a **core autogynephilia scale** which was constructed to have face validity for autogynephilia. The instrument asks transwomen subjects to rate how often they feel various concepts of themselves as a woman. But responses to these questions, as in all concept recall, necessitates recall and visualization of attributes (Bruner, Goodnow, & Austin, 1967). This means that if the subject learned sexual arousal to these attributes as stimuli (say, ladies' dresses or lipstick), then they would become sexually aroused by the attributes but not the concepts. Moser (2009) constructed a natal *female* autogynephilia scale according to the methods used by Blanchard. Results with this scale indicated the same sort of results with transwomen, but according to the autogynephilia proponents, autogynephilia should only apply to natal males.

Moser (2010) also conducted a peer review of the literature on autogynephilia and found:

- No reports of any substantial difference between older, nonhomosexual transwomen who supposedly had autogynephilia and younger homosexual transwomen.
- A substantial proportion of homosexual transwomen (15–36 percent report sexual arousal to crossdressing and presentation.
- A substantial proportion of nonhomosexual transwomen report no sexual arousal to crossdressing and presentation.
- The clinical importance of the distinction of those supposedly with and without autogynephilia is undetermined.
- Many of the tenets of autogynephilia are not supported by evidence or in some cases both supporting and refuting evidence exists.

It seems clear that the idea of autogynephilia does not rise to the level of a scientific theory and is unsupported by scientific evidence. There is thus no scientific basis for autogynephilia that justifies the continuing pathologization and sexualization of transgender people through the use of this idea.

Treatment of Transgender Children Using Puberty-Blocking Drugs

Current practice under the affirmative treatment approach in treating transgender children involves the use of puberty-blocking drugs to provide time for transkids to determine their congruent gender before unwanted, irreversible effects of puberty occur. Treatment of transgender children with puberty-blocking drugs is currently being examined under high-profile studies because of the concerns about the potential side effects of such drugs. The puberty-blocking drugs were originally used in cases of precocious puberty in children to allow them to go through puberty at a later age, which was considered normal. They were used for limited periods of several years, and then the child with precocious puberty was allowed to later go through a normal puberty based on their sex at birth. The results for these cases were generally good with reversible effects on female reproduction after medication ceased (Pasquino et al., 2008).

Puberty-blocking drugs are considered off-label by the FDA for use in delaying puberty for transkids. Current use of puberty blockers with transkids may extend from the onset of puberty at ages 7–11 to age 16, which is somewhat longer than these drugs have been typically administered for precocious puberty.

Several potential side effects of these drugs have been hypothesized (Hruz, Mayer, & McHugh, 2017) without scientific evidence and these and many others are being addressed by current studies. There is concern that the puberty blockers may prevent development of adequate bone growth and external genital tissue because growth of these tissues is normally regulated by sex hormones. Having adequate genital tissue makes TGPS easier to perform for transwomen. The experience with precocious puberty in female children indicated that bone density temporarily decreased but that it reverted to normal after termination of the administration of depot triptorelin after approximately four years (Pasquino et al., 2008). This and other studies have concluded that blocking agents were safe and its effects reversible with respect to height, reproductive function, and bone density growth. These concerns have been addressed by administering low doses of sex hormones along with the blocking drugs.

There are also concerns about transkids being unable to give informed consent, but most children learn about gender behavior categories by the time they are two to three years old, and transkids start to emerge at ages four to six. Transkids are not confused about their congruent gender (Olson, Key, & Eaton, 2013). Candidate transgender children for blockers are usually evaluated by a team of parents, medical doctors, endocrinologists, and mental health professionals, and the children must be consistent, insistent, and persistent about their congruent gender. This does not happen until signs of the beginning of puberty, Tanner stage 2.

Long-term outcomes and any side effects for the transkids on blockers awaits future research reporting because this procedure has only been used in the past few years. The risks associated with *not* blocking puberty include rejection, depression, isolation, and suicide. The attempted suicide rate in transgender people is approximately 40 percent, primarily in youth at 31 percent (see Chapter 6).

Effects are positive. Positive effects are observed immediately in terms of increased authenticity and reduced anxiety about incipient puberty with its irreversible effects on gender presentation.

Continuation/Discontinuation of Being Transgender over the Lifespan

The issue of whether transgender children spontaneously, without treatment, cease their transgender behavior in their teenage years and adulthood has been raised in connection with criticism of the affirmative treatment approach and in support of the "watchful waiting approach" (see Chapter 2). The criticism asks, "Why pursue affirmative treatment if the child is going to stop their transgender behavior due to maturation and social rejection anyway?"

The terms frequently used in this argument are "persister" and "desister." These words have pathological and antisocial behavioral connotations as used in psychiatry, pathology, and sociology. They were deliberately repurposed from pathological psychiatric disorders, because they had previous pathological behavioral connotations (Zucker, 2018). In sociology, they are used in conjunction with juvenile delinquency or juvenile offending, which involves the commission of crimes. Of course, being transgender does not involve commission of crimes since public crossdressing laws were repealed or not observed starting in the 20th century. These terms are no more descriptive of the behavior of interest than **continuation** and **discontinuation**, used here, and these come without the baggage of negative connotations. They are mentioned here for information purposes.

Although one might hypothesize that transgender behavior is discontinued during the lifespan due to not wanting to risk social rejection because the transgender person has increased responsibilities for family and job, the evidence supports these factors only as they drive transgender behavior into secrecy. Some researchers take the "out of sight, out of mind" position, indicating that if clients do not show up in gender clinics, the behavior does not continue. But the later public emergence of transgender people who have lived in secret, sometimes for many years, has accelerated in recent years, belying this position. In addition, there are those who join support groups that preserve secrecy.

We do not know how long a transgender child continues with transgender behavior for three reasons:

- Evidence cited for this contention mainly comes from clinical studies of children who were *not transgender;* many were prehomosexual or had other problems.
- The cited *clinical studies all involved treating the children under study,* so it is not clear that any children who did cease their transgender behavior did so spontaneously.
- *Many transgender children and adults continue their transgender behavior in secret,* likely the great majority.

As cited in Chapter 2, the established existence of prehomosexual children complicates the identification of transgender children. (Notice that the use of the term "differential diagnosis" would be inappropriate here since neither homosexuality nor being transgender are pathological.) The evidence most often cited to prove discontinuation comes from the gender clinic at the Canadian Center for Addiction and Mental Health, which was recently closed. Subsequent analysis of these case records indicates that 63 percent were prehomosexual/pre-bisexual in fantasy behavior and 47 percent in interpersonal behavior, and *only 12 percent actually were transgender* (Singh, 2012). The remaining "patients" were either heterosexual or asexual. The children in the Singh study received treatment varying from jawboning and operant conditioning to "watchful waiting" with counseling, so they cannot be said to have achieved their outcomes spontaneously.

Other studies cited explicitly state that they were dealing with prehomosexual children or their outcomes were measured as homosexual/bisexual (Davenport, 1986; Steensma, McGuire, Kreukels, Beekman, & Cohen-Kettenis, 2013; Wallien & Cohen-Kettenis, 2008; Whitam 1977; Zuger & Taylor 1969). These patient reports in these studies included 167 participants, 102 of whom were prehomosexual and only 5 of whom were transgender. The reason for this confusion is that, even after homosexuality was eradicated from the DSM, prehomosexual children were diagnosed and treated under categories seemingly intended for transgender people.

We do not know how many transgender children go into secrecy, but we do know that many transadults emerge from secrecy, sometimes in middle age or later. The number of those emerging in adulthood has recently been increasing, based on survey results. However, the frequency of being transgender from these survey results is just now approaching those of earlier estimation studies based on support group membership and throughput of doctors providing transgender transition services including TGPS. The increased emergence numbers in the survey data is probably due to the increased acceptance of transgender people and essentially that there is a backlog of those in secret, hiding during the eras of nonacceptance.

Rapid Onset Gender Dysphoria (ROGD)

ROGD stands for **rapid onset gender dysphoria**, which refers to the idea that being transgender can rapidly emerge during teenage years without warning, at least without warning to parents. ROGD was reported in a controversial research paper by Lisa Littman (Littman, 2018 and revised by Littman in 2019 under pressure) who contends that transgender emergence like this is a new phenomenon and that it is triggered by social "contagion" from peer groups. The basis for being transgender, she contends, is early trauma and psychodynamics.

The paper is clearly an attempt to critique the affirmative treatment approach and bring psychoanalysis as a potential "cure" for being transgender back into consideration. In 1972, the American Medical Association indicated that psychoanalysis was ineffective for curing transgender behavior (AMA, 1972). The data for the Littman paper ostensibly comes from a community of parents who support reparative therapy and psychoanalysis on various websites. Ostensibly is the word, because there is no confirmation that all the people claiming to be parents are real. Former prominent providers, who are now disaffected, are often cited to tout the psychodynamic explanation of being transgender as involving an autogynephilia fetish, supporting reparative therapy, and early trauma. They reject the affirmative approach.

While the affirmative treatment approach for both children and adults has grown in acceptance, there are still critics of the approach. The use of puberty blockers for transkids has made this approach even more controversial (see Chapter 8). The use of blockers has only been followed for a few years, but parents and children have judged it to be preferred to the stress of secrecy or "toughing it out," which facilitates depression and anxiety, resulting in suicide attempts. Although affirmative treatment seems to be winning, competing treatments and causal ideas for transgender people never disappeared completely even though they had been found to be ineffective and sometimes dangerous.

The ROGD story begins with several websites started ostensibly by parents of teenage transkids who were unhappy with the treatment they got from mental health and medical providers, most of whom were aligned with the affirmative approach. (No confirmation is offered that these were actually parents of teenage transkids.) They reported that their children, without warning, abruptly came out to them as transgender in adolescence. Discarded and dangerous alternative treatments and associated causal ideas have been featured on these websites. Reparative therapy is championed based on cultural cisgenderism and can feature both operant and classical conditioning as well as jawboning or bullying to try to discourage transgender behavior. The rationale is that cisgenderism is the natural state of affairs;

transgender children must be disciplined or trained to behave in a gender category assigned by natal sex and reduce sexual arousal, or they will greatly suffer in later life. The idea is that being transgender is due to sexual arousal pathologizes and causes people to view transgender people as being sexually perverted and pathological. This is a common basis for misinformed public rejection. After the Littman ROGD paper, we can now add psychodynamics as a nonscientific causal idea and psychoanalysis to the list of the ineffective and discarded approaches that appear on these websites.

Littman proceeded to send out an Internet link through these websites, which spread around the Internet. The link was to a survey site for ostensible parents to fill out a survey to provide information on respondent experiences. According to her report, she received about 250 responses, ostensibly from parents of transboys. The dissemination of this link was not controlled so anyone could have responded to the survey, not just parents, and parents with positive experiences were not recruited for the survey. Littman refers to this as an available sample but scientifically this could be considered an uncontrolled, biased sample.

The collected data showed that the children involved were clearly transgender as indicated by reports of changes of presentation involving dress, hair, and behavior, by their verbal statements, and by their requests to consult with providers about their suspected transgender status. The children were mostly above average or average in intelligence (many were in gifted and talented programs). They consulted their peers and Internet websites to find information on being transgender. Even though Littman termed this information gathering "contagion," she stated that she did not believe that this contagion was the cause of their being transgender. She left that for psychodynamics.

"Contagion" to most people connotes disease caused by germs or other agents and signifies pathology or a poison. The third meaning of contagion is "rapid communication of an influence or doctrine." It is possible that Littman intended the latter, but that connotation implies that children can be indoctrinated into being transgender. There is no empirical evidence for that. Whatever meaning is assumed, the word was clearly inappropriate for general audiences and wrong scientifically. If it was chosen to be sensational, it is totally inappropriate on ethical grounds.

Her obvious *a priori* psychodynamic belief is that transkids had undergone early trauma and that this trauma was responsible for them being transgender. She collected trauma information based on her belief, but did not collect information on alternative hypotheses. Sexualized trauma causation is a staple of psychodynamics, even though many times the patient cannot initially remember a trauma. Scientifically, it has been shown that in the course of certain types of analysis, false memories can be "recovered." Her psychodynamic interpretation was that being transgender resulted from an ineffective coping mechanism to deal with the trauma. As Littman defined it:

> A maladaptive coping mechanism is a response to a stressor that might relieve the symptoms temporarily but does not address the cause of the problem and may cause additional negative outcomes. . . . Transition as a drive to escape one's gender/sex, emotions, or difficult realities might also be considered when the drive to transition arises after a sex or gender-related trauma or within the context of significant psychiatric symptoms and decline in ability to function. Although trauma and psychiatric disorders are not specific for the development of gender dysphoria, these experiences may leave a person in psychological pain and in search of a coping mechanism. (Littman, 2018)

Of course, these statements are unprovable because they involve internal mental processes and intervening variables that are not observable. Respondents reported that some of the children had received trauma, but there were no comparisons made to the frequencies of occurrence for non-transgender children or the population. It should also be pointed out that one child's trauma is another child's growth experience. It is not just the event; it is the injurious effect on a person that makes it traumatic.

Littman asked the respondents to judge their children on psychiatric criteria, which mental health providers use for the diagnosis of childhood and adult transgender gender dysphoria. Gender dysphoria is a recent billing code for treatment of people who meet certain criteria in the *Diagnostic and Statistical Manual* of the American Psychiatric Association (2017). This code is mainly used for transgender transition treatment billing. Only about 1–2 percent of transgender people meet the requirements for gender dysphoria. Littman included most of the criteria except for one—whether the transgender children were debilitated or in distress because they were transgender. This latter criterion is a *sine qua non* criterion and usually makes the difference between those who are just transgender and those who want to seek medical treatment to change their bodies through transgender transition. Littman evidently simplified the criteria for respondents, but did not post these simplified criteria in her paper. Littman interpreted the data to mean that the children were not transgender in childhood, but were transgender in adolescence and adulthood.

However, if the DSM criteria are followed strictly, none of the children met the requirements for gender dysphoria in adolescence and adulthood because the requirement of distress or debilitation was not considered. Although from incidental reporting it is clear that some children desired to go into an affirmative program and perhaps transition, a diagnosis of gender dysphoria is not indicated both because of not meeting all the required criteria and because the parents were given simplified criteria. But the biggest reason is that *the criteria are intended to be evaluated by trained providers, not parents.* Littman cannot confirm that any of the transgender kids were gender dysphoric, which is a major assumption of the concept of rapid onset gender dysphoria.

One of the interesting reported findings is that most of the transkids previously had been formally diagnosed with anxiety and depression by providers. These are frequently effects of secrecy. Were the children living in secret about being transgender from earlier childhood? We do not know from the report. The transkids were not asked.

Another overlooked finding is that parents reported that most (64 percent) of the female children had been previously diagnosed as bi, lesbian, or pansexual. There were no reports that parents found coming out in these sexual orientation categories as abrupt or shocking. Do children come out first with their queer sexual orientation before coming out with being transgender because it is more socially acceptable and may not require body changes as in transgender transition? When a child comes out as transgender, there is typically a "grieving" process for a lost child. Is this why parents reject coming out as transgender and not as queer? It is a hypothesis that Littman should have considered.

The Littman paper was deemed scientifically unsound by several professional societies and authorities, and its assertions negatively impact transgender kids, particularly the assertions that appear to be made to be sensational like "contagion." The immediate impact is that parents may be hesitant to bring transkids to qualified providers if being transgender is suspected. (There have already been reports of parental hesitancy to admit their children to affirmative treatment programs because of this controversy.) Children should not be restricted from finding out about being transgender from their peers and the Internet, but they can get the best information from trained providers. Since many parents frequently do not know much about being transgender, those sources are the only way that children can become informed patients when it comes to meeting with a provider.

The long-term negative impact of this report and the disgruntled parent websites is that they will continue branding transgender children and adults as pathological. They already suffer greatly from cultural rejection, and pathology provides some handy reasons for that cultural rejection.

OBSTACLES

Cultural Change to Reduce Transgender Rejection and Homelessness

The greatest obstacle to the advancement of the health and welfare of transgender people is rejection by parents, relatives, and communities, which puts transgender children and youth on the street, homeless. Although antidiscrimination laws may help, in order to overcome this obstacle, it will be necessary to change culture. Parents and families reject their own children whom they love because their relatives and communities tell them that doing so is the right thing to do. As children, the outcasts have limited occupational skills and end up living on the street and engaging in some of the worst street economies, such as prostitution and drug pushing. If convicted of sex-related crimes and put on sex registries, they will forever be rejected for future jobs. Many cisgender people drive by these unfortunates on the street and see that as the face of being transgender. But it is not. The vast majority of transgender people live in secret, have jobs, support families, contribute to society, and contribute to national defense. The biggest employer of transgender people in the world is the U.S. military (at the time of writing). There are prominent transgender people who contribute to society in the arts, the sciences, and the helping professions.

Cultural change is difficult, but not impossible. It requires people of goodwill to understand the truth about being transgender and to propagate that truth. The truth is that transgender people were born with particular genes and experienced an epigenetic environment that did not change them or block their expression. They were not responsible for their genetic gender predisposition. They were also not responsible for being born into a Western culture that is cisgender, binary, and rigid.

The primary way that the culture can be changed is for individuals to have positive relationships with transgender people, but only 16 percent of the population actually knows a transgender person (Adam & Goodman, 2015). Often, they know the transgender person before they come out and observe that they are the same people that they already knew but just look a little different. Some come to know transgender people after they emerge. Loving parents who have transgender children usually become instant transgender advocates if culture does not intervene. Some cultures teach parents that their transgender children are diseased, disordered, and living a delusion, and that they must separate themselves from these children, lest they be contaminated too. Community religious and political organizations use transgender wedge issues to fund their organizations and get elected. Many people, otherwise of goodwill in community organizations, are afraid to advocate for tolerance and acceptance because they fear that they will lose financial support and membership.

As more and more transgender people emerge, cultural change is inevitable, but it can be accelerated by providers advocating for transgender people. As community leaders, they can stop rejection by changing opinions through vocalizing the scientific evidence of the basis for transgender causation. Providers also need to advocate for increased scientific funding to explore transgender causation and how best to change culture. And as science progresses, providers need to take informed positions with regard to such issues as identification of individuals as transgender from their genomes and epigenomes, and potential gene "therapy." It has been said that being transgender has the power to change society like a nuclear explosive. And like nuclear power, knowledge of being transgender can be used for good or ill. It requires knowledge of both science and the humanities to make informed decisions.

Pathologization

Culture uses pathologization to reject transgender people. In the past, providers, in attempting to help reduce the suffering that results from cultural rejection, took them under the protection of medical and mental health authorities. This started with Magnus Hirschfeld at the turn of the last century. Since then, we have learned that being transgender is a feature of natural diversity, and transgender people are ready to assume the responsibility for their own welfare. In order to clear the way for this, pathologization of being transgender must end. Being transgender must not reflect ideas about how it might be a mental health disorder when there is no evidence for that.

No doubt medical and mental health providers will still be involved in treating transgender people. One way they can help is to stop using pathological terms. Transgender people have demonstrated that they have the power to depathologize and change the definition of pathological terms. Transgender people have demonstrated that they could depathologize and repurpose formerly pathological terms like transsexual, gender identity, and transgender itself.

Just as the DSM was depathologized with regard to homosexuality, so must the DSM be purged of pathological categories related to being transgender. As for homosexuals, if transgender people need counseling, there are innumerable billing categories for that in the DSM. No pathological category needs to be included in the DSM for transgender people. The ICD-11 has solved the problem by devising a nonpathological category to cover such things as TGPS and dropping other categories like gender identity disorder. All DSM billing is actually converted to ICD billing through computer pointers in a process known as "harmonization." Since all providers are encouraged to use ICD codes anyway, DSM codes will be irrelevant with regard to being transgender once ICD-11 is implemented.

There is a need for new terms and approaches that accurately reflect the realities of transgender people, and some are offered in this book. But they are only temporary. Transgender people are good at inventing new terms or repurposing old terms. Given this track record, the term transgender itself is likely to be replaced eventually.

Bullying and Public Transgender Rejection

Transgender people often report both bullying in school and on the job as well as public rejection. **Bullying** involves both physical and nonphysical aggression that is designed to humiliate and dominate others. These actions involve both verbal and physical abuse. U.S. schools and workplaces have generally failed to deal with the problem of bullying despite laws and several federal school programs designed to reduce bullying. Transgender people are especially vulnerable because being transgender is a violation of culture. Western culture sanctions bullying because transgender people are cultural outlaws. Many people think they are defending the culture by bullying transgender people or use this as an excuse.

In the early years of this century, bullying was recognized as a significant problem in U.S. schools. Many of them started to address this in 2012–2013 by establishing antibullying programs and student training. Students were taught what constituted bullying and urged to refrain from doing it. Unfortunately, the results of these well-meaning programs were that they actually *increased* bullying. They made bullies into better bullies and taught teachers to look the other way because of liability issues. The only remaining thing of value in these programs is that some did establish anonymous ways to report bullying. These unsuccessful U.S. programs were followed by programs designed to change the "school environment." Everyone, including bus drivers, janitors, and administrators, now receives training on how to improve the interpersonal environment. Bullying has not stopped.

While workplace bullying is illegal in the United States, cases of bullying are hardly ever solved on the job. In spite of its being illegal and in spite of the required employee training, bullying continues to occur. The person being bullied is almost sure to part ways with their employers and will likely be tagged as a troublemaker by the employer and other workers. Employers may allow bullying to continue or find some subtle way to lay off a complaining transgender employee. For those transgender people being bullied on the job, the best advice is to formally complain, and in doing so be sure to quantify the costs to the employer of replacement. However, complaining does not always work, and the person should also start looking for another job. They should not just let the bullying continue, because it is injurious to their mental and physical health. When people are bullied, their body reacts emotionally, and these emotions and their memories can lead to depression, PTSD, and suicide.

Transgender bullying both inside and outside of jobs and school is often ignored by law enforcement although it constitutes battery (verbal) and assault (physical). In some cases, it can be a felonious assault and battery and a hate crime. Transgender people are reticent about pressing charges and sometimes law enforcement personnel are the abusers. The best solution found so far for bullying is **bystander training**, which involves preparing potential bystanders with information about how to recognize bullying as well as clear procedures as to what to do when they observe it. The science for this approach was developed by John Darley at Princeton University in 1968 (Darley & Latané, 1968) when it was found that bystanders were reticent to help people in distress unless they had appropriate training. This research was triggered by press reports about the Kitty Genovese murder case in Newark, New Jersey, in 1964, which became highly publicized. There were reports that large numbers of people heard Kitty being repeatedly stabbed over the course of an hour, but no one called the police. Kitty died of those injuries. Initially, Darley replicated group conformity studies in which an emergency was simulated with college students and found that they would not report even obvious signs of physical danger such as a room filling up with smoke. However, when Darley used people outside of the college community, he found that those trained in responding to emergencies would immediately respond. This result was replicated with ship captains and first responders.

People in the Finnish school system had been reading Darley's social psychology reports and developed a program they call "KiVa" (which simply means "against bullying" in Finnish) to teach student bystanders to recognize and deal with bullying (Sainio et al., 2018). The idea is to teach bystander students to recognize bullying situations and how to intervene to stop them.

And the program worked. Ninety-eight percent of those who had previously been subject to bullying in test schools reported that the bullying was reduced. The program later demonstrated bullying reduction in a study that involved 30,000 students. The KiVa program was implemented in 117 schools in Finland. The program was not implemented in an additional 117 schools that served as controls. As of now, over 90 percent of Finnish schools and some U.S., Japanese, and German schools have enrolled in KiVa. In order to be maximally effective for transgender people on the job, at school, or in public, the bystander must be trained on what constitutes abuse of transgender people, why it must be stopped, and how to report it.

But what if a particular school does not adopt KiVa? How should a transgender person deal with bullying? Although it takes some courage, one way that seems to work is to form networks of friends in school and in the community who could intervene. This takes courage because many people who are subject to bullying retreat into themselves and do not reach out to form new friendships. What is needed is continuing peer pressure to stop bullying. Gay-Straight Alliances and other student groups can spread the word about recognizing and dealing with bullying if a student is a bystander. There is no guarantee that this will work without school support.

Significantly, while some religions reject transgender people, some churches and the Tyler Clementi Foundation have launched programs to eliminate bullying in religion, such as the Truth Faith Doesn't Bully Campaign (Tyler Clementi Foundation, 2018). This effort describes the problem:

> LGBTQ individuals are particularly vulnerable to religion-based bullying because of the history of religious groups condemning LGBTQ people. Treating LGBTQ people as less valued, preaching at LGBTQ people, and calling LGBTQ people's sexual orientation or gender identity "sinful" are all potential examples of religion-based bullying.
>
> We believe that all people should have a place in their chosen faith communities, and that no person should be made to feel that who they are is a sin, whether or not they belong to a faith community. (Tyler Clementi Foundation, 2018)

Of course, bullying has now gone high tech through cyberbullying on social media. Cyberbullying has been shown to cause psychological and emotional effects including suicidal ideation, depression, lower self-esteem, and lower school grades (Abreu & Kenny, 2018). Programs to alert transgender people and youth in general about this problem have been put forward. Their effectiveness has not been established.

Provider Education

Consistent provider education about being transgender is still not established. In the past, most provider schools provided only a few hours of instruction in the entire LGBT curriculum. That has improved, but there is still contention over whether it should be provided as one block or distributed over the broader curriculum. Short courses for continuing education credit are now provided by WPATH, and other organizations for transgender treatment, but are still not perfected. Even those who do not specialize in transgender procedures need to have familiarity with being transgender. WPATH has recommended that providers should intern for 6–12 months with an experienced provider, but no large-scale organized program for this currently exists. Treating transgender people is not a formal medical specialty that one can train and apply for when coming out of medical school as one can for internal medicine, cardiology, or surgery. Many doctors are "board certified" in specialties such as internal medicine or OB-GYN, which take considerable time and effort. There are no recognized transgender specialties in any of the provider disciplines. WPATH has established a route to certification including their CEU course and other voluntary activities, but it is only a first step and has no legal standing.

Evidence-Based Treatment

Ideally, provider treatments should be based on scientific evidence as far as possible. There are several barriers to obtaining such evidence for treating transgender people.

The first barrier is that being transgender is not a disease and most countries and institutions only fund provider research that pertains to a recognized disease. Many politicians regard research on transgender and other similar matters such as homosexuality, sex, and love as being frivolous because "we already know the answers" and because they are not considered to be politically correct.

This is especially true for basic research on transgender causal factors. Such transgender scientific research usually comes from providers outside the United States and/or is collected in conjunction with clinical intake and treatments. Only a few countries can fund "big science," the United States being one of them, yet there is a lack of grants in the United States for research aimed at such basic research as full genome scans to look for genetic markers of being transgender, even though large quantities of genetic data are already available (Polderman et al., 2018). Private institutions often fund such "controversial" research but even they are limited by the political climate and government restrictions. Yet knowing why people are transgender is critical to treatment approaches and advocacy.

Transgender treatment research is *often attacked as being "unscientific" because most studies are unable to be designed with control groups.* However, *research ethics, laws, and policies in the United States and elsewhere often forbid withholding established beneficial treatments to people in control groups.* There are strategies for dealing with this ethics imperative, including such things as using unintended delay of treatment to form a control group. This might be considered for research on the initial effects of HT. But, as has been seen in the United Kingdom, at least 22 percent of those delayed for HT because of inadequate NHS resources resort to taking unprescribed hormones. This would compromise any control group formed to research HT using the delay approach. Such study design problems do not just apply to HT but to other transgender treatments. Many of the critics do not understand or ignore such ethical restrictions, thinking that human research is akin to animal research in which control groups can be formed without ethical qualms. But there are no animal models for being transgender.

Politicization of Being Transgender

Paradoxically, one of the barriers to transgender treatment and progress comes from some in the academic community and elsewhere who ostensibly support transgender advocacy. They encourage confrontation with providers over pronouns and honorifics and take offense for what they see as transgender issues when most transgender people may not. They define gender as a social construct but deny any biological involvement in behavior such as genetic gender behavior predispositions. They also refuse to acknowledge scientific discourse and debate. Rather than debate the issues, their tactic is to shun or physically confront those with whom they disagree. Their goal in doing this is to achieve social power by misrepresenting themselves as representatives of transgender people. Providers should avoid supporting such factions, which are starting to be seen as misguided because of their ineffectiveness and perfidy.

REFERENCES

Abreu, R. L., & Kenny, M. C. (2018). Cyberbullying and LGBTQ youth: A systematic literature review and recommendations for prevention and intervention. *Journal of Child & Adolescent Trauma, 11*(1), 81–97.

Adam, S., & Goodman, M. (2015). *Number of Americans who report knowing a transgender person doubles in seven years, according to new GLAAD survey.* GLAAD. https://www.glaad.org/releases/number-americans-who-report-knowing-transgender-person-doubles-seven-years-according-new

American Medical Association. (1972). *Human sexuality.* American Medical Association.

Blanchard, R. (2005). Early history of the concept of autogynephilia. *Archives of Sexual Behavior, 34*(4), 439–446.

Blanchard, R., Racansky, G., & Steiner, B. W. (1986). Phallometric detection of fetishistic arousal in heterosexual male cross-dressers. *Journal of Sex Research, 22*(4), 452–462.

Both, S., Brauer, M., & Laan, E. (2011). Classical conditioning of sexual response in women: A replication study. *Journal of Sexual Medicine, 8*, 3116–3131.

Both, S., Spiering, M., Laan, E., Belcome, S., van den Heuvel, B., & Everaerd, W., (2008). Unconscious classical conditioning of sexual arousal: Evidence for the conditioning of female genital arousal to subliminally presented sexual stimuli. *Journal of Sexual Medicine, 5*, 100–109.

Bruner, J., Goodnow, J. J., & Austin, G. A. (1967). *A study of thinking.* New York: Science Editions.

Buhrich, N. (1978). Motivation for cross-dressing in heterosexual transvestism. *Acta Psychiatric Society of Scandinavia, 57*(2), 145–152.

Cogle, C. R., Yachnis, A. T., Laywell, E. D., Zander, D. S., Wingard, J. R., Steindler, D. A., & Scott, E. W. (2004). Bone marrow transdifferentiation in brain after transplantation: A retrospective study. *The Lancet, 363*(9419), 1432–1437.

Darley, J. M., & Latané, B. (1968). Bystander intervention in emergencies: Diffusion of responsibility. *Journal of Personality and Social Psychology, 8*, 377–383.

Davenport, C. W. (1986). A follow-up study of 10 feminine boys. *Archives of Sexual Behavior, 15*(6), 511–517.

Diamond, M. (2002). Sex and gender are different: Sexual identity and gender identity are different. *Clinical Child Psychology & Psychiatry, 7*(3), 320–334.

Ford, C. S., & Beach, F. A. (1952). *Patterns of sexual behavior.* Harper and Brothers.

Hirschfeld, M. (1910/1991). *The transvestites: The erotic drive to cross-dress* (M. A. Lombardi-Nash, Trans.). New York: Prometheus Books.

Hoffman, H. (2012). Considering the role of conditioning in sexual orientation. *Archives of Sexual Behavior, 41*, 63–71.

Hoffman, H., Janssen, E., & Turner, S. (2004). Classical conditioning in sexual orientation. *Archives of Sexual Behavior, 33*, 43–53.

Hruz, P. W., Mayer, L. S., & McHugh, P. R. (2017, Spring). Problems of puberty suppression in treating gender dysphoria. *New Atlantis*, 3–36.

Janssen, E., Everaerd, W., Spiering, M., & Janssen, J. (2010). Automatic processes and the appraisal of sexual stimuli: Toward an information processing model of sexual arousal. *Journal of Sexual Research, 37*, 8–23.

Koksal, F., Domjan, M., Kurt, A., Ozlem, S., Orung, S., Bowers, R., & Kumru, G. (2004). An animal model of fetishism. *Behaviour Research Therapy, 42*, 1421–1434.

Lalumiere, M., & Quinsey, V. (1998). Pavlovian conditioning of sexual interests in human males. *Archives of Sexual Behavior, 27*, 241–252.

Levis, D., & Castelda, B. (2007). Stampfl's therapist directed implosive (flooding) therapy. In M. Hersen & J. Rosqvist (Eds.), *Encyclopedia of behavior modification and cognitive behavior therapy.* Thousand Oaks, CA: Sage.

Levitt, H. M., & Ippolito, M. R. (2014). Being transgender: The experience of transgender identity development. *Journal of Homosexuality, 61*(12), 1727–1758.

Littman, L. (2018, August 16). Rapid-onset gender dysphoria in adolescents and young adults: A study of parental reports. *PLOS One*, 0202330. https://journals.plos.org/plosone/article?id=10.1371/journal.pone.0202330

McHugh, P. R., & Mayer, L. S. (2016). Sexuality and gender. *New Atlantis, 30.*

Money, J., Hampson, J. G., & Hampson, J. L. (1955). An examination of some basic sexual concepts: The evidence of human hermaphroditism. *Bulletin of the Johns Hopkins Hospital, 97*(4), 301–319.

Moser, C. (2009) Autogynephilia in women. *Journal of Homosexuality, 56*(5), 539–547.

Moser, C. (2010). Blanchard's autogynephilia theory: A critique. *Journal of Homosexuality, 57*, 790–809.

Olson, K. R., Key, A. C., & Eaton, N. R. (2013). Gender cognition in transgender children. *Psychological Science, 26*(4), 467–474.

Pasquino, I. M., Pucarelli, I., Accardo, F., Demiraj, V., Segni, M., & Di Nardo, R. (2008). Long-term observation of 87 girls with idiopathic central precocious puberty treated with gonadotropin-releasing hormone analogs: Impact on adult height, body mass index, bone mineral content, and reproductive function. *Journal of Clinical Endocrinology & Metabolism, 93*(1), 190–195.

Polderman, T. J. C., et al. (2018). The biological contributions to gender identity and gender diversity: Bringing data to the table. *Behavioral Genetics, 48*, 95–108.

Sainio, M., Herkama, S., Turunen, T., Rönkkö, M., Kontio, M., Poskiparta, E., & Salmivalli, C. (2018). Sustainable antibullying program implementation: School profiles and predictors. *Scandinavia Journal of Psychology, 12487.*

Singh, D. (2012). A follow-up study of boys with gender identity disorder. Doctoral thesis, Department of Human Development and Applied Psychology, University of Toronto.

Steensma, T. D., McGuire, J. K., Kreukels, B. P. C., Beekman, A. J., & Cohen-Kettenis, P. T. (2013). Factors associated with desistence and persistence of childhood gender dysphoria: A quantitative follow-up study. *Journal of the American Academy of Child & Adolescent Psychiatry, 52*(6), 582–590.

Tyler Clementi Foundation. (2018). *True faith doesn't bully.* https://tylerclementi.org/true-faith/

Wallien, M. S. C., & Cohen-Kettenis, P. T. (2008). Psychosexual outcome of gender-dysphoric children. *Journal of the American Academy of Child & Adolescent Psychiatry, 47*(12), 1413–1423.

Whitam, F. L. (1977). Childhood indicators of male homosexuality. *Archives of Sexual Behavior, 6*(2), 89–96.

Zucker, K. (2018). The myth of persistence: Response to "A critical commentary on follow-up studies and 'desistance' theories about transgender and gender nonconforming children" by Temple Newhook et al. *International Journal of Transgenderism,* https://doi.org/10.1080/15532739.2018.1468293

Zuger, B., & Taylor, P. (1969). Effeminate behavior presentation in boys from early childhood. II. Comparison with similar symptoms in non-effeminate boys. *Pediatrics, 44*(3), 375–380.

PART 3

Research and Looking Ahead

11

Classic Research

This chapter presents important research studies that have influenced transgender understanding and treatment and sent research in new directions.

MAGNUS HIRSCHFELD AND TRANSVESTISM (1911)

As one of the first sexologists and following the methodologies of biological classification, Magnus Hirschfeld tried to identify various types of "sexual intermediaries" or behavioral categories of people including those that we would later call transgender. He was looking at people through the eyes of sex, not gender. The idea of gender behavior categories distinct from sex had not yet been conceived. These included homosexuality and heterosexuality, but also masculine and feminine gender roles. Most important for this discussion, one of these intermediary categories was

Research on a Shoestring

None of the classic research studies cited in this chapter received "big science" funding. All but one were on a shoestring budget as offshoots of clinical practice or were funded by private donors like Reed Erikson, who funded Harry Benjamin so he could write up his results. Only one received research funding support, but it was a very small-scale anatomical study involving six transgender people who donated their brains. It has not been replicated in 23 years.

How can it be that important basic research studies that give us insights into human behavior are rejected for funding?

One clue may come from the experience of Ellen Berscheid. She is a social psychologist who in 1974 won a small grant from the National Science Foundation to study why people fall in love. But Senator William Proxmire called Berscheid's study a waste of money and gave it his "Golden Fleece" award, a satirical award usually given to government "pork barrel" projects. The case sent a chill through the ranks of researchers and discouraged them from applying for government and private grants for understanding human connection behavior. Berscheid lost any hope of future research funding and retreated into administrative management. It has only been recently that her contributions to social psychology have been recognized with the Presidential Award from the APA. In 2018 her study was again attacked on the floor of the U.S. Senate. Also in 2018, in a country with a divorce rate of 50 percent, a study of newlywed behavior was defunded by Congress.

We can never fully anticipate the impacts of basic research into the human condition, and clearly the insights gained through research about gender behavior should be valuable.

transvestism, meaning those who had the urge to dress in the manner associated with the opposite sex.

Hirschfeld's methodology was the case study. In his seminal book *The Transvestites* (Hirschfeld, 1911), he presented 18 cases, only one of whom was a transman; the rest were transwomen. The general approach was to capture as much information as seemed important on the background of each case study person: their history and demographics, their sex lives and sexual orientations, their fetishes, and their behavior, including what today we would call their gender behavior. He captured detailed inventories of clothing that the subjects used when in transvestite mode.

Analysis of the cases presented in his book revealed the strong desire to crossdress and their feelings of "peace, security, exaltation, happiness and well-being that overcomes them." They also reported discomfort with having to wear clothing associated with their birth sex (Hirschfeld, 1911, p. 125). Hirschfeld noted that the urge began in early childhood and increased during puberty. Most started in childhood using the clothing of mothers or sisters. Some only wore opposite-gender clothing in secret but many wore it in public. Some would stop their transvestite behavior for long periods and then resume. Some would go away from home for trips or vacations to places where they could crossdress for longer periods of time. Some closely followed feminine fashion magazines or crafts. They speculated on how they got this way and what the future might hold.

From his studies, Hirschfeld concluded that transvestites were different from homosexuals because the latter's sexual orientation was aimed at the opposite birth sex. There was little evidence in his case studies that would support the idea that transvestitism was an extension of homosexuality, even though feminine behavior could be observed in each.

Furthermore, *not all of his cases experienced sexual arousal when crossdressed, and he distinguished transvestism from fetishism because fetishist interest was in a specific body part or object.* Likewise, he distinguished transvestism from masochism, although transvestites tolerated some discomfort from opposite-gender clothing in order to experience the emotional comfort that crossdressing provided. Transvestites were under no illusion that their sex had been changed when crossdressed, so they were not delusional, nor were they hallucinating. Finally, he did not consider sexual intermediaries, including transvestism, to be pathological, nor did he believe that the transvestic drive could be made to disappear. It was a facet of personality.

In retrospect, the views of Hirschfeld were not radically different from our understanding today. Although he started out believing that transgender people were motivated by sexual arousal, by the end of his studies he had found evidence to the contrary. Although the word transvestite is currently out of fashion because it is tinged with the ideas of sexual arousal and fetishism, it appears that Hirschfeld did not originate this connotation, although he included transgender people in this taxonomy of "sexual intermediaries." The association may have originated because sexologists studied all three phenomena and the work of Hirschfeld on transvestism was most prominent. Another potential factor is that his book *The Transvestites* did not receive an adequate translation from German until 1991.

HARRY BENJAMIN AND *THE TRANSSEXUAL PHENOMENON* (1965)

By 1965, Harry Benjamin had worked with over 300 transgender and transitioning transgender (transsexuals) people to provide HT and to find surgeons who would perform TGPS and other procedures. He documented his experience in a book entitled *The Transsexual Phenomenon* (Benjamin,

1966), which included descriptive commentary from case histories. His views have impacted what we believe today.

He believed that transgender people did not necessarily have a sexual deviation or perversion. Some transvestites crossdressed strictly for emotional relief without sexual arousal and mainly did it in private. Benjamin popularized the word transsexual for those who were deeply unhappy with the sex to which they were assigned at birth and wanted to change their bodies. Therefore, transsexuals sought "corrective surgery," which had only become available in the previous decades. He found them to be intense and likely to commit suicide if untreated. He referred to the case of Christine Jorgensen, who had managed to obtain transgender genital plastic surgery in Denmark because her family was originally from there. (Denmark refused to provide TGPS to non-Danish citizens.)

As Hirschfeld had done, he struggled to categorize his patients into a taxonomy of six groups using the criteria of sexual behavior, crossdressing and gender behavior, sexual orientation, and the likelihood of wanting to transition. The six categories included three for transvestites (using Hirschfeld's definition) and three for transsexuals (using Cauldwell's definition of transsexual).

He speculated that all six groups might have actually been transsexual and that the three transvestite categories might just be at a low intensity of the same transsexual phenomenon, believing that "nature does not abide by rigid systems" (Benjamin, 1966, p. 8). He termed this condition "sex or gender role disorientation and indecision" (Benjamin, 1966, p. 4).

Benjamin took a position on sexual orientation that caused rejection of many transsexuals for surgery and deception on the part of some of those who got surgery. He believed that transsexuals were basically homosexuals; that is, if they were male their sexual orientation initially was toward other males. Many transsexuals got the word, and when requesting surgery learned to lie by saying that they were attracted to people of the same sex. Benjamin believed that "the transsexual feels himself to be a woman trapped in a man's body and is attracted to men" (Benjamin, 1966, p. 7). Today we accept transgender people for transition of any sexual orientation (see Chapter 5). Benjamin knew about marriage flight, in which transgender people become heterosexually attracted and form relationships to try to lead a normal life, but he was skeptical that such arrangements were lasting.

Benjamin speculated about transgender causation, citing several factors and concluding that in research "we will most likely have to concern [ourselves] with work in two areas: genetics and neurophysiology" (Benjamin, 1966, p. 4).

In 1965, he foresaw that in the future, the legal change of sex and identification would be guided by common sense, and some things have changed only slowly since then:

> As far as the legal change of sex after a conversion operation is concerned, the respective patient in the United States in 1965 has to be lucky. He has to have been born in a state that proceeds from good will, cuts through red tape, and issues a new birth certificate on application accompanied by medical testimony. If he is not lucky and has been born . . . [in a state not like that] . . . he has to have money, swallow his sugar-coated pill of disappointment, entrust his fate to a judge, and hope for the best. (Benjamin, 1966, Appendix A, p. 4)

And finally, he predicted that "sex reassignment surgery, that is to say a conversion operation, will be accepted eventually as a legitimate treatment for a selected group of transsexuals" (Benjamin, 1966, p. 2).

ZHOU ET AL.: A SEX DIFFERENCE IN THE BRAIN AND TRANSSEXUALITY (1995)

This short paper, published in 1995, set off the hunt for brain anatomy and mechanisms that are different in transgender people versus controls. The idea was that if the theories of biological causation factors are correct, then there might be detectable structures and mechanisms in the brain involved in being transgender. Since this paper was published, there have been a plethora of research studies performed to look for anatomical and neurophysiological correlates using conventional neuroanatomy techniques, MRI, and fMRI studies (which were described in Chapter 3).

The Zhou study was performed by neuroanatomists in the Netherlands at the Netherlands Institute of Brain Research and the Free University in Amsterdam, Netherlands. The objective of this study was to look for neuroanatomical correlates in humans of being transgender. They used postmortem specimens of transitioned transwomen.

The structure under study was a small nucleus just dorsal to the anterior commissure between the fornix and the internal capsule. The nucleus is called the basal nucleus of the stria terminalis pars C (BNSTc), which contains cell bodies of fibers that wrap around through lateral ventricles to connect the hypothalamus with the amygdala. From the size of the axons, the bundle of the stria terminalis is believed to have evolved earlier than other connections between these two structures such as the amygdalofugal pathways. It has been well established that many structures in this area are sexually dimorphic (Swaab & Hofman, 1995) and the BNSTc is one of them, being larger in males than females.

There were six postmortem specimens used in the study, which were stained using vasoactive intestinal polypeptide stains. The controls were 42 specimens, matched for chronological and specimen preparation age.

The size of BNSTc was measured; the size of the transwomen's structures were closer to the female controls than the male controls on average, and two of the specimens were actually smaller than the female range. The authors provided evidence from other specimens that the effect was probably not due to the estrogen the transgender group had been taking, nor to the reduction of testosterone. Homosexual transgender specimens were not different from heterosexual transgender specimens. The sizes of the control males and homosexual groups were not statistically different, indicating that the effect could not be attributed to homosexuality.

Photomicrograph images from this study are commonly used in articles and textbooks as evidence for biological transgender causation factors (for an example, see Carlson, 2004).

LYNN CONWAY AND POPULATION FREQUENCIES (2001)

Lynn Conway, a computer hardware engineer, did some preliminary estimates of transgender population frequencies (see Chapter 6). The accepted estimates at the time for transwomen, 1:7200 to 1 in 42,000 (Kaplan, 2010), had led some to underestimate the need for transgender research and treatment based on the number of people affected. But the published estimates were based primarily on clinical presentation to gender clinics, not on transgender people "in the wild." Conway's calculations concluded that such estimates were orders of magnitude in error.

Conway built engineering estimation models of transwomen and transitioning transwomen, which indicate that the actual population frequencies were at least three orders of magnitude higher than the accepted estimates. As inputs to this model, she used numbers of transgender people in support groups and the capacities of those treating transitioning transgender people and surgeons who performed TGPS. She estimated a lower bound of 1 percent of the male population were transgender and .1 percent were transitioning transwomen, and those completing TGPS at .025 percent. Her results for support group estimates were confirmed by Reed et al. in 2009 (Reed, Rhodes, Shofield, & Wylie, 2009).

Since then, surveys have been conducted that seem to confirm her estimates. Although the U.S. government bans the collection of population frequency data for transgender people in its census, one CDC survey provides estimates and demographic data that can be used to extrapolate those estimates. In such surveys, the population frequency of being transgender has risen from .3 percent to almost .8 percent (Flores, Herman, Gates, & Brown, 2016). These results include transwomen, but also include transmen whose population frequency is believed to be lower than transwomen's, lowering the overall frequency number. The population frequency of "reported being transgender" has been gradually increasing because of the improved tolerance and acceptance of transgender people.

Conway's research opened up the issue of transgender population frequencies and gave transgender people more hope that they were numerous enough to be understood and treated.

JOAN ROUGHGARDEN: *EVOLUTION'S RAINBOW* (2004)

As an evolutionary biologist, Joan Roughgarden exhaustively studied sex and gender behavioral science about a wide variety of species, including humans, with regard to their gender behavior and concluded that the Darwin/Wallace theory of **sexual selection** is wrong.

This theory of sexual selection has resulted in stereotyping of the sexes and social injustice for transgender people, women, and others. Her analysis was documented in her book *Evolution's Rainbow* (Roughgarden, 2004) (see Chapter 5). The other theory by Darwin/Wallace, the theory of **natural selection**, seems to be on the right track as we are learning from the biological and behavioral sciences. However, the Darwin/Wallace theory of evolutionary sexual selection indicated that females selected those that they mated with on the basis of attraction and that males competed with each other to be most attractive and did not cooperate in mating. Each of the sexes supposedly had behavioral and personality traits that were compatible with this model of sexual selection.

The Darwin/Wallace theory of sexual selection contributes to modern sex and behavior stereotypes for males and females, which Roughgarden found to contradict the scientific evidence. Using anthropomorphic thinking about animals, males were supposed to have stronger passions and the females were supposed to be coy and less eager than males to have sex. Although Darwin/Wallace knew about cases of sexual diversity from the study of barnacles and sex role reversal in birds, the theory ignored them as exceptions to the rules of the theory. Animal models of same-sex sexuality were left out altogether. The only positive was that Darwin/Wallace stood up for the ability of females to be intelligent enough to make choices. Much of the behavioral stereotyping appears to have been inspired by ideas embedded in the society of the British Empire, with idealized strong male soldiers and sexually weak and frigid wives. Modern versions of sexual selection further characterized males as being promiscuous and constantly looking to mate. But in many species, females are the ones cheating on their male mates, particularly if the male is willing to take care of their offspring.

The evidence that Roughgarden used to criticize the Darwin/Wallace sexual selection theory came from her research about sex and gender. Sex is not always binary and the ability to reproduce does not persist throughout life. Biological gender behavior does not conform to binary categories. Sex and gender roles can be reversible, as has been demonstrated in recent history in which more males contribute to child rearing, some full-time. Some males refuse offers of sexual relations, instead looking to establish relationships that go beyond the sex act. The sexual selection theory postulated that deceit between competing males occurs. However, there is no evidence that social deceit in mating exists. She provides animal examples of cooperation. Same-sex relationships and mating are common both in animals and humans. Much more sex goes on than is required for reproduction, particularly in humans.

She concludes by saying:

> The true story of nature is profoundly empowering for peoples of minority gender expression and sexualities. Yet, this truth has been suppressed by biologists, and the few accounts that do surface are embedded in pejorative language. *To remove the conceptual rot,* we've had to excavate deep into the foundation of evolutionary theory, identifying the collapsing member—Darwin's theory of sexual selection—and replace it with new ideas that may be better able to carry the load as the future unfolds. (Roughgarden, 2004, p. 181)

VIRGINIA ERHARDT: *HEAD OVER HEELS* (2007)

In her clinical psychology practice, Virginia specialized in relationships involving LGBT people. The culmination of her work with transwomen and their wives was the book *Head over Heels.* This study is a first step toward understanding how to keep marriages and committed relationships together if one of the parties is revealed or comes out to the other as being transgender. This study is important because over half of transgender people get married (Crissman, Berger, Graham, & Dalton, 2014) and form families. Most transgender spouses never come out publicly or transition, but being transgender can impact marital relations. This is particularly true if the revelation of being transgender occurs suddenly by, for example, the accidental discovery of hidden opposite-gender clothing by the nontransgender spouse. So, her study provides information on how to keep marriages together if at all possible, but analyzes those successful marriages in which one spouse is transgender. In previous work by others, the focus had always been on the transgender partner, but in this book the nontransgender partner is given equal treatment.

The analysis is based in part on 30 case histories of a wide variety of transwomen and their partners who decided to stay together and maintain their marriages. All of the natal female partners were unaware that their spouse was transgender before marriage. Their case histories are presented in the book, as well as commentary from Erhardt's expert experience in such matters. For many years, Virginia Ehrhardt served as the leader of the significant-other track at Southern Comfort Conventions, and she held workshops at many other transgender events. This gave her access to many wives of transwomen. In her book, she provided a running commentary for each case history of ways in which counseling helped or could have helped.

The initial shock of revelation can become a traumatic stress event. After initial shock, the natal females go through a process of questioning their own gender and sexual orientation and through a grieving process of "losing" their man, at least on a part-time basis. Most natal female spouses feel the need to keep their partner's transgender behavior a secret, yet this places a burden on them similar to the burden that the transgender partner carries. Power struggles may ensue over limits on transgender behavior because of the natal female's fear of discovery. Rules about what the transgender partner wears during sex are common. Most important is that trust is broken and must be repaired. Some natal female partners actually benefit from the experience, which makes them stronger people.

With regard to marital therapy, expressing and discussing personal needs between the two parties seems to be a fruitful process of understanding and self-discovery. This research provides a start on marital therapy involving transgender partners. But clearly research needs to continue in this area because improvement would benefit, by far, the greatest number of transgender people.

POLDERMAN ET AL.: THE POLYGENETIC THRESHOLD MODEL (2018)

Evidence has been mounting for a genetic causative factor in being transgender. But the Polderman et al. (2018) study provides the first comprehensive genetic analysis of heritability and DNA marker research as well as application of the first sophisticated genetic model of being transgender—the polygenetic threshold model. Recognition of a biological genetic factor in being transgender is essential to reducing pathologization and health disparities among transgender people.

The polygenetic threshold model seems to be applicable to many complex traits (Visscher & Wray, 2015). In this model, multiple genes contribute to a given trait and there is a threshold which, if reached, instantiates the trait. The model seems to fit the trait of being transgender.

The Polderman et al. analysis of 11 of the transgender heritability studies, including monozygotic and dizygotic twins, indicate heritabilities of 30–60 percent, which is the range of many complex traits (Polderman et al., 2015).

Although DNA marker studies have been conducted for individual genes with regard to being transgender, they advocated for a genome-wide association study (GWAS) to determine if the polygenetic threshold model or another model best fits the results. Future GWAS research is needed to identify marker genes from across the entire genome, and Polderman indicated that extensive genetic data is available from transgender and non-transgender people for comparison.

REFERENCES

Benjamin, H. (2018). The transsexual phenomenon. (Originally published by the Julian Press, 1966.) Dusseldorf: Electronic Edition by Symposium Press Publishing. http://www.mut23.de/texte/Harry%20Benjamin%20-%20The%20Transsexual%20Phenomenon.pdf

Carlson, N. R. (2004). *Physiology of behavior* (p. 329). Boston: Pearson.

Crissman, H. P., Berger, M. B., Graham, L. F., & Dalton, V. K. (2014). Transgender demographics: A household probability sample of US adults. *American Journal of Public Health: Transgender Health, 107*(2), 213–215.

Erhardt, V. (2007). *Head over heels.* Binghamton: Haworth Press.

Flores, A. R., Herman, J. L., Gates, G. J., & Brown, T. N. T. (2016). *How many adults identify as transgender in the United States?* Los Angeles, CA: Williams Institute.

Hirschfeld, M. (1911/1991). *Transvestites: The erotic urge to cross-dress* (M. Lombardi-Nash, Trans.). New York: Prometheus.

Kaplan, A. B. (2010). Discussions of mental health issues for gender variant and transgender individuals, friends and family: Basic issues in transgender mental health. *Transgender Mental Health.* https://tgmentalhealth.com/2010/03/31/the-prevalence-of-transgenderism/

Polderman, T. J., Benyamin, B., de Leeuw, C. A., Sullivan, P. F., van Bochoven, A., Visscher, P. M., & Posthuma, D. (2015). Meta-analysis of the heritability of human traits based on fifty years of twin studies. *Natural Genetics, 47*(7), 702–709.

Polderman, T. J., et al. (2018). The biological contributions to gender identity and gender diversity: Bringing data to the table. *Behavioral Genetics, 48,* 95–108.

Reed, B., Rhodes, S., Shofield, P., & Wylie, K. (2009). Gender variance in the UK: Prevalence, incidence, growth and geographic distribution. GIRES.

Roughgarden, J. (2004). *Evolution's Rainbow.* Berkeley: University of California Press.

Swaab, D. F., & Hofman, M. A. (1995). Sexual differentiation of the human hypothalamus in relation to gender and sexual orientation *Trends in Neuroscience, 18*(6), 264–270.

Visscher, P. M., & Wray, N. R. (2015). Concepts and misconceptions about the polygenic additive model applied to disease. *Human Heredity, 80*(4), 165–170.

Zhou, J. N., Hofman, M. A., Gooren, L. J., & Swaab, D. F. (1995). A sex difference in the human brain and its relation to transsexuality. *Nature, 378*(6552), 68–70.

12

New and Emerging Research

Based on the science in this book, this chapter provides an overview of emerging and needed future research to understand transgender causation, develop treatments, and contribute to the resolution of other issues. The purpose of this book is to provide a snapshot of existing transgender scientific evidence because of provider commitment to evidence-based treatment, but future research will undoubtedly improve our understanding of being transgender.

CAUSATION

Understanding causation is important for approaching treatment and explaining transgender behavior to patients and SOFFAs. However, some transgender people, antitransgender people, and others do not want causation to be explored. For example, some transgender people are afraid that

Community Research Participation

WPATH and USPATH want to be sure that community organizations participate in research studies on being transgender. And it looks like these policies will have some real teeth.

A group of providers that studied the issue (Adams et al., 2017) made some recommendations to involve community organizations in research. These recommendations include early and continuous involvement with research studies, ensuring that the studies use the right language, ensuring that the results are disseminated back to the community, making sure that informed consent is understood, ensuring patient privacy, and eliminating gender change efforts. The guidelines will be disseminated to institutional review boards, which govern most research in the United States.

WPATH is in alignment with these guidelines and discourages research studies in its flagship journal, *The International Journal of Transgenderism,* that do not include adequate community involvement.

This approach should improve research quality, make possible research that has difficulty recruiting transgender subjects, and improve community acceptance of the results. It also should reduce the stigma of pathologization by eliminating terms and words that are no longer used in the community. Although researchers say that they will report the results back to their subjects, they now *must* do that. Informed consent is pretty tricky to obtain, particularly for minor transgender children. Parents have legal control but every effort should be made to ensure that minors understand, insofar as they can at their age and maturity.

Because transgender people and groups may be leery of approaches by researchers, the new policy needs to be widely understood by the trans community.

knowing causation will lead to genetic testing, discrimination against transgender people, or genetic engineering to eliminate being transgender. Some antitransgender people believe that sex and gender are the same thing based on their philosophical beliefs, and that being transgender is somehow a pathological delusion. Others, while not being transgender, want to take advantage of transgender people to gain political power, and scientific evidence may interfere with their plans.

Although Western culture has defined a binary, cisgender, and inflexible gender system, it also has a tradition of supporting scientific investigation as a means to avoid societal problems and to solve those problems based on facts, in so far as science can discover them. That is the basis for the development of modern medicine and mental health practice. Protections such as the Genetic Information Nondiscrimination Act (GINA) can be put in place to keep genetic information private with regard to employment (EEOC, 2018). Protections could easily be put in place to control testing and genetic therapies. But future safeguards will require a body of knowledge for construction and implementation.

GENETICS

Emerging genetic research has focused on heritability studies, finding DNA markers for being transgender and understanding related DNA mechanisms. This is expected to continue as genomic analysis becomes less expensive and faster to perform, stimulated by medical research in other areas. Much of the samples have already been collected, and they are gradually being exploited, but "big science" support could greatly expedite this line of investigation.

Now that transgender people are more visible and tolerance and acceptance has improved, it becomes possible to begin genealogical research to look for patterns of transgender genetic inheritance. Geneticists have already hypothesized models of inheritance based on the existing data, which can be tested through genealogical research on family trees. For example, the recent Polderman et al. study (Polderman et al., 2018) which summarized existing evidence, postulated a defined polygenetic threshold model that would predict that the probability of another family member being transgender would depend on how close the family genealogical relationship was. This is a testable scientific hypothesis resulting from a genetic theory that can stimulate future research. Other models exist and with improved transgender visibility, genealogical evidence can be used to compare their predictive power.

It is important to compare genetic evidence with evidence of other phenomena such as sex and homosexuality to tease these phenomena apart based on genetics. This should also be performed to compare with the genetics of phenomena that are suspected of co-occurrences with being transgender such as handedness, ADHD, the autism spectrum, and multiple sclerosis. Similar comparisons in the epigenetics domain will further clarify whether co-occurrences actually exist and if there are overlapping mechanisms involved.

EPIGENETICS

Although the science of epigenetics has made progress in defining and understanding basic epigenetic mechanisms, and although there were a few studies in the past, no emerging studies have been projected in the literature for transgender causation. Studies of genetic imprinting and diethylstilbestrol (DES) were done in the past, but they have not been replicated with better samples.

Green and Keverne (2000) found that transwomen had more maternal aunts than uncles, which suggested that the mother of the aunts and uncles had inherited a non-DNA chemical that selectively reduced the survival of prenatal males but not females. This was passed on to the mother of the transwomen. The possible nature of this chemical is that it might be an epigenetic mechanism that acts with the X chromosome, or it might be an immune system antibody. Although this study involved a sample of 417 people, it has never been replicated nor has this phenomenology been explored since then. Future research could easily be performed to replicate these results, which might open up the science in this area. Since we now realize that many of the children classified as being transgender were really prehomosexual, the results of replication may affect our knowledge of homosexuality causation, rather than transgender causation.

With regard to DES, Kerlin and Beyer (2002) and Kerlin (2005) published survey results indicating that DES sons' exposure might be associated with being transgender. However, this study had some methodological problems because the survey was based on data from volunteers on the Internet and no proof or quantification was provided about exposure. There are more robust database "cohorts" that the CDC, National Cancer Institute, and NIH have access to (2,600 males and 5,000 females), which are vetted for exposure, but the people in these cohorts have never been asked if they were transgender. Since this drug has been banned for pregnant women, time is running out to question these cohorts who were exposed as they drop out or pass away.

The prenatal testosterone theory of being transgender (PTTT) is described in Chapter 3. This theory postulates that prenatal testosterone levels in the fetus may cause being transgender. Prenatal testosterone levels have also been hypothesized in other phenomena including homosexuality and the autism spectrum. Chapter 3 presented evidence that currently does not support the PTTT theory, but measuring prenatal testosterone levels in fetuses is currently beyond the state of the art. Future medical technology research is needed to provide a definitive test of this theory by having the technical capability to make such measurements.

The most salient epigenetic issue concerns why the identical twin of a transgender person is only transgender about 50 percent of the time. Epigenetic mechanisms are known to change the outcomes of traits for identical twins in this way by mutating DNA genes and by modifying how they are expressed. Future research is needed to understand the mechanism that blocks or promotes the formation of the genetic predisposition for being transgender.

EARLY LEARNING AND EMERGENCE

Research is needed to explore why *parents sometimes disown transgender children* and throw them out of the household. This is a salient societal issue that impacts public health, transgender poverty, drug addiction, and crime. *Do parents do it because their family, community, and culture teach them to do this?* Does this rejection reflect itself in violence? What interventions would help to prevent parents from rejecting transgender children and reunite parents and their transgender children?

Future research should be performed to understand how individual transgender and cisgender children react to various gender behaviors. This would help us to understand how they determine the "fit" with gender categories to find their congruent gender category and to determine if there are more natural clusterings of behaviors other than binary categories. This requires conducting a task analysis of behaviors deemed to be gender behaviors by Western culture. Cross-subcultural studies are indicated because subcultures vary in egalitarianism, which might reduce the impact of culture on responses.

It has been established at a top level that transgender people differ in personality (Lippa, 2001) and childhood activity level (Zucker & Bradley, 1995) but these finding have not been explored further to date. We know that personality varies from genetic males to genetic females (Lippa, 1998), and genetic markers for activity have been found (Rankinen & Bouchard, 2012). Lippa is able to categorize people-versus-things personalities, which bears on the co-occurrence of the autism spectrum. Personality and activity of transgender children/people should be compared in childhood between transgender and cisgender children and later as adults. Also of interest is whether transgender people experience personality changes as a result of transition, as many report that they become more extroverted.

There are several phenomena that appear to be associated with being transgender in childhood. In this section, we have already mentioned two of them—personality and activity level. But several others might help explain interactions between genetic and epigenetic influences. Handedness is a third phenomenon discussed in Chapter 3. Three medical problems have also been detected: being on the autism spectrum, ADHD, and multiple sclerosis. Research in these areas has been hampered by difficult definitions and lack of validated behavioral scales. An overlap with multiple sclerosis (Pakpoor, Wotton, Schmierer, Giovannoni, & Goldacre, 2016) has been reported. There is also the problem of clinical bias in accepting difficult cases with multiple problems. Some negative results have also been reported. All these phenomena are worthy of study to try to clarify their relationship to being transgender and potentially similar mechanisms (if any).

SEXUAL AROUSAL LEARNING

Although it may start in late childhood, normal puberty is the period when males and females learn about sexual arousal, but this process remains unexplored. It is relevant to explaining why transgender people initially are aroused by stimuli provided by presentation in their congruent gender, which is not the one associated with their sex at birth. Later the arousal declines because of crosspresentation episodes that result in classical conditioning extinction. How are sexually conditioned reflexes formed? Do some transgender people form conditioned reflex stimuli associated with genders? What conditioned reflexes are formed by prehomosexual children?

CULTURE

Culture defines gender behavior categories based on behaviors considered to be in one of two gender categories. Future research should define those behaviors through task analysis. Task analysis involves observation-interviews with people to define the tasks they perform (McNeese & Vidulich, 2002), in this case, gender-related tasks. This will open up new research opportunities for understanding the reactions of transgender versus cisgender children and adults, which are a factor in being transgender. Clustering analysis of these tasks will help define existing gender categories and establish alternatives to binary gender categories, which would be more natural. The tasks of today and their clustering can be compared with the tasks of tomorrow to detect changes in culture.

Research is needed to develop cultural change methods to reduce transgender rejection. Mechanisms for cultural change are already practiced within large organizations and societies. Some of these are applicable to cultural change regarding being transgender. Cultural change methods were also used by GLB people to achieve legislation and policy changes restoring their rights. For example, there was a concerted effort by lesbian couples to invite key political figures including members of Congress to dinner at their homes to show that they were living perfectly normal lives. We already know that personal contact and friendship can reduce rejection. We hypothesize that knowing a transgender person is important, and about 16 percent of people (Adam & Goodman, 2015) say that they know a transgender person, as compared with 8 percent a few years ago. Even brief personal educational contact about the issue has an effect. Many people seem to instantly change their attitudes when they find that a child or relative emerges as being transgender. We hypothesize that transgender visibility is important, and it has been increasing. Educational resources with correct information are increasing (Taylor &

Haider-Markel, 2014), and 76 percent of people can correctly define transgender (Cox & Jones, 2011).

Transgender people are often criticized for having a "transgender ideology," yet transgender people are so diverse that there is really no accepted ideology and plans for progress cannot always be agreed upon. Judging from organizational cultural change efforts, we hypothesize that transgender people need champions and allies, and together we should identify short measurable steps and celebrate accomplishments. We hypothesize that efforts to depathologize being transgender has helped the cultural change process, but more efforts are needed. Specifically, gender dysphoria and all transgender-related categories need to be deleted from the DSM. However, social psychology research is needed to understand cultural change and prioritize efforts related to changing attitudes about tolerance and acceptance. Social science is also needed to determine how best to change policy once attitudes are changed (Flores, 2015). This can contribute to other cultural change efforts besides those for being transgender.

There are several examples of a prevailing religion in a region or country working out ways of living in harmony, *vivre ensemble,* with established cultural traditions of local transgender people. Examples include the Bugis in Indonesia and their spiritual gender category (one of five categories) versus Islamic clerical practice, and the Muxe in Mexico who are blessed by the Catholic church (see Chapter 1). We need to know how such harmonious relationships are formed for transgender people with societal groups with philosophies that do not initially accept being transgender.

PARENTAL RELATIONS AND CHILD REARING

Parental relations and child rearing have been examined extensively with no indication that they contribute to transgender causation. However, there are two needed areas of research concerning parents.

It has been reported that transgender people appear to be overrepresented among adopted children (Shumer, Abrha, Feldman, & Carswell, 2017; Spack et al., 2012; Zucker & Bradley, 1998) They are overrepresented in the range of 7–8 percent. There are several possible explanations for these findings. They may just be a "presentation bias" artifact in that adoptive parents more rapidly seek provider care for their adopted children and typically have more financial resources to do so. Or they could be due to clinical selection bias, because university clinics get the most difficult cases including children with multiple problems. Maternal stress could play a factor, in that mothers who are planning to put their child up for adoption may be under stress before delivery. Research in this area is needed to clarify the factors involved because, if real, this phenomenon has ramifications for anticipatory guidance for adoptions and expectations for those who treat transgender children.

Greater research attention is needed to deal with parental rejection of transgender children. Rejecting parents exhibit violence toward transgender children, both verbal and sometimes physical (Bandini et al., 2001). Parental violence affects health outcomes (Ryan, Huebner, Diaz, & Sanchez, 2009). Intervention methods need to be explored to prevent such violence. There are often racial, ethnic, linguistic, religious, immigrant, and other cultural forces that seem to be involved in rejection. They seem to be funneled through family and local community organizations. Greater inquiry into familial acceptance-rejection among people of color is needed (Koken, Bimbi, & Parsons, 2009).

GENDERQUEER

Genderqueer transgender people are understudied because they are a relatively recent phenomenon. Genderqueer is an umbrella term for those who cannot find a congruent gender behavior category and are outside of the Western culture binary. These are subjective self-assigned categories and may include being agender (having no gender), having two or three genders, or having a third gender. Genderqueer individuals may present in a mixture of masculine, feminine, or gender neutral clothing and behavior that is relatively consistent. Gender fluid individuals present in varying combinations of masculine and feminine and neutral clothing and behavior. Genderqueer is independent of sex and sexual orientation. Genderqueer phenomena are so recent that outcomes are not well characterized.

Genderqueer individuals manifest health disparities resulting from negative health care encounters (Baldwin et al., 2018; Eisenberg et al., 2017; Lykens, LeBlanc, & Bockting, 2018; Puckett, Cleary, Rossman, Newcomb, & Mustanski, 2018). Negative encounters include misgendering, not understanding how to get care, lack of permission from parents not recognizing their gender category, or co-occurring high-risk behaviors. Genderqueer patients may have communication difficulties with providers because of their wide terminology and because many of them use nontraditional pronouns.

The difficulty in studying genderqueer individuals is one of definition because they are subjectively defined and may encompass a wide range of presentations and behaviors (Gower et al., 2018). The definition of gender behaviors based on task analysis is one approach to this problem. Analysis of genderqueer behaviors may provide insight into treatments and how to reduce health disparities. Performing task analysis and task categorization on genderqueer individuals may enlarge the behavioral taxonomy.

There are an increasing number of genderqueer children and adolescents who are on puberty blockers, but they cannot continue after age 16. They will need to determine whether they want the gender associated with their sex assignment at birth or whether to go through transgender transition to the sex not assigned at birth.

EXISTENTIAL CRISIS

Case histories indicate that transgender people sometimes radically change their behavior as a result of life crises, sometimes described as life/existential crises or spiritual struggle (Grossoehme, Teeters, Jelinek, Dimitriou, & Conard, 2016). Such crises are triggered by realization of mortality, meaninglessness, isolation, and freedom of action/free will (Yalom, 1980). They can be triggered by external events or internal thoughts, such as the death of a loved one (mortality), being alone and isolation (need for love), freedom of action (the world's problems are my problems), or meaninglessness (life has no intrinsic meaning). For some, these realizations can be interpreted as spiritual struggles.

As a result of such crises, transgender people may show reactive depression and after resolution of the crisis, report sudden increases in transgender behavior, emergence of being transgender, coming out, and desire for transition.

Existential crises that change behavior were first studied by Victor Frankl, an Austrian neurologist and psychiatrist who found that radical behavioral changes occurred after life crises. (Yalom, 1980). Frankl would try to provoke existential crises in his patients who were having difficulty changing their behavior. For example, he would bring up the recent death of a relative in order to put such a patient into an existential crisis involving mortality.

Providers should be aware that such crises result in depression until resolved and that they may trigger visits to providers for transgender services and procedures. However, there is little scientific data to understand this critical aspect of being transgender and other phenomena, and future research should explore this phenomenon.

AUTHENTICITY VERSUS SEXUAL AROUSAL

Future research is needed to understand the motivation for transgender behavior, which includes the controversy over authenticity versus sexual arousal. Some still believe that the motivation for transgender behavior is exclusively sexual arousal, but studies of transgender people indicate that the motivations are authenticity with their congruent gender and relaxation (Buhrich, 1978; Hirschfeld, 1911; Levitt & Ippolito, 2014). Although transgender people initially report sexual arousal from presenting in their congruent gender because of novelty and previous classical conditioning, sexual arousal declines due to extinction.

This issue deserves continuing research because of antitransgender arguments that sex and gender are the same thing, with the clear implication that being transgender is motivated by sexual arousal and therefore is to be considered as a fetish or perversion.

EXPLORATION OF CO-OCCURRENCES WITH POSSIBLE GENETIC OR EPIGENETIC INVOLVEMENT

There is evidence to show that being transgender, handedness, the autism spectrum, and multiple sclerosis have genetic bases, but their co-occurrences indicate possible epigenetic involvement rather than DNA involvement. Transgender people are less right-handed than controls (Green & Young, 2001; Orlebeke, Boomsma, Gooren, Verschoor, & Van Den Bree, 1992; Watson & Coren, 1992; Wisnewski et al., 2005; Zucker et al., 2001), and research has indicated that being transgender and being on the autism spectrum overlap by 8–20 percent (de Vries, Noens, Cohen-Kettenis, van Berckelaer-Onnes, & Doreleijers, 2010; reviewed in Strang et al., 2018). People on the autism spectrum are less right-handed (Gillberg, 1983). Those exposed to DES are less right-handed (Schachter, 1994; Scheirs & Vingerhoets, 1995), and there is weak evidence that DES may be involved in facilitating being transgender (Kerlin, 2005; Kerlin & Beyer, 2002). One study has reported an overlap between being transgender and multiple sclerosis (Pakpoor et al., 2016). Genes that govern the immune system and environmental factors such as flu are implicated. Although these are correlations and do not imply causation, they may form the basis for future research hypotheses into the commonality of genetic or epigenetic mechanisms or their interactions involved with these phenomena.

TREATMENT

Due to increased tolerance of transgender people, transgender treatment procedures are being researched by clinicians at an accelerated rate. What was once considered politically incorrect research is now deemed to be lifesaving. The driver for this research is, of course, the high rate of transgender attempted suicide, approximately 40 percent. Research extends from how to treat transkids and adults to widening the alternatives and associated treatments for transgender genital plastic surgery (TGPS). This area deserves increasing research study.

TRANSGENDER NOT CHIEF COMPLAINT

Little research has been performed for those whose chief complaint does not require transgender procedures, although they make up the largest proportion (90 percent) of transgender people. They may call themselves crossdressers and may not even want to be under the transgender umbrella. They often suffer from loneliness and isolation due to secrecy. Their main expressed need is for trans-knowledgeable marital therapy. These issues were discussed in Chapters 6 and 7, but there are undoubtedly deeper issues associated with depression resulting from secrecy. How can the suffering of these people be reduced? Research must be accompanied by outreach to give support to individuals and community groups.

TRANSKIDS

Research on the appropriate treatment for transgender children is accelerating, in part due to the high frequency of attempted suicide among transgender young people and the desire to prevent suicide. Future research is underway to evaluate the affirmative model and puberty blockers for treating transkids. These are relatively recent developments, but within the next few years we should know the results of outcomes and identified side effects and limitations.

The question still remains whether transgender children continue to perform transgender behavior into adulthood and whether it continues in secret despite cultural rejection and social pressures. Such research will not automatically be performed because most transkids that can be observed are already in clinics for treatment and there is currently no means to study them "in the wild." Adult support groups can be used for retrospective studies, but most adults in these groups experienced more severe rejection from a time when culture encouraged pathologization and rejection.

In light of the ROGD results, an interesting research hypothesis is that some transgender children first come out to their parents as homosexual and only later as transgender. This is a "break it to me gently" approach since the impact on parents of homosexuality is not as severe as the impact of being transgender. To parents, their children being transgender is perceived as losing a child, grieving, and learning to deal with the child's congruent gender.

HORMONE THERAPY

Research studies on hormone therapy have not addressed important considerations such as choice of drugs, dosages, targeted blood concentrations, and outcomes, leaving it up to the clinician to try to achieve "normal" sex hormone levels of the opposite birth sex in the hope that appropriate bodily changes will occur. *So the clinician may need to tinker with medications and dosages until the desired sex hormone blood levels are reached.* It is not possible to set up control groups for comparison because they would violate ethical principles of denying effective treatment, and do-it-yourself administration would corrupt control variables. It may be possible to collect useful evidence from those in the university and hospital clinics and those "in the wild" whose providers are not associated with clinics. Standards for measuring outcomes and identification of side effects would be required. For example, for transwomen, standardized measurements of breast development would require use of laser metrology scanners, which are now available. These studies would help resolve some of the issues associated with HT, which include whether progesterones should be prescribed, and appropriate dose in terms of body weight rather than just weight. This would require collection and analysis of large amounts of data, but modern statistical random effects models and other statistical and artificial intelligence tools for "big data" could be used.

SURGERIES

Future research on various transgender surgeries is expected and there are two areas of importance. The first area pertains to vaginoplasty versus the newer vulvoplasty procedures for TGPS. Who chooses vulvoplasty over traditional vaginoplasty and are they satisfied with the result?

The second line of inquiry is whether body mass index (BMI) cutoffs for TGPS really are required to improve outcomes. Body mass index has no empirical basis; it was developed in the 19th century by Quetelet, a mathematician, who even said that it was not an indicator of fatness (Eknoyan, 2008). BMI makes no allowance for the relative proportions of bone, muscle, and fat in the body. Some transgender people believe it is used to stop surgeries to save insurance companies money, and it is regarded as "fat-shaming" by some providers in the medical profession. However, this issue is nontrivial. Transgender people denied surgery are at greater risk for suicidal ideation and attempted suicide. There is currently no published research that indicates that a particular BMI should be required for TGPS with regard to outcomes and infection, although some clinics have set arbitrary limits with no evidentiary basis—this in spite of the fact that there is evidence that being denied TGPS can increase the probability of attempted suicide (Testa et al., 2012).

PATIENT POPULATIONS

Research is needed to deal with issues connected with various transgender subpopulations, including seniors and those in the military. Research has started on identifying the needs of senior transgender people because of the increase in general senior populations. Research indicates that transgender seniors are plagued by discrimination, social isolation, disproportionate poverty, health disparities, and a lack of access to culturally competent providers (Adams & Tax, 2017). Lack of social resources may lead to personal neglect (Burnett et al., 2006). Senior transgender people have significant fears about their future life and are ill-prepared (Witten, 2014, 2015). Cultural competency training is underway for senior providers (Yang, Chu, & Salmon, 2018) and should continue. Finding the right ways to develop cultural competency is an important research issue. Little is known about HT drugs and dosages for senior transgender people with regard to DVT and thromboembolic events or osteoporosis with or without TGPS.

However the challenged ban on transgender people in the U.S. military turns out, there will be some 15,000 to 20,000 transgender people who will have lasting psychological effects because, as current or retired members of the military, they are likely to see themselves as being stigmatized and deemed unworthy. These effects, combined with PTSD from combat, will be a challenge for the military medical establishment and the U.S. Veterans Administration in the future.

REFERENCES

Adam, S., & Goodman, M. (2015). Number of Americans who report knowing a transgender person doubles in seven years, according to new GLAAD survey. GLAAD. https://www.glaad.org/releases/number-americans-who-report-knowing-transgender-person-doubles-seven-years-according-new

Adams, M., & Tax, A. D. (2017). Assessing and meeting the needs of LGBT older adults via the Older Americans Act. *LGBT Health, 4*(6), 389–393.

Adams, N., Pearce, R., Veale, J., Radix, A., Castro, D., Sarkar, A., & Thom, K. C. (2017). Guidance and ethical considerations for undertaking transgender health research and institutional review boards adjudicating this research. *Transgender Health, 2*(1), 165–175. https://www.liebertpub.com/doi/pdfplus/10.1089/trgh.2017.0012

Baldwin, A., Dodge, B., Schick, V. R., Light, B., Scharrs, P. W., Herbenick, D., & Fortenberry, J. D. (2018). Transgender and genderqueer individuals' experiences with health care providers: What's working, what's not, and where do we go from here? *Journal of Health Care for the Poor and Underserved, 29*(4), 1300–1318.

Bandini, E., et al. (2001). Childhood maltreatment in subjects with male-to-female gender identity disorder. *International Journal of Impotence Research, 23*(6), 276–285.

Buhrich, N. (1978). Motivation for cross-dressing in heterosexual transvestism. *Acta Psychiatric Society of Scandanavia, 57*(2), 145–152.

Burnett, J., Regev, T., Pickens, S., Prati, L. L., Aung, K., Moore, J., & Dyer, C. B. (2006). Social networks: A profile of the elderly who self-neglect. *Journal of Elder Abuse and Neglect, 18*(4), 35–49.

Cox, D., & Jones, R. P. (2011, November 3). Most Americans favor rights and legal protections for transgender people. https://www.prri.org/research/american-attitudes-towards-transgender-people/

Eisenberg, M. E., Gower, A. L., McMorris, B. J., Rider, G. N., Shea, G., & Coleman, E. (2017). Risk and protective factors in the lives of transgender/gender nonconforming adolescents. *Journal of Adolescent Health, 61*(4), 521–526.

Eknoyan, G. (2008). Adolphe Quetelet (1796–1874)—the average man and indices of obesity. *Nephrology Dialysis and Transplantation, 23*(1), 47–51.

Equal Employment Opportunity Commission. (2018). The Genetic Information Nondiscrimination Act. https://www.eeoc.gov/laws/types/genetic.cfm

Flores, A. R. (2015). Attitudes toward transgender rights: Perceived knowledge and secondary interpersonal contact. *Politics, Groups, and Identities, 3,* 3. http://dx.doi.org/10.1080/21565503.2015.1050414

Gillberg, C. (1983). Autistic children's hand preferences: Results from an epidemiological study of infantile autism. *Psychiatry Research, 10*(1), 21–30.

Gower, A. L., Rider, G. N., Coleman, E., Brown, C., McMorris, B. J., & Eisenberg, M. E. (2018). Perceived gender presentation among transgender and gender diverse youth: Approaches to analysis and associations with bullying victimization and emotional distress. *LGBT Health, 5*(5), 312–319.

Green, R., & Keverne, E. (2000). The disparate maternal aunt-uncle ratio in male transsexuals: An explanation invoking genomic imprinting. *Journal of Theoretical Biology, 201,* 55–63.

Green, R., & Young, R. (2001). Hand preference, sexual preference, and transsexualism. *Archives of Sexual Behavior, 30*(6), 565–574.

Grossoehme, D. H., Teeters, A., Jelinek, S., Dimitriou, S. M., & Conard, L. A. (2016). Screening for spiritual struggle in an adolescent transgender clinic: Feasibility and acceptability. *Journal of Health Care Chaplains, 22*(2), 54–66.

Hirschfeld, M. (1911/1991). *The transvestites: The erotic drive to cross-dress* (M. A. Lombardi-Nash, Trans.). New York: Prometheus Books.

Kerlin, S. (2005). Prenatal exposure to diethylstilbestrol (DES) in males and gender-related disorders: Results from a 5-year study. Paper presented for the International Behavior Development Symposium. http://e.hormone.tulane.edu

Kerlin, S., & Beyer, D. (2002). The DES Sons online discussion network. *Transgender Tapestry, 100,* 18.

Koken, J. A., Bimbi, D. S., & Parsons, J. T. (2009). Experiences of familial acceptance-rejection among transwomen of color. *Journal of Family Psychology, 23*(6), 853–860.

Levitt, H. M., & Ippolito, M. R. (2014). Being transgender: The experience of transgender identity development. *Journal of Homosexuality, 61*(12), 1727–1758.

Lippa, R. A. (1998). Gender-related individual differences and the structure of vocational interests: The importance of the "People-Things" dimension. *Journal of Personality and Social Psychology, 74*, 996–1009.

Lippa, R. A. (2001). Gender-related traits in transsexuals and non-transsexuals. *Archives of Sexual Behavior, 30*(6), 603–614.

Lykens, J. E., LeBlanc, A. J., & Bockting, W. O. (2018). Healthcare experiences among young adults who identify as genderqueer or nonbinary. *LGBT Health, 5*(3), 191–196.

McNeese, M. D., & Vidulich, M. A. (2002) *Cognitive systems engineering in military aviation environments*. Human Systems Information Analysis Center, Wright-Patterson Air Force Base, Ohio.

Orlebeke, J., Boomsma, D. I., Gooren, L. K. G., Verschoor, A. M., & Van Den Bree, M. J. M. (1992). Elevated sinistrality in transsexuals. *Neuropsychology, 6*, 351–355.

Pakpoor, J., Wotton, C. J., Schmierer, K., Giovannoni, G., & Goldacre, M. J. (2016). Gender identity disorders and multiple sclerosis risk: A national record-linkage study. *Multiple Sclerosis, 22*(13), 1759–1762.

Polderman, T. J., et al. (2018). The biological contributions to gender identity and gender diversity: Bringing data to the table. *Behavioral Genetics, 48*, 95–108.

Puckett, J. A., Cleary, P., Rossman, K., Newcomb, M. E., & Mustanski, B. (2018). Barriers to gender-affirming care for transgender and gender nonconforming individuals. *Sex Research and Social Policy, 15*(1), 48–59.

Rankinen, T., & Bouchard, C. (2012). Genetic differences in the relationships among physical activity, fitness and health. In C. Bouchard, S. N. Blair, & W. Haskell (Eds.), *Physical activity and health*. New York: Human Kinetics.

Ryan, C., Huebner, D., Diaz, R. M., & Sanchez, J. (2009). Family rejection as a predictor of negative health outcomes in white and Latino lesbian, gay, and bisexual young adults. *Pediatrics, 123*(1), 346–352.

Schachter, S. C. (1994). Handedness in women with intrauterine exposure to diethylstilbestrol. *Neuropsychologia, 32*(5), 619–623.

Scheirs, J. G., & Vingerhoets, A. J. (1995). Handedness and other laterality indices in women prenatally exposed to DES. *Journal of Clinical and Experimental Neuropsychology, 17*(5), 725–730.

Shumer, D. E., Abrha, A., Feldman, H. A., & Carswell, J. (2017). Overrepresentation of adopted adolescents at a hospital-based gender dysphoria clinic. *Transgender Health*, 2(1), 76–79. http://online.liebertpub.com/doi/10.1089/trgh.2016.0042

Spack, N. P., Edwards-Leeper, L., Feldman, H. A., Leibowitz, S., Mandel, F., Diamond, D. A., & Vance, S. R. (2012). Children and adolescents with gender identity disorder referred to a pediatric medical center. *Pediatrics, 129*(3), 418–425.

Strang, J. F., et al. (2018). Initial clinical guidelines for co-occurring autism spectrum disorder and gender dysphoria or incongruence in adolescents. *Journal of Clinical Child & Adolescent Psychology, 47*(1), 105–115.

Taylor, J. K., & Haider-Markel, D. P. (2014). Conclusion and future directions in transgender politics and policy. In J. K. Taylor & D. P. Haider-Markel (Eds.),

Transgender rights and politics: Groups, issue framing, and policy (pp. 273–282). Ann Arbor, MI: University of Michigan Press.

Testa, R. J., Sciacca, L. M., Wang, F., Hendricks, M., Goldblum, P., Bradford, J., & Bongar, B. (2012). The effects of violence on transgender people. Manuscript submitted for publication to *Professional Psychology: Research and Practice, 43*(5), 452–459.

Watson, D. B., & Coren, S. (1992). Left-handedness in male-to-female transsexuals. *Journal of the American Medical Association, 267*(10), 134.

Wisniewski, A. B., Prendeville, M. T., & Dobs, A. S. (2005). Handedness, functional cerebral hemispheric lateralization, and cognition in male-to-female transsexuals receiving cross-sex hormone treatment. *Archives of Sexual Behavior, 34*(2), 167–172.

Witten, T. M. (2014). It's not all darkness: Robustness, resilience, and successful transgender aging. *LGBT Health, 1*(1), 24–33.

Witten, T. M. (2015). Elder transgender lesbians: Exploring the intersection of age, lesbian sexual identity, and transgender identity. *Journal of Lesbian Studies, 19*(1), 73–89.

Yalom, I. (1980). *Existential psychotherapy.* Basic Books.

Yang, J., Chu, Y., & Salmon, M. A. (2018). Predicting perceived isolation among midlife and older LGBT adults: The role of welcoming aging service providers. *Gerontologist, 58*(5), 904–912.

Zucker, K. J., & Bradley, S. J. (1995). *Gender identity disorder and psychosexual problems in children and adolescents* (pp. 189–193). New York: Guilford Press.

Zucker, K. J., & Bradley, S. J. (1998). Adoptee overrepresentation among clinic-referred boys with gender identity disorder. *Canadian Journal of Psychiatry, 43*(10), 1040–1043.

Zucker, K. J., Beaulieu, N., Bradley, S. J., Grimshaw, G. M., & Wilcox, A. (2001). Handedness in boys with gender identity disorder. *Journal of Child Psychology and Psychiatry, 42*(6), 767–776.

13

The Future

Predicting future behavior is always risky business. One can project from current trends into the future, but there will be unexpected events and scientific discoveries that affect the future behavior of people, culture, and societies. In this chapter, we identify established trends and possible scenarios, and aim to anticipate some unanticipated events and scientific discoveries.

MOMENTUM FOR VISIBILITY, TOLERANCE, AND ACCEPTANCE OF TRANSGENDER PEOPLE

There is clearly current momentum for increasing the visibility, tolerance, and acceptance of transgender people. This momentum has been gradually building for the past 50 years, based primarily on the initiatives of transgender people themselves but with help from providers and

Being Transgender in the Future

Being transgender has been described as an atomic bomb that could change society. The implication was that any change to society that recognizes diversity would be a bad thing. As Milton Diamond is fond of saying about gender, "nature loves diversity, society hates it."

But the results from increased visibility and acceptance of transgender people may well result in a positive cultural change that extends beyond transgender people. This change would relieve the burden of rigid gender behavior categories that stifle authenticity and bring anxiety and fear to millions of people. It also would help us understand the origin of some human behaviors that can serve as an example to understand other behaviors.

As the Western gender system is relaxed, people will be free to explore and express whatever gender behaviors they recognize "fit" them. Each individual reacts to each gender behavior in their own way. Clusters of gender behaviors may well be recognized that are different from the arbitrary clustering imposed by culture into a binary, cisgender, inflexible system. In other cultures, some of these behavior clusters, although probably not perfectly grouped, were realized and three, four, and even five gender categories received formal recognition. What we will ultimately realize is that each individual has a cluster of their own, freeing them to express themselves authentically. This actually supports the basis of Western individualism and protection against government intrusion into personal lives.

These changes, recognizing diversity, will bring us closer to the recognition of science to deal with seemingly intractable societal issues. This comes from using science to understand our own behavior.

SOFFAs like those addressed in Chapter 1. Recent events have contributed to this buildup, but others have weakened it. Advocacy will need to continue, just as the drives for equal rights for females and minorities have needed to be continued. Visibility, tolerance, and acceptance contribute to each other in complicated cultural forces.

Visibility has progressed from both the top down and the bottom up in terms of numbers of people that become aware of transgender people. From the top down, it started with the visibility of celebrities like Christine Jorgensen, Caitlyn Jenner, Janet Mock, Laverne Cox, Renee Richards, Jennifer Finney Boylan, and Jazz. They became highly visible for their life histories and talents. Lesser known transgender people who have made major contributions to society and are visible in their own niches can be seen on Lynn Conway's excellent website (http://ai.eecs.umich.edu/people/conway/TSsuccesses/TSsuccesses.html).

Transgender support groups and advocates, and sometimes their leaders, became increasingly visible, like Virginia Prince and Dallas Denny.

Support group meetings grew into conventions, some with thousands of participants, meetings so big and unique that they piqued journalistic attention. The journalists, seeing the opportunities for feature articles, have continued to describe and, unfortunately, sometimes stereotype, transgender people.

Filmmakers and writers, always looking for new stories of interest, found transgender stories to have the heroic conflicts they were looking for as well as the possibility of titillating transgender tropes such as obligatory makeup application and boudoir dressing. To be sure, such creators were following long Western traditions since the Enlightenment with low excursions into English Pantomime. Although most people may only be aware of *The Crying Game, Boys Don't Cry, Transamerica, La Cage aux Folles, The Danish Girl, Orange Is the New Black,* and, more recently, *A Fantastic Woman,* entertainment with transgender and crossdressing themes have long been embedded in Western culture from early films such as *Some Like It Hot* and TV drag comedians such as Milton Berle.

From the bottom up, transgender people became more visible because of significant others, friends, families, and advocates (SOFFAs) who found that they knew someone who was transgender. They suddenly found that the person they knew did not change after they came out as transgender except that they flourished. Many of these SOFFAS are providers as well. In 2015, it was found that the number of people who personally knew a transgender person had gone up from 8 to 16 percent of the U.S. population in seven years (Adam & Goodman, 2015), and by now is probably nearing 20 percent. Organizations such as PFLAG provided information and helped people deal with situations through the related experiences of peers. As their transgender family members and acquaintances suffered discrimination and violence, they became vocal advocates in churches and communities. What was a base of 1 percent of transgender people advocating for themselves became a visible advocacy base several times that size. The Texas legislature tried to pass a discriminatory restroom law and there were over 11 hours of testimony. Much of the testimony came from mothers of transkids who had become advocates, known as "Momma Bears" for their tenacity. This visible advocacy of transgender people and their SOFFAs has been repeated in local, state, and federal legislation and rule-making proceedings.

Visibility increases the chances of tolerance and acceptance because people become used to seeing transgender children and adults, but tolerance and acceptance also requires cultural change. There are people and institutions who profit from opposing cultural change, both in terms of money and power, by making people afraid of transgender people and telling their followers what they should do. Hatemongers can provide a populist base for getting elected. Transgender people and their SOFFAs never cease to be amazed by these activities. Most transgender people only want to be left alone and to have the same rights as other people because their transgender behavior hurts no one. They have become grist for the populist mill.

Recently, the National Center for Transgender Equality published a list of 38 discriminatory federal actions against transgender people since 2016, many of which have gone unnoticed by the public (NCTE, 2018). Similar discriminatory proposals have been pursued by populists at the local and state levels, but many of them have been defeated. And recently the U.S. Department of Health and Human Services leaked language to be used by all federal agencies that would have defined being transgender out of existence. Pushback was swift in the "We will not be erased" reaction.

No matter how many discriminatory laws are defeated or repealed, there is still a need for cultural change to increase tolerance and bring about acceptance. This will require transgender people and their SOFFAs to be even more visible and for organizations to take a stand. Many large corporations now take stances against discrimination, figuring that discrimination prevents them from hiring qualified people, both transgender and cisgender. It also impacts attracting customers. Many businesses have exerted leverage on state and local organizations and governments against discriminatory legislation. It is true that civil freedoms go hand in hand with economic freedoms.

Some churches, community groups, and businesses have lined up in favor of these populist moves to deny transgender people their rights, but others have not, citing the positive aspects of their religions and beliefs, such as "love thy neighbor." Seeing a decline in church attendance, many churches have changed their policies at the local level and some at the national level with regard to homosexuality and being transgender. And some churches, like the Episcopal Church, have broken up, and more, like the Methodist Church, are likely to break up over transgender and LGB issues.

It will take continuing mobilization of transgender people, SOFFAs, businesses, churches, and community organizations to gain tolerance and acceptance. The need for change is most pressing in preventing parents from rejecting and disowning their own children. Such rejection results in many transgender children ending up homeless, which provides negative visibility. Such parents reject their children because they are following the cultural dictates to which they have been exposed.

THE FUTURE OF THE EVOLUTION OF THE WESTERN GENDER SYSTEM

The future of the evolution of the Western gender system is largely in the hands of young people. Current indications are that young people increasingly violate gender categories and do not care about enforcing them on others. Breakdowns in the gender system occur out of economic necessity. Most are too focused on making a living and on their personal lives to bother with following and enforcing cultural rules, which they identify as belonging to previous generations. Because of slowdowns in wages, members of opposite sex couples both work, which means that more and more young people come to see the value of economic and political freedom. Many have grown up and gone to school with visible homosexual and transgender people, and the diversity continues with sexual orientation and heritage. Being genderqueer or gender fluid is no longer shocking. Diversity is an economic and creative strength of the human race, and transgender people are visible examples of this diversity.

A likely scenario is that the Western binary gender system will continue as is, but people will be allowed the freedom to present and practice gender behaviors as they wish without cultural rejection or reprisal and ignoring their sex at birth. Extreme feminine and masculine presentations will mostly be reserved for dating or finding a mate and for ceremonies such as weddings and proms. In such a scenario, gender behavior predisposition is more likely to be revealed and we will see how behaviors cluster according to biology, not according to an artificial cultural system. At this point, it should become obvious that gender does not appear to be a spectrum, but rather an incremental gender function that looks like a spectrum in low resolution. It is based on reactions to individual gender behaviors. Regroupings of behaviors may occur as they do now for genderqueer and gender fluid individuals. Categorization may no longer be possible or useful, but its remnants will die hard.

There should be less stigma attached to transgender behavior, and transgender transition as it is constituted now may be less in demand. However, individual procedures that are now included in transition may be requested as individual preference dictates. Regroupings of behaviors may occur as they do now for genderqueer and gender fluid individuals.

Relaxation of the gender system of categories should allow people to be freer to express their predispositions through their vocations and avocations. Being free to choose one's gender behaviors should contribute to economic prosperity as individuals contribute according to their authentic talents.

ASSOCIATIONS AND FAMILIES WE CHOOSE

We have already seen that transgender people are having trouble making connections with educational opportunities, vocations, social groups, and relationships in particular areas of the United States. Transgender people are having trouble making dating and pair-bonding connections with cisgender people. So, for a time, transgender people may continue to migrate to states and cities where they are accepted for schools and jobs and choose families with other transgender people. Migration and choosing nontraditional families are consistent with the way the United States developed, because there were minimal restrictions on moving. Families with one parent or children with nonbiological connections to a family have always existed in the United States and elsewhere.

So, in the short term, one could imagine that transgender people will migrate to places where they are accepted, which in the United States are mainly states on the East and West Coasts, and cities such as Atlanta in the South. Schools, organizations, and businesses in the South and Heartland will be deprived of the diverse capabilities of transgender people. Given market forces, we should expect that this migration will stop within a few decades. Established connections may keep some transgender people in those locations, but market forces will facilitate movement to the locations where expertise is needed.

In the past, many transgender people have formed families with other transgender people. Transgender people are aware of one another's struggles, and since they go to support groups, meetups, and other social activities, relationships and pair bonding among them are more likely. Still, transgender people are a diverse lot, having in common only a few genes that form a genetic gender predisposition that does not match their culturally assigned gender behavior category. As more transgender people become visible, tolerated, and accepted, they are increasingly trying to date cisgender people, but there are difficulties. The most obvious is that even though transgender people have transitioned, they may still appear to be different from other people in the same gender. Once revealed, being sexually attracted to someone who once was of a different sex sets off questioning of one's own sexual orientation. When to reveal one's transgender history in dating is under considerable debate among transgender people.

Transgender people sometimes have not lived in their congruent gender long enough to know how to act or to understand cisgender people of the same gender. They do not have shared experiences. For instance, many adult transwomen may never have gone to a prom, formal party, or pajama party during their teenage years as women. They may have gone as men and learned the wrong lessons. They would also not have learned makeup application or dressing when they were teenagers.

Transgender people may misinterpret social signals because of incomplete learning about their congruent gender. Cisgender women may open up to transwomen and tell them things about their sex lives and loves as they do with other cisgender women. This may be misinterpreted by transwomen as a green light for a relationship and/or sex because they have limited experience with norms of their congruent gender. Likewise, transmen may misinterpret masculine norms. These types of encounters create misunderstanding and embarrassment and may destroy some incipient friendships and relationships, but they are learning experiences.

DEPATHOLOGY

In future we should expect the DSM and ICD to eliminate all mention of transgender pathology. Indeed, the ICD-11 in 2019 has eliminated gender identity disorder but include a billing code in the normal sexual health category for transition treatments. The ICD is the master coding scheme, because the DSM actually maps to it before the bill processing. This should be conclusive in depathologizing being transgender. Since changes in the DSM are now possible between versions, there are movements underway to eliminate gender dysphoria and any other transgender pathological codes within the next two years. This would make the DSM more "harmonized" with the ICD. If transgender people need counseling, there will still be billing codes for this in either the ICD or DSM, just as there are for people who are homosexual, who were once pathologized.

However, there are still a few mental health providers that have been fighting depathologization. As we saw in the ROGD controversy, such providers are quick to assume pathology with psychodynamic interpretations. Since psychodynamic interpretations and ideas do not rise to the level of scientific theory, they provide no evidence to support old or new pathological categories. However, we should expect continuing backlash over the next few years.

PROVIDER EDUCATION

We can expect provider education about transgender people to increase in the future. Those dealing directly with a chief complaint unrelated to being transgender will still need to know the basics about being transgender, because transgender people now realize that they need to be open with their providers in order to get accurate treatment. Even specialties such as dermatology will need to know about transgender status. For example, transmen are prone to acne from HT, which complicates drug treatment (Boos, Ginsberg, & Peebles, 2018; Campos-Muñoz, López-De Lara, Rodríguez-Rojo, Conde-Taboada, A., & López-Bran, 2018; Ginsberg, 2017; Motosko, Zakhem, Pomeranz, & Hazen, 2018; Sabra, Fang, & Kundu, 2018). The complications arise from FDA rules that do not allow a female who is capable of having a child to get the acne drug isotretinoin. Rigid FDA rules do not cover transwomen whose ability to have children is blocked by HT temporarily, but with the cession of HT they can conceive and deliver. The decision to prescribe isotretinoin is complicated and requires the dermatologist to consider FDA rules as well as transgender patient autonomy (Yeung, Chen, Katz, & Stoff, 2016).

Those dealing with a chief complaint of being transgender will, of course, need specific education and training on transgender-specific treatments as well as experience working with a recognized expert. In the future, these will need to be developed into recognized subspecialties.

SECRECY OF THE 90 PERCENT

From the work of Lynn Conway (Conway, 2001–2002; Olyslager & Conway, 2007) we have estimates of the population frequency of being transgender and the population of transitioning transgender people of approximately 9:1. This means that the vast majority of transgender people do not transition and practice transgender behavior part-time and in secret. They show up on surveys, contributing the most to the 1 percent of the population that are transgender. Some of them do not want to be under the transgender umbrella but consider themselves to be crossdressers quite apart from other transgender people. Little research is conducted on the situation of these people, but we do know a few things.

We know that many live in secret and we know that there are corrosive effects of such secrecy (Kelly, 2002). Some of them have confided in their spouses and others that they trust about being transgender. This makes their spouses and SOFFAs also vulnerable to the corrosive effects of secrecy. Unlike some other lesser secrets, exposure of being transgender can have severe effects on families, jobs, and relationships.

We know that being transgender sometimes interferes with or is involved in spousal and other relationships, yet the transgender person feels that they cannot be forthright about it. Most never see a provider about being transgender. This segment of transgender people does not want to share their secret with providers, which may interfere with treatment of medical, family, and marital problems. This includes covert do-it-yourself HT and other treatments.

This group is starting to express their needs, and transgender providers must be aware of them. First of all, most want to keep their marriages intact. Marital therapists must try to understand transgender people, although, like the rest of the provider community, most have little training. The same goes for family therapists, who also need to understand about transgender children.

We know that most of the people in this group do not want to transition because they do not feel strongly enough about coming out full-time and changing their bodies. They may prefer to avoid causing pain to themselves and their SOFFAs, or they may just look forward to part-time crossdressing as sort of a hobby. Providers should avoid urging them to transition or overtreat them. History has shown that they do serve as a reservoir of people who potentially want to transition, but it is up to the individual.

In the future, advocacy should be pursued to protect those who lose their jobs due to transgender discovery, just as for transgender people who are out voluntarily.

Although we are currently concentrating on integration of knowledge about transgender people into professional schools and education of providers who will provide direct transgender treatments, in the future, all providers need to know about being transgender, including those who may only deal with transgender issues peripherally.

RESTROOM AND LOCKER ROOM DESIGN

Transgender people should be free to use restroom and locker room facilities that are compatible with their congruent gender or to use gender neutral facilities as long as they are not stigmatized for using gender neutral facilities. The real problem is the design of such facilities. Current design of restrooms and locker rooms, particularly in the United States, is based on making them cheap to build and easy to clean, not for privacy. Current designs are baked into U.S. but not international plumbing codes. To accommodate the particular requirements of transgender people, families, people with dementia, and others will require great improvements in the design of these facilities.

Alternative restroom designs are commonplace in Europe and elsewhere that offer privacy as well as cleanliness. In many European countries, sinks, diaper changing tables, and other facilities are provided in an outer common area with cubicles to accommodate individual toilet and bidet needs. The cubicles lock and have floor to ceiling walls, offering maximum privacy. In the United States, partitions between toilet facilities are several inches above the floor to allow for convenience in hosing down the floor. These partitions offer very little privacy as do the doors, which have cracks that allow visibility into the area. They are designed to allow people from outside each toilet area to determine whether there is a current occupant. This can easily be remedied with door indicators. Door locks are not secure, deliberately designed to be easily opened from outside. All this is coded in U.S. architectural standards for public plumbing.

In the United States, some single-occupant restrooms are set aside for families and sometimes as all-gender restrooms. Such facilities comply with international building codes for public facilities such as airports.

However, they are inefficient with respect to getting large numbers of people to use them over time.

Locker rooms are designed to be cheaply configured. They typically have communal showers and floors that breed fungus and bacteria. Unless individual stalls are included, there is no privacy whatsoever. Stalls with shower curtains provide only a little privacy.

The first times that children and teenagers are introduced to such restrooms and locker rooms and are embarrassed by the lack of privacy are regarded as rites of passage into society. These times may be the first times that children have seen other people's naked bodies, and they become fixated and curious about anatomical variations. Parents assume that these rooms have to be designed this way for privacy, but they are only designed to be inexpensive.

To provide a tissue of privacy, many restrooms and locker rooms are segregated by sex. Of course, this does not address the privacy problems that occur in the similar designs for both male and female restrooms. This also does not solve the problem that user throughput is slower in female restrooms because there are usually fewer stalls than urinals.

Most transgender people are afraid to go into restrooms at all, and this results in health problems for transgender children and adults. And they are afraid for good reason; they have suffered violence in such facilities.

The current debate is over how restrooms should be assigned, according to sex or gender, but the real debate should be about how we upgrade facility designs to make them cleaner and more private, even if it costs a little more. This would benefit all people, including transgender people.

CONTRIBUTIONS OF TRANSGENDER SCIENCE TO BIOPSYCHOLOGY

Being transgender provides a striking example of how behavior results from multiple factors, beginning with genetics and epigenetics, early learning, and unconscious "fit" with cultural behavior categories and norms. Other behaviors and phenomena follow these patterns, but being transgender is the most prominent at the moment. We are just beginning to understand the biological mechanisms involved in these factors for being transgender and to separate them for different behaviors and phenomena.

While we tend to focus on the evolution of anatomy and physiology, there is much to be learned about the evolution of behavioral predispositions, which also contribute to human diversity. Human diversity, as it functioned in the past, is needed to solve future human problems.

Many transgender people are in the unique position of experiencing more than one gender category, which gives them broader insights into the human condition. In the future, this knowledge should be captured by science and continue to be explored in art and the humanities.

Providers need to know that transgender people report that transgender emergence is a profound spiritual experience. Providers need to know this to understand the basis for the commitment of transgender people to their congruent gender. This discovery process serves as an example for other behaviors.

REFERENCES

Adam, S., & Goodman, M. (2015). Number of Americans who report knowing a transgender person doubles in seven years, according to new GLAAD survey. GLAAD. https://www.glaad.org/releases/number-americans-who-report-knowing-transgender-person-doubles-seven-years according-new

Boos, M. D., Ginsberg, B. A., & Peebles, J. K. (2018). Prescribing isotretinoin for transgender youth: A pledge for more inclusion. *Pediatric Dermatology,* https://www.sciencedirect.com/science/article/pii/S2352647516300338

Campos-Muñoz, L., López-De Lara, D., Rodríguez-Rojo, M. L., Conde-Taboada, A., & López-Bran, E. (2018). Transgender adolescents and acne: A cases series. *Pediatric Dermatology, 35*(3). e155–e158.

Conway, L. (2001–2002). How frequently does transsexualism occur? http://www.lynnconway.com

Ginsberg, B. A. (2017). Dermatologic care of the transgender patient. *International Journal of Women's Dermatology, 3*(1), 65–67.

Kelly, A. E. (2002, January). *The psychology of secrets.* Springer Science and Business Media.

Motosko, C. C., Zakhem, G. A., Pomeranz, M. K., & Hazen, A. (2018). Acne: A side-effect of masculinizing hormonal therapy in transgender patients. *British Journal of Dermatology,* 18(1), 26–30.

NCTE. (2018). The discrimination administration. https://transequality.org/the-discrimination-administration.

Olyslager, F., & Conway, L. (2007). *On the calculation of the prevalence of transsexualism.* Presentation at 2007 WPATH Symposium, Chicago, IL.

Sabra, J. J., Fang, C. X., & Kundu, R. V. (2018). A knowledge-based assessment of dermatological care for transgender women. *Transgender Health, 3,* 1. https://doi.org/10.1089/trgh.2018.0001

Yeung, H., Chen, S. C., Katz, K. A., & Stoff, B. K. (2016). Prescribing isotretinoin in the United States for transgender individuals: Ethical considerations. *Journal of the American Academy of Dermatology, 75*(3), 648–651.

Glossary

Affirmative approach
Procedures that allow transgender people to find and support their congruent gender.

Androgen insensitivity syndrome
Genetic intersex condition in which body cells do not respond to testosterone during development.

Aptic structure
Brain mechanism making one more apt to feel or behave in a certain way.

AR
Androgen receptor gene.

Aromatase
Enzyme that catalyzes the conversion of testosterone to estrogen.

Asexual
Not attracted to either sex in sexual orientation.

Authenticity
Behaving in a genuine manner.

Autism spectrum
Group of neurodevelopmental differences.

Autogynephilia
Controversial idea that some transwomen are motivated by sexual arousal to be transgender; does not qualify as a scientific theory.

BDSM
Bondage, discipline, sadism, masochism producing sexual arousal from unusual stimuli; refers generally to support group philosophy.

Being transgender
Displaying transgender behavior including verbal behavior; not behaving in one's assigned gender behavior category, which was assigned at birth based solely on sex assigned at birth.

Binary gender system
System with two cultural gender categories.

Biomarkers
Structural and functional differences between humans.

Biopsychology
Science of using biology and biological techniques to explain generation of behavior.

Bisexual
Person attracted to people of both sexes.

BNSTc
Bed/basal nucleus of stria terminalis in brain, part C.

Boy/Man/He/Sir
Words associated with Western culture masculine gender category.

Bullying
Minor assaults and batteries intended to coerce or dominate.

Buserelin
Puberty-blocking drug.

Bystander training
Training bystanders to recognize bullying and how to deal with it.

CAH
Congenital adrenal hyperplasia; genetic condition resulting in high levels of testosterone produced and released by adrenal glands.

Chief complaint
Presenting complaint; initial step in medical history taking in provider-patient encounter.

Chromosome
Division of DNA.

Cisgender
Gender system rule that automatically assigns people to gender behavior categories based on natal sex; males assigned masculine category, females assigned to feminine category.

Coolidge effect
Renewed interest in sex from introduction of new, receptive sex partner.

Crossdressing
Presenting in clothes and behavior of nonassigned gender behavior category.

Culture
Rules, values, and customs for behavior of a group.

Cyproterone acetate
Testosterone-blocking drug used in HT in Europe but not approved in United States due to side effects.

DES
Diethylstilbestrol, a drug formerly given to prevent miscarriage that modifies DNA or its expression.

Dihydrotestosterone
Form of testosterone with high activity.

Drag
Crossdressing for theatrical purposes, dressed as a girl.

DSD
Differences in sexual development; intersex.

DSM
Diagnostic and Statistical Manual of Mental Disorders; list of diseases used for diagnosis and insurance reimbursement.

Electrolysis
Hair removal using electrolytic and/or radio frequency current to destroy hair follicles through a small electrode.

Epigenetics
Non-DNA influences on development that modify DNA or its expression.

Estradiol valerate
Estradiol type currently used in hormone therapy.

Ethinyl estradiol
Estradiol type formerly used in HT but no longer used because of potential for DVT and pulmonary clots.

Evidence-based diagnosis and treatment
Use of best available scientific research for diagnosis and treatment.

Existential crisis
One of four life realizations that tend to change behavior.

Feminine
One of two gender behavior categories of Western culture gender system.

Fetishism
Sexual arousal to unusual stimuli, usually nonhuman stimuli.

Finasteride
Drug that blocks conversion of testosterone to dihydrotestosterone (propecia).

Follicle-stimulating hormone
Hormone released from anterior pituitary to trigger sex hormone production and release from gonads.

Fraternal twins
Dizygotic twins with nonidentical DNA at conception.

FSH
Follicle-stimulating hormone that helps trigger manufacture and release of sex hormones from the gonads.

Gay
Male attracted to another male; also used as female attracted to another female.

GCE
Gender change efforts.

Gender
Gender behavioral category determined by culture; contains tasks, rules, and norms.

Gender behavior
Behaviors identified by culture as belonging to gender.

Gender behavior predisposition
Biological genetic tendency with regard to gender behaviors.

Gender change efforts
Use of psychological procedures to attempt to change gender; also called reparative or conversion "therapy."

Gender dysphoria
Pathological term for people who experience debilitation and distress because of being transgender.

Gender fluid
Self-assigned term referring to moving between or combining gender behaviors from gender behavior categories.

Gender identity
Self-described gender.

Gender identity disorder (GID)
Now defunct pathological diagnosis for person who experiences debilitation or distress from being transgender.

Genderqueer
Self-assigned term referring to being unable to find a congruent gender behavior category.

Gender system
System of rules for gender behavior including defined gender behavior categories developed by culture.

Genetic gender predisposition
Formation of brain mechanisms that emotionally react to exposure and learning about gender behaviors.

Genetic markers
Features of the DNA molecule that are associated with particular traits.

Girl/Woman/She/Ma'am
Words associated with Western culture feminine gender behavior category.

Goserelin
Puberty-blocking drug.

GWAS
Genome-wide association study.

Handedness
Preference for use of left or right hand for a range of tasks.

Heritability
Proportion of the variance accounted for by genetics of a trait.

Histrelin
Puberty-blocking drug.

Homosexuality
Sexual orientation toward same-sex person.

HT
Hormone therapy; procedure involving cross-sex hormones and other drugs to change bodies to make them more compatible with expectations of culture for congruent gender.

Hypercalcemia, hyperkalemia
Excess potassium levels in blood serum.

ICD
International Classification of Diseases; list of categories for diagnosis and health insurance reimbursement.

Identical twins
Monozygotic twins whose DNA is the same at conception.

INAH3
Interstitual nucleus of the anterior hypothalamus number 3.

Intersex
Differences in sexual development.

Kegel
Isometric exercise designed to strengthen the perineum muscles.

Kinship theory of gender evolution
Theory that human survival depends on the fitness of a group that shares some of the same genes.

Lesbian
Female attracted to another female.

Leuprolide acetate
Puberty-blocking drug.

Luteinizing hormone
Hormone that helps trigger manufacture and release of sex hormones from the gonads.

Marriage flight
Getting married in an attempt to deal with being transgender.

Medroxyprogesterone
Synthetic progestin drug

Metioplasty
A type of TGPS for transmen.

Military flight
Joining the military in an attempt to deal with being transgender.

Misgendering
Using incorrect gender pronouns and honorifics.

Natal
Assigned at birth.

Neovagina
Anatomy created for transwomen in vaginoplasty surgery.

Operant conditioning
Use of reinforcement and/or response contingent withdrawal of reinforcement to change behavior.

Orchiectomy
Removal of testicles by surgery; type of TGPS for transwomen.

Paraphilia
Intense sexual arousal triggered by various stimuli.

PCOS
Polycystic ovary syndrome, a phenomenon that occurs in some natal females, resulting in high levels of testosterone.

Perlutal
Drug combination manufactured in Mexico consisting of estradiol enanthate combined with dihydroxyprogesterone acetophenide used for birth control; not approved for use in United States. Estrogenic drug manufactured in Mexico and brought to the United States; not FDA approved

Phalloplasty
Surgical construction of penis for transmen.

Polycythemia
Condition in which the volume percentage of red cells in the blood is elevated.

Population frequency
Percentage of occurrence in the population; nonpathological equivalent of prevalence.

Pre-op/Post-op
Respectively, before and after TGPS.

PrEP
Pre-exposure prophylaxis for HIV/AIDS protection.

Prometrium
Micronized progesterone used by oral route of administration in HT.

PTTT
Prenatal Testosterone Theory of being Transgender; theory that extreme levels of testosterone cause being transgender.

Puberty blockers
Drugs to prevent puberty.

Putamen
One of the brain structures for sensation and movement.

Queer
Those who are neither cisgender nor heterosexual.

Questioning
Those unsure of congruent gender and/or sexual orientation.

Real-life test/Real-life experience
Living in congruent gender for one year to prove that one could function in job and social life.

ROGD
Rapid onset gender dysphoria. Controversial, hypothesized syndrome of transgender emergence in teenage years due to psychodynamics.

Salpingo-oophorectomy
Surgical removal of fallopian tubes (salpingectomy) and ovaries (oophorectomy).

Sex
Sexual organs usually indicating the ability to reproduce sexually; generally determined at birth by inspection of external genitalia.

Sexual arousal
Physiological changes in anticipation of sexual behavior.

Sexual fetish
Obtaining sexual arousal from various stimuli.

Sexual orientation
Attraction based on a person's sex.

SOC
Standards of Care for transgender health developed by WPATH.

SOCE
Sexual orientation change efforts.

SOFFA
Significant others, friends, family, and allies of transgender people.

Spironolactone
Testosterone-blocking drug; potassium-sparing diuretic.

Stealth
Changing identity and living in secret at the completion of transgender transition.

Tetragametic chimera
Person with two types of DNA due to cell merger shortly after conception; one's own twin.

Traditional sex-based theory of gender
Theory that sex determines gender behaviors.

Transgender
Not behaving in one's culturally defined gender behavior category.

Transgender genital plastic surgery (TGPS)
Surgical procedures that change anatomy of genital organs for transitioning transgender people to appear like the anatomy of cisgender sex associated with congruent gender.

Transgender transition
Process by which a person changes their body to be more compatible with cultural expectations of their congruent gender; formerly transsexual transition.

Transman
Transgender person who was determined to be female at birth but has congruent gender of masculine.

Transsexual
Older term for transgender person undergoing transgender transition.

Transvestite
Term for transgender person, popularized by Magnus Hirschfeld.

Transwoman
Transgender person who was determined to be male at birth but has congruent gender of feminine.

Triptorelin
Puberty-blocking drug.

Vulvoplasty
Form of TGPS for transwomen to create realistic vulva from the outside.

WPATH
World Professional Association for Transgender Health; formerly HBIGDA, Harry Benjamin International Gender Dysphoria Association.

Resources

ADVOCACY

Gay and Lesbian Medical Association
Advocates for LGBT health.
http://www.glma.org

GLAAD
Advocacy for appropriate media (e.g., film, TV) depiction of transgender people.
https://www.glaad.org

Human Rights Campaign
Lobbying group for LGBT people; maintain indices of businesses who support LGBT.
https://www.hrc.org

National Center for Transgender Equality
Advocacy for wide variety of transgender issues.
https://transequality.org

National LGBTQ Task Force
Instruction on advocacy.
http://www.thetaskforce.org

Organization Intersex International Australia
Advocates for intersex issues.
http://oiiinternational.com

Trans Advocate
News on transgender issues and advocacy.
https://www.transadvocate.com

CONFERENCES

Esprit
Conference in Port Angeles, WA.
https://www.espritconf.com

Fantasia Fair
Conference in Provincetown, MA.
http://fanfair.info

First Event
Conference in Boston, MA.
http://firstevent.org

Gender Odyssey
Conferences in Seattle and California.
http://www.genderodyssey.org

Keystone Conference
Transgender conference in Pennsylvania.
http://www.keystone-conference.org/index.cfm

Sparkle
U.K. transgender conference.
https://www.sparkle.org.uk

Trans Wellness Conference
Philadelphia health conference.
https://www.mazzonicenter.org/trans-wellness

EDUCATION

European Transgender Network
Association of transgender advocacy organizations in Europe.
http://www.tgeu.net

Female to Male
Transmen newsletter.
https://www.femaletomale.org/overview/

Gender Identity Research and Education Society (GIRES)
Information on transgender science.
https://www.gires.org.uk

Gender Spectrum
Transgender information and organization training.
https://www.genderspectrum.org

Gender Talk
Podcast by Nancy Nangerone.
http://www.gendertalk.com

International Foundation for Gender Education
Oldest transgender information organization; source for books.
http://www.ifge.org

Susan's Place
Blog site for transgender support.
https://www.susans.org

TGForum Online Bibliography
Blog site bibliography section.
https://tgforum.com/wordpress/bibliography/

Trans Central IPA
Information and support group.
http://transcentralpa.org/connect_spouses.cfm

Transgender Archives, University of Victoria
Transgender library and historical research.
https://www.uvic.ca/transgenderarchives/

Trans-man.Org
Sources of equipment and surgery for transmen.
http://www.trans-man.org

FAMILY

Family Acceptance Project
Support group for transgender people and SOFFAs.
https://familyproject.sfsu.edu

PFLAG
Support group for transgender people and SOFFAs.
https://pflag.org

HEALTH CARE

American Psychiatric Association
Research and counseling for transgender people.
https://www.psychiatry.org/patients-families/gender-dysphoria

American Psychological Association
Research and counseling for transgender people.
https://www.apa.org/topics/lgbt/transgender.aspx

Center of Excellence for Transgender Health, UCSF
Counseling and medical treatment of transgender people.
http://www.transhealth.ucsf.edu

Endocrine Society
Research and guidelines for HT.
https://www.endocrine.org/advocacy/priorities-and-positions/transgender-issues

National Coalition for LGBT Health
Training for providers of transgender care.
http://healthhiv.org/certificate-programs/national-coalition-for-lgbt-health-lgbt-health-training-and-certificate-program/

SYPP at Children's Hospital, Los Angeles
Research and treatment of transgender children.
https://www.chla.org/profile/johanna-olson-kennedy-md

Transgender Surgery Guide
Identification and contact information for surgeons.
http://www.tssurgeryguide.com

Trans Health
News on transgender health.
http://www.trans-health.com

UCSF Transgender Care
Transgender medicine and surgery source.
https://transcare.ucsf.edu

World Professional Association for Transgender Health
Develops Standards of Care for transgender health.
https://wpath.org

LEGAL

Lambda Legal
Legal advocacy.
https://www.lambdalegal.org

Sylvia Rivera Law Project
Legal advocacy.
https://srlp.org

Transgender Law Center
Legal advocacy.
https://transgenderlawcenter.org

Transgender Legal
Legal advocacy.
http://www.transgenderlegal.com

MEDIA

GLAAD
Media watchdog and advocacy for appropriate media (e.g., film, TV) depiction of transgender people.
https://www.glaad.org

SCIENCE

Bevan, T. (2015). *The psychobiology of transsexualism and transgenderism.* Santa Barbara, CA: Praeger.

Bevan, T. (2017). *Being transgender.* Santa Barbara, CA: Praeger.

Brill, S., & Pepper, R. (2008). *The transgender child: A handbook for families and professionals.* Berkeley, CA: Cleis Press.

Colapinto, J. (2001). *As nature made him: The boy who was raised as a girl.* New York: HarperCollins.

Ehrensaft, D. (2008). *Gender born, gender made: Raising healthy gender non-conforming children.* Kindle/Amazon Digital Services.

Ehrensaft, D. (2016). *The gender creative child.* New York: The Experiment Publishing Company.

Erhardt, V. (2007). *Head over heels: Wives that stay with cross-dressers and transsexuals.* London: Haworth.

Eugenides, J. (2002). *Middlesex.* New York: Picador.

Krieger, I. (2011). *Helping your transgender teen: A guide for parents.* Kindle/Amazon Digital Services.

Kuklin, S. (2014). *Beyond magenta: Transgender teens speak out.* Kindle/ Amazon Digital Services.

Lev, A. (2004). *Transgender emergence.* New York: Seven Stories Press.

Morris, J. (1974). *Conundrum.* New York: Signet.

National Center for Transgender Equality (NCTE). (2009). *Injustice at every turn.* https://transequality.org/issues/resources/national-transgender-discrimination-survey-executive-summary

Roughgarden, J. (2004). *Evolution's rainbow.* Berkeley: University of California Press.

Stryker, S. (2008) *Transgender history.* Berkeley: Seal Press.

Tannenhill, B. (2018). *Everything you wanted to know about trans.* New York: KJP.

World Professional Association for Transgender Health. (2018). *Standards of Care Version 7.* https://www.wpath.org/media/cms/Documents/Web%20Transfer/SOC/Standards%20of%20Care%20V7%20-%202011%20WPATH.pdf

SENIORS

FORGE
LGBT senior information.
https://forge-forward.org

SAGE (Service & Advocacy for GLBT Elders)
http://sageusa.care
https://lgbtagingcenter.org

University of Washington LGBT Senior Care
Research and treatment of LGBT seniors.
https://csde.washington.edu/news-events/karen-fredriksen-goldsen-publishes-research-on-aging-in-lgbt-populations/

SUPPORT GROUPS

Baltimore Transgender Alliance
Support group in Baltimore, MD.
http://www.bmoretransalliance.com

Beaumont Society
Support group in United Kingdom.
https://www.beaumontsociety.org.uk

Renaissance
Support group near Philadelphia, PA.
http://ren.org/index.html

Seahorse Society, NSW, Australia
Transwoman support.
http://www.seahorsesoc.org/index.html

Tiffany Club of New England
Transgender support group; holds First Event Conference.
https://tcne.org

Trans Family Support Group
Support for SOFFAs.
http://www.transfamily.org

Transgender Education Association of Greater Washington, DC
Transgender support group.
http://www.tgeagw.org/?page_id=54

Tri-Ess
Heterosexual, married transgender support.
https://www.tri-ess.org

VOICE

Authentic Voices
Advocacy for transgender voice therapy.
https://speech.steinhardt.nyu.edu/blog/voice-modification-in-the-transgender-community/

Exceptional Voice
Voice therapy treatment.
https://www.exceptionalvoice.com

Index

About the Author

Dana Jennett Bevan, PhD, is a research psychologist and an expert on transgender science. Bevan has published three books on transgender science: *The Transsexual Scientist, The Psychobiology of Transsexualism and Transgenderism,* and *Being Transgender,* the latter two writing as Thomas E. Bevan. She received her PhD from Princeton University and BA degree from Dartmouth College, both in research psychology. Recently, she was elected to the Board of Directors of the United States Professional Association for Transgender Health, which encourages transgender science research and advocates for transgender people. She received an Innovation Achievement Award from the Department of the Army for her medical training research. Dana held the rank of professor at the Georgia Institute of Technology and currently conducts artificial intelligence research. She is a member of WPATH and the APA. She audio podcasts *The Transgender Scientist,* blogs monthly at Tgforum.com, and videoblogs on YouTube as *The Transgender Scientist.*